SIGNS & SYMPTOMS IN PEDIATRICS

Urgent and Emergent Care

Editor-in-Chief
KAREN D. GRUSKIN, MD
Instructor, Department of Pediatrics
Harvard Medical School;
Assistant in Medicine and Director of Network Services
Division of Emergency Medicine
Children's Hospital Boston
Boston, Massachusetts

Editors
VINCENT W. CHIANG, MD
Assistant Professor, Department of Pediatrics
Harvard Medical School;
Assistant in Medicine and Chief of Inpatient Services,
    Department of Medicine
Children's Hospital Boston
Boston, Massachusetts

SHANNON MANZI, PharmD
Department of Pharmacy
Children's Hospital Boston;
Adjunct Clinical Faculty
Northeastern University and Massachusetts College of Pharmacy and
    Allied Health Sciences
Boston, Massachusetts

Series Editor
MARK A. DAVIS, MD, MS
Institute for International Emergency Medicine and Health
Department of Emergency Medicine
Brigham and Women's Hospital
Harvard Medical School
Boston, Massachusetts

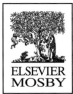

ELSEVIER
MOSBY

ELSEVIER
MOSBY

The Curtis Center
170 S Independence Mall W 300E
Philadelphia, Pennsylvania 19106

SIGNS AND SYMPTOMS IN PEDIATRICS

NOTICE

Pediatrics is an ever-changing field. Standard safety precautions must be followed, but as new research and clinical experience broaden our knowledge, changes in treatment and drug therapy may become necessary or appropriate. Readers are advised to check the most current product information provided by the manufacturer of each drug to be administered to verify the recommended dose, the method and duration of administration, and contraindications. It is the responsibility of the licensed prescriber, relying on experience and knowledge of the patient, to determine dosages and the best treatment for each individual patient. Neither the publisher nor the author assumes any liability for any injury and/or damage to persons or property arising from this publication.

Library of Congress Cataloging-in-Publication Data

Sign and symptoms in pediatrics: literature-based approach to pediatric conditions/ editor-in-chief, Mark A. Davis . . . [et al.].
    p. cm.
    ISBN 0-323-01898-x
    1. Pediatrics–Handbooks, manuals, etc. 2. Children–Diseases–Diagnosis–Handbooks, manuals, etc. 3. Symptoms–Handbooks, manuals, etc. I. Davis, Mark A.

RJ48.S645 2005
618.92–dc22   2004055176

Acquisitions Editor: James Merritt

Printed in the United States of America

Last digit is the print number: 9   8   7   6   5   4   3   2   1

I would like to dedicate this book to the memory of my parents, Alberta "Peachie" and Alan Burton Gruskin, who were the two best teachers I knew. They taught me much of what I know, how to admit to what I don't know and most importantly how to find the answers to my questions.

SIGNS & SYMPTOMS
IN PEDIATRICS

Urgent and Emergent Care

Contributors

Dewesh Agrawal, MD
Attending Physician, Emergency Medicine
Children's National Medical Center;
Assistant Professor of Pediatrics and Emergency Medicine
George Washington University School of Medicine and Health Sciences
Washington, DC

Jennifer Audi, MD
Clinical Instructor Emergency Medicine—Emory Healthcare;
Fellow in Medical Toxicology—Emory/Centers for Disease Control &
Prevention;
Georgia Poison Center—Grady Health System
Atlanta, Georgia

Richard Gary Bachur, MD
Associate Chief and Fellowship Director, Division of Emergency
    Medicine
Children's Hospital Boston
Boston, Massachusetts

Mary Christine Bailey, MD, FAAP
Director of Pediatric Emergency Medicine, Department of Emergency
    Medicine
Newton-Wellesley Hospital
Newton, Massachusetts

Theresa Moore Becker, DO
Clinical Fellow in Pediatrics, Department of Pediatrics
Beverly Hospital
Beverly, Massachusetts

Marisa Brett-Fleegler, MD
Instructor in Pediatrics, Harvard Medical School;
Division of Emergency Medicine
Children's Hospital Boston
Boston, Massachusetts

Michael J. Burns, MD, FACEP, FACMT
Co-Director, Division of Medical Toxicology
Department of Emergency Medicine
Beth Israel Deaconess Medical Center;
Assistant Professor of Medicine, Harvard Medical School
Boston, Massachusetts

Andrew J. Capraro, MD
Division of Emergency Medicine
Children's Hospital Boston
Boston, Massachusetts

Michelle M. Carlo, MD
Instructor in Pediatrics (2002-2003), Department of Emergency Medicine
Children's Hospital Boston
Boston, Massachusetts

Sarita A. Chung, MD
Instructor in Pediatrics, Harvard Medical School;
Attending Physician, Division of Emergency Medicine
Children's Hospital Boston
Boston, Massachusetts

Jacqueline Bryngil Corboy, MD
Instructor in Pediatrics, Harvard Medical School;
Children's Hospital Boston
Boston, Massachusetts

Atima C. Delaney, MD, FAAP
Instructor in Pediatrics, Harvard Medical School;
Assistant in Medicine and Attending Physician
Division of Emergency Medicine
Children's Hospital Boston
Boston, Massachusetts

Laura A. Drubach, MD
Instructor in Pediatrics, Harvard Medical School;
Division of Pediatric Emergency Medicine
Department of Medicine
Children's Hospital Boston
Boston, Massachusetts

Karen Eileen Dull, MD
Instructor in Pediatrics, Harvard Medical School;
Division of Emergency Medicine
Children's Hospital Boston
Boston, Massachusetts

Alexandra Epee-Bounya, MD
Clinical Instructor in Pediatrics, Division of Emergency Medicine
Children's Hospital Boston
Boston, Massachusetts

David Greenes, MD
Assistant Professor of Pediatrics, Harvard Medical School;
Department of Medicine
Children's Hospital Boston
Boston, Massachusetts

Marvin B. Harper, MD
Assistant Professor of Pediatrics, Harvard Medical School;
Attending in Infectious Diseases and Emergency Medicine
Children's Hospital Boston
Boston, Massachusetts

Joeli Hettler, MD
Attending Physician, Departments of Emergency Medicine and Pediatrics
University of Michigan Health System
Ann Arbor, Michigan

Ron Kaplan, MD
Assistant Professor of Pediatrics
University of Washington School of Medicine;
Attending Physician, Emergency Services
Children's Hospital & Regional Medical Center
Seattle, Washington

Yiannis L. Katsogridakis, MD, MPH
Instructor, Department of Pediatrics
Northwestern University Feinberg School of Medicine;
Attending Physician
Division of Pediatric Emergency Medicine
Children's Memorial Hospital
Chicago, Illinois

Lois K. Lee, MD, MPH
Instructor in Pediatrics, Harvard Medical School;
Attending Physician
Division of Emergency Medicine
Children's Hospital Boston
Boston, Massachusetts

Katherine F. McGowan, MD, MPH
Assistant Professor of Pediatrics and Emergency Medicine
University of Connecticut School of Medicine
Connecticut Children's Medical Center
Hartford, Connecticut

Mark I. Neuman, MD, MPH
Instructor in Pediatrics, Harvard Medical School;
Staff Physician
Division of Emergency Medicine
Children's Hospital Boston
Boston, Massachusetts

Ana Maria Paez, MD
Attending Physician, Emergency Physicians Department
Miami Children's Hospital
Miami, Florida

Barbara M. Garcia Peña, MD, MPH
Director, Pediatric Emergency Medicine Research;
Assistant Director, Pediatric Emergency Medicine Fellowship
Miami Children's Hospital
Miami, Florida

Catherine E. Perron, MD
Instructor in Pediatrics, Harvard Medical School;
Attending Physician, Division of Emergency Medicine
Children's Hospital Boston
Boston, Massachusetts

Cara Pizzo, MD
Pediatrician and Director of Pediatric Urgent Care
Palo Alto Medical Foundation
Palo Alto, California

Sara Ann Schutzman, MD
Assistant Professor of Pediatrics, Harvard Medical School;
Division of Emergency Medicine
Children's Hospital Boston
Boston, Massachusetts

Andrea E. C. Shah, MD
Instructor of Pediatrics, Harvard Medical School;
Department of Emergency Medicine
Children's Hospital Boston
Boston, Massachusetts

Michael W. Shannon, MD, MPH
Chief, Division of Emergency Medicine
Children's Hospital Boston;
Associate Professor of Pediatrics, Harvard Medical School
Boston, Massachusetts

Sujit Sharma, MD
Education Director and Staff Physician
Division of Emergency Medicine
Children's Healthcare of Atlanta at Scottish Rite
Atlanta, Georgia

Anne M. Stack, MD
Assistant in Medicine, Children's Hospital Boston;
Assistant Professor of Pediatrics, Harvard Medical School
Boston, Massachusetts

Andrea Stracciolini, MD
Division of Sports Medicine and Division of Emergency Medicine
Harvard Medical School;
Children's Hospital Boston
Boston, Massachusetts

Susan B. Torrey, MD
Assistant Clinical Professor of Pediatrics, Harvard Medical School;
Staff Physician, Emergency Medicine
Children's Hospital Boston
Boston, Massachusetts

Kevin J. Walsh, MD
Instructor in Pediatrics, Harvard Medical School;
Division of Emergency Medicine
Children's Hospital Boston
Boston, Massachusetts

Mark L. Waltzman, MD
Assistant Professor of Pediatrics, Harvard Medical School;
Attending Physician, Division of Emergency Medicine
Children's Hospital Boston
Boston, Massachusetts

Debra L. Weiner, MD, PhD
Assistant in Medicine, Children's Hospital Boston;
Assistant Professor of Pediatrics
Harvard Medical School
Boston, Massachusetts

Ben M. Willwerth, MD
Clinical Instructor in Pediatrics, Harvard Medical School;
Division of Emergency Medicine
Children's Hospital Boston
Boston, Massachusetts

Preface

Although most literature-based textbooks are designed around diseases, children generally present to emergency departments and clinics with symptoms for evaluation and care. The Signs and Symptoms Series is designed to stimulate the practitioner to consider many of the important conditions that could be responsible for the presenting problems of our patients. In most cases, chapters are organized so that the most life threatening, and not the most common, diagnoses are listed first. Although we always consider the most serious conditions before the most common, in most cases all that is required to effectively rule out a life- or limb-threatening diagnosis is history and examination. We have been gratified and appreciative of the wonderful feedback we have received from readers of the *Signs and Symptoms in Emergency Medicine* text. We hope this next volume in the series is as useful to students and practitioners and look forward to your comments and suggestions.

This text is not a "cook-book" for care, nor is it possible in a text of this size to list a complete differential diagnosis. It is intended to be useful in clinical care settings and as a study guide to urgent and emergent pediatric conditions. For each diagnosis listed within a symptom chapter, symptoms, signs, workup, and treatment considerations are addressed. The authors and editors have tried, where possible, to provide a literature-based assessment of the frequency with which findings and tests will be present/positive where the disease is present (i.e., sensitivity). The following system has been used:

+	(<5%)
++	(6%-30%)
+++	(31%-69%)
++++	(70%-94%)
+++++	(95%-100%)

If a test is highly sensitive, it is likely to be positive when the disease is present. However, as sensitivity rises, specificity (the frequency of negative results in those without the disease) usually falls, which increases the likelihood of false positive results. It is also important to remember the importance of "pre-test probability" of disease on our decision to order and final interpretation of the results of a test. By definition, most medical tests show a high frequency of false positive results in populations of patients with low prevalence of disease (and conversely high frequency of false negative results in populations with high prevalence of disease) because of imperfect specificity and sensitivity of tests.

Therefore, experienced practitioners and medical decision scientists alike understand that the thoughtful application of literature-based decision-making requires a thorough understanding of the literature with recognition of patterns in presentation that allows us to bring order to the seeming chaos of medical diagnosis and treatment. We hope that the information "framing" each discussion of symptoms and diagnoses in this text will help in this regard (thank you, Dr. Jerry Hoffman, my good friend and mentor).

I want to express my sincere thanks and appreciation to the faculty at the Boston Children's Hospital at Harvard Medical School for their outstanding work on this volume. In particular, the focus of the Emergency Medicine Group in leading and providing most of the material for this text has been inspiring. The faculty, fellows and residents are incredibly talented individuals who have made this book possible. Dr. Karen Gruskin, the Editor-in-Chief for this edition, managed to find the balance between our desire for consistency in the series and the special circumstances of Pediatric Medicine and its literature basis. Shannon Manzi, PharmD, showed a remarkable depth of knowledge and attention to detail that added a tremendous amount, and Dr. Vinny Chiang demonstrated leadership and insights that are found throughout. It was Dr. Gary Fleisher, Division Chief of Emergency Medicine at Boston Children's (now Pediatrician-in-Chief of the hospital), who first supported Boston Children's taking on this project. All of us at Harvard admire and appreciate Gary's unparalleled academic leadership and warm personal style. In addition, Dr. Michael Shannon, now Chief of Emergency Medicine at Boston Children's, has been so very generous in sharing his personal time and thoughts in reviewing this manuscript. And as always, thanks to Sigalit, Eric, Michael, Ruth, and Joe.

Caring for children is an awesome responsibility and a wonderful opportunity. We hope that this text may add to your ability to provide comfort, diagnosis, and treatment for our children (and their parents) in their time of need.

Mark A. Davis, MD, MS

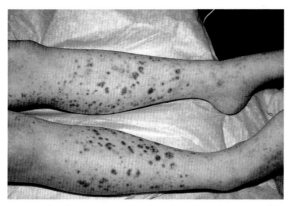

Fig. 6-2 Skin lesions of Henoch-Schönlein purpura in its typical symmetric distribution—on the lower extremities. (From Shah B, Laude T: *Atlas of pediatric clinical diagnosis,* Philadelphia, 2002, WB Saunders.)

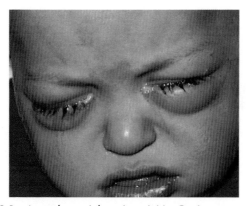

Fig. 12-3 Acute bacterial conjunctivitis. Copious amounts of mucopurulent discharge have made the upper and lower eyelids adhere to each other. Chemosis of the upper and lower lids may also make opening the eyelids difficult. (From Zitelli B, Davis H: *Atlas of pediatric physical diagnosis,* 4th ed, St. Louis, 2002, Mosby.)

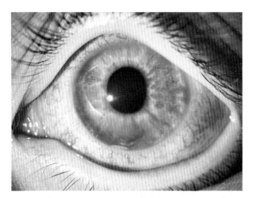

Fig. 12-5 Viral conjunctivitis with hyperemia and a watery discharge. (From Zitelli B, Davis H: *Atlas of pediatric physical diagnosis,* 4th ed, St. Louis, 2002, Mosby.)

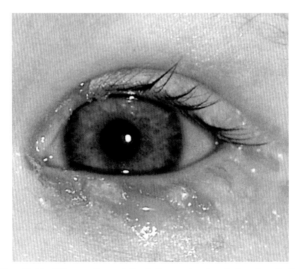

Fig. 12-7 Obstruction of the left nasolacrimal duct has led to the development of mucopurulent discharge and tearing. (From Zitelli B, Davis H: *Atlas of pediatric physical diagnosis,* 4th ed, St. Louis, 2002, Mosby.)

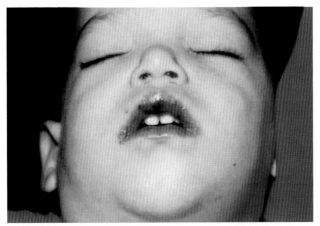

Fig. 14-2 Patient with Kawasaki disease. **A,** Dry, fissured lips. (Courtesy Anthony J. Mancini, MD, Chicago.)

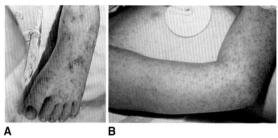

A   **B**

Fig. 29-1   Rocky Mountain spotted fever. **A,** The exanthem characteristic of this disease first appears distally on wrists, ankles, palms, and soles. **B,** In this child the rash has become generalized. Both petechial and blanching erythematous lesions are present. (From Zitelli B, Davis H: *Atlas of pediatric physical diagnosis,* 4th ed, St. Louis, 2002, Mosby. Courtesy Ellen Wald, MD, Children's Hospital of Pittsburgh, Pittsburgh, PA.)

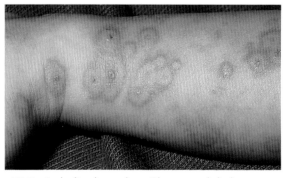

Fig. 29-2   Early fixed papules with a central dusky zone on the dorsum of the forearm of a child with erythema multiforme caused by herpes simplex virus. (From Weston W, Lane A, Morelli J: *Color textbook of pediatric dermatology,* 3rd ed, St. Louis, 2002, Mosby.)

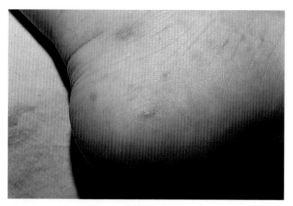

Fig. 29-3 Scabies. Papules and burrows on the foot of an infant. (From Weston W, Lane A, Morelli J: *Color textbook of pediatric dermatology,* 3rd ed, St. Louis, 2002, Mosby.)

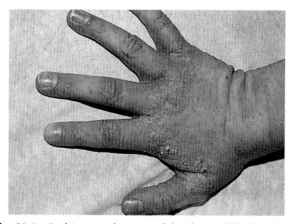

Fig. 29-4 Scabies. Involvement of the dorsa of the hands and interdigital webs in a child. (From Weston W, Lane A, Morelli J: *Color textbook of pediatric dermatology,* 3rd ed, St. Louis, 2002, Mosby.)

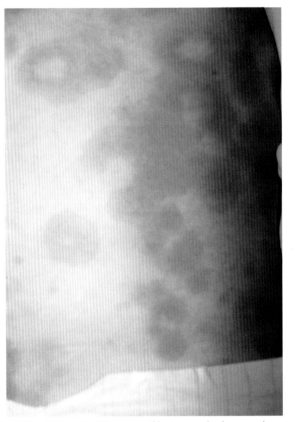

Fig. 29-6 Urticaria. Close-up of lesions, which are pale edematous plaques with irregular margins and a surrounding erythematous flare. (From Shah B, Laude T: *Atlas of pediatric clinical diagnosis*, Philadelphia, 2002, WB Saunders.)

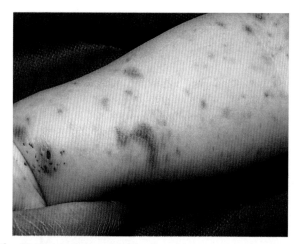

Fig. 29-7 Meningococcemia. Petechiae are more apparent in this close-up of an infant. Gram stain of petechial scrapings may reveal organisms. (From Zitelli B, Davis H: *Atlas of pediatric physical diagnosis,* 4th ed, St. Louis, 2002, Mosby.)

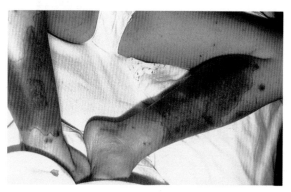

Fig. 29-8 Meningococcemia. Purpura may progress to form areas of frank cutaneous necrosis, especially in patients with disseminated intravascular coagulation. (From Zitelli B, Davis H: *Atlas of pediatric physical diagnosis,* 4th ed, St. Louis, 2002, Mosby. Courtesy Kenneth Schmitt, MD.)

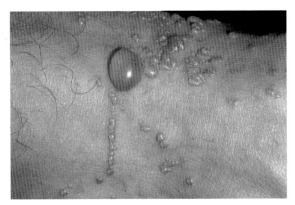

Fig. 29-9 Poison ivy. A classic presentation with vesicles and blisters. A line of vesicles (linear lesions) caused by dragging the resin over the surface of the skin with the scratching finger is a highly characteristic sign of plant contact dermatitis. (From Habif T: *Clinical dermatology,* 3rd ed, St. Louis, 1996, Mosby.)

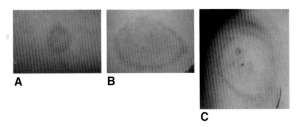

Fig. 29-12 Erythema migrans. **A,** This 2- to 3-cm lesion is just starting to clear centrally. **B,** This larger plaquelike lesion had a bluish center the day before, which has faded to pink. **C,** Central clearing is nearly complete, and within the erythematous border the puncta of two tick bites are evident. (From Zitelli B, Davis H: *Atlas of pediatric physical diagnosis,* 4th ed, St. Louis, 2002, Mosby. **A** and **B,** Courtesy Sylvia Suarez, MD, Centerville, VA; **C,** Courtesy Ellen Wald, MD, Children's Hospital of Pittsburgh, Pittsburgh, PA.)

Contents

CHAPTER 1

Abdominal Pain

BARBARA M. GARCIA PEÑA

Abdominal pain is one of the most common complaints of pediatric patients coming to the emergency department (ED). Although in most cases the cause is benign, one must be cautious not to miss the life-threatening conditions that require immediate diagnosis and treatment. Clues to abdominal pain that may be caused by acute abdominal emergencies include the intensity of the pain, acuity of onset, and positive physical findings. In addition, there are many extraintestinal causes of abdominal pain that should be considered when evaluating abdominal pain in children.

GASTROINTESTINAL DISORDERS

MALROTATION AND VOLVULUS

Malrotation of the intestines is a congenital condition with abnormal fixation of the bowel mesentery. This causes a propensity for the bowel to "volvulize," or twist, causing obstruction and bowel ischemia (Fig. 1-1). Volvulus from malrotation often presents during the first few weeks of life but may commonly be seen in children up to 1 year of age and less commonly later in life. A complete volvulus of the bowel for even 1 hour can cause ischemia and necrosis.

Symptoms
- Severe, constant abdominal pain if complete and ischemic +++++
- Bile-stained vomiting +++
- Abdominal distention
- Constipation

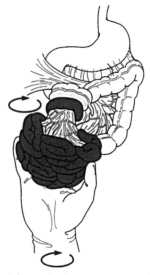

Fig. 1-1   Schematic showing intestinal volvulus.

Signs
- Diffuse abdominal tenderness
- Bloody stool ++
- Peritoneal signs if ischemia has developed

Workup
- Flat and upright films of the abdomen may show evidence of bowel obstruction with dilated loops of bowel, air-fluid levels, gastric dilation, and/or limited gas distal to the obstruction ++ (Fig. 1-2).
- Upper gastrointestinal (UGI) series is the study of choice.

Comments and Treatment Considerations
Intravenous (IV) fluid and electrolyte replacement should begin immediately. Immediate surgical correction is mandatory if volvulus is present.

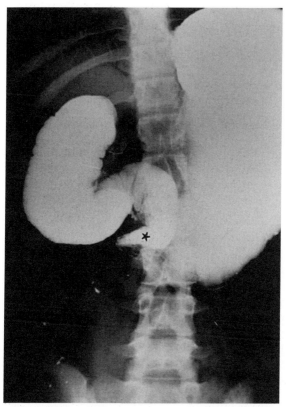

Fig. 1-2   This upper gastrointestinal contrast study shows malrotation with volvulus. The "beak" (asterisk) is illustrated.

INTUSSUSCEPTION

Intussusception is the telescoping of one segment of bowel into a more distal segment, usually occurring at the junction of the terminal ileum and the ileocecal valve (Fig. 1-3). It is the most common cause of acute intestinal obstruction in infants and usually occurs between 3 and 24 months of age.

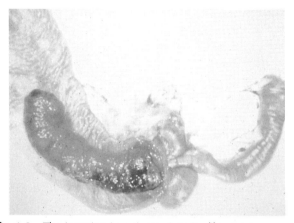

Fig. 1-3 The intestine invaginates into itself in intussusception. The ileum is pulled through the ileocecal valve into the colon, the most common pattern seen in infancy.

Symptoms
- Episodic, crampy abdominal pain +++++
- Vomiting ++++
- Episodes of crying and drawing up legs followed by periods of quiet and/or lethargy ++++
- Poor oral feeding
- Bloody (currant jelly) stool (often a late finding) ++

Signs
- Sausage-shaped abdominal mass usually palpated in the right upper quadrant +++
- Abdominal distention +++
- Abdominal tenderness +++
- Dehydration
- Occult blood in the stool +++
- Currant jelly stool ++

Workup
- Plain films of the abdomen are variable and depend on the duration of the intussusception. Findings range from normal

++ to distended bowel with air-fluid levels to a soft tissue mass +++ (Fig. 1-4).

- Air enema +++++ is replacing barium enema (BE) ++++, which has long been the gold standard for diagnosing and treating intussusception. Air enemas are considered safer and more efficacious in reduction. Surgical consultation should be considered, because some children with intussusception require surgery if the reduction is unsuccessful or incurs complications, such as perforation or if the child shows evidence of gangrenous bowel.
- Routine laboratory tests are not helpful in intussusception.
- Ultrasound ++++ is proving to be useful in diagnosing intussusception; however, the patient would have to undergo air enema or BE to attempt reduction of the intussusception.

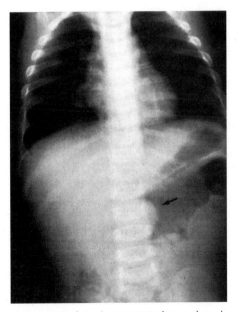

Fig. 1-4   Intussusception. Anteroposterior supine view of abdomen demonstrates soft tissue density (*arrow*) in distended small bowel. (From Rosen P: *Diagnostic radiology in emergency medicine,* St Louis, 1992, Mosby.)

Comments and Treatment

The recurrence rate of intussusception is 1% to 3% after BE or air enema reduction. When there is a second recurrence many practitioners suggest that a second BE/air enema reduction be performed. With a third event, surgical correction is recommended. Some experts recommend IV antibiotic administration before reduction with air enema or BE.

APPENDICITIS

Acute appendicitis is the most common abdominal surgical emergency seen in children. It is particularly difficult to diagnose in infants and young children and in its early stages. Expedient diagnosis of appendicitis is urgent because appendiceal perforation can occur within 24 to 48 hours of symptom onset.

Symptoms

- Periumbilical abdominal pain that migrates to the right lower quadrant within 12 to 48 hours of onset ++++
- Anorexia ++++
- Nausea and vomiting +++
- Diarrhea ++

Signs

- Right lower quadrant abdominal tenderness ++++
- Low-grade fever +++
- Rebound tenderness +++
- Guarding +++
- Psoas sign (abdominal pain with passive extension of the right hip or active flexion against resistance) ++
- Rovsing's sign (right lower quadrant pain with palpation of the left lower quadrant) ++
- Obturator sign (pain with passive internal rotation of the right hip) +++
- Pain with hopping on right foot or coughing

Workup

Appendicitis is considered to be a clinical diagnosis, although abdominal computed tomographic (CT) scanning, particularly with rectal contrast, has shown significant success in decreasing the number of patients taken to the operating room (who do not have appendicitis).

- Abdominal CT scanning, particularly with rectal contrast, has a sensitivity and specificity of 94% to 100% +++++.
- White blood cell (WBC) count is usually mildly elevated (between 10,000 and 15,000) but has low accuracy and discriminates poorly between appendicitis and other conditions.
- Plain x-rays may show a fecalith in 8% to 10% of patients; however, x-ray findings are normal in most patients with appendicitis.
- Ultrasound (US) has accuracy rates that vary according to radiologist's experience; not helpful in obese children ++++.

Comments and Treatment Considerations

Children are more likely to have atypical presentations of appendicitis than adults and are also more likely to have perforated appendicitis at the time of ED presentation. IV antibiotic therapy may be indicated and should be discussed with the consultant surgeon.

BOWEL OBSTRUCTION

Small-bowel obstructions are caused mainly by postoperative adhesions, incarcerated hernias, and neoplasms. In the newborn, congenital malformations of the intestinal tract will also present as bowel obstruction.

Symptoms

- Abdominal pain +++
- Nausea and vomiting +++
- Inability to pass stool or flatus ++++
- Bloating
- Incarcerated hernias present with inguinal pain or bulge or mass in scrotum

Signs

- Diffuse abdominal tenderness
- Abdominal distention +++

- Low-grade fever
- Tender mass in scrotum with inguinal hernias

Workup

- Flat and upright abdominal films looking for air-fluid levels and distention of the small bowel +++. A "double-bubble" sign is pathognomonic for duodenal atresia +++++ (Fig. 1-5).
- Laboratory tests are not helpful.

Comments and Treatment Considerations

Surgical consultation should be considered if there is suspicion of complete or partial bowel obstruction. The patient should be NPO, a nasogastric tube (NGT) inserted, and IV fluids started. There may be a role for CT scanning when obstruction is not clearly demonstrated on x-rays and for further diagnostic evaluation.

INFLAMMATORY BOWEL DISEASE

Patients with inflammatory bowel disease (IBD) often have severe colicky abdominal pain and diarrhea with or without blood. The pain may localize in the right lower quadrant, especially with Crohn's disease, necessitating consideration of acute appendicitis. Rarely, massive colonic distention (toxic megacolon) may develop with ulcerative colitis (UC) or Crohn's disease. This is a life-threatening emergency that has a mortality rate as high as 25% (see Chapter 16, Gastrointestinal Bleeding).

PEPTIC ULCER DISEASE

Peptic ulcer disease (PUD) is becoming a more recognized disorder in pediatrics because of the increasing use of endoscopy in children. Primary duodenal ulcers are far more common than primary gastric ulcers in children. *Helicobacter pylori* infection is strongly associated with antral gastritis and duodenal ulcer disease in children. Perforated ulcers can lead to severe peritonitis and may not be overtly symptomatic upon initial presentation.

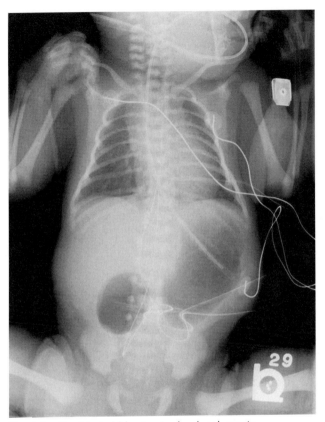

Fig. 1-5 Double-bubble sign in duodenal atresia.

Symptoms
- Generalized abdominal pain in younger children and epigastric abdominal pain in older children +++
- Nausea or vomiting ++
- GI bleeding (hematemesis or melena)

Signs

- Diffuse poorly localized abdominal tenderness in younger children and epigastric tenderness in older children +++
- Weight loss
- Hemoccult-positive stools +++
- Acute peritonitis with rigid abdomen if perforated ++++

Workup

- Esophageal endoscopy is the most accurate method of diagnosing PUD in children.
- *H. pylori* titers may be helpful.
- If perforation is suspected, flat and upright abdominal films should be obtained to look for free air ++++.
- CT scan is highly sensitive in identifying free air in the abdomen ++++.

Comments and Treatment Considerations

Emergency medical treatment of children with PUD should focus on detecting and treating the life-threatening complications of perforation and GI bleeding (see Chapter 16, Gastrointestinal Bleeding).

GASTROENTERITIS

The abdominal pain seen with acute gastroenteritis is commonly crampy and colicky. Vomiting and diarrhea are the hallmarks of this disease. Ninety percent of children with gastroenteritis have a viral etiology. There may be diffuse mild abdominal tenderness on physical examination (see Chapter 38, Vomiting).

GASTROESOPHAGEAL REFLUX DISEASE

Gastroesophageal reflux disease (GERD) presents with mid-epigastric abdominal pain and vomiting or spitting up after eating. Complications seen with GERD include failure to thrive, esophagitis, esophageal ulceration, and stricture (see Chapter 38, Vomiting).

CONSTIPATION

Constipation is one of the most common causes of abdominal pain seen in pediatrics. Although it is usually benign, more serious conditions that may present as constipation must be considered, including the following: mechanical obstruction, dehydration, lead ingestion, and infantile botulism. Also, on rare occasions constipation may indicate a more serious non-acute abdominal condition. No tests may necessarily be required, but a thoughtful evaluation with follow-up is needed for patients discharged with a diagnosis of constipation.

Symptoms
- Hard, infrequent stools associated with pain
- Nonspecific abdominal pain
- Encopresis (stool soiling in the otherwise toilet-trained child)

Signs
- Diffuse abdominal tenderness
- Distended abdomen
- Palpable stool in the abdomen
- Hard stool on rectal examination

Workup
- History and physical examination are diagnostic.
- Flat and upright abdominal films can be done to evaluate the quantity of stool in the bowel, although this is not usually necessary.

Comments and Treatment Considerations
Simple constipation should be treated initially with dietary changes. Increasing fluids and fiber intake may be enough to alleviate the symptoms. If not, bulk stool softeners, lubricants, and enemas can be used initially. In addition, psychosocial issues may be present in children with constipation and should be addressed for the benefit of the child. Consistent follow-up is strongly recommended because constipation may be a long-term problem for many children.

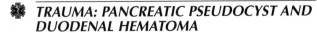

TRAUMA: PANCREATIC PSEUDOCYST AND DUODENAL HEMATOMA

Many children suffer from minor abdominal trauma during the course of play or after accidents. Those with a significant mechanism or worrisome physical examination results should be evaluated by abdominal CT and consultation with a pediatric surgeon (see Chapter 36, Trauma). Sometimes children with abdominal trauma do not show evidence of injury on initial evaluation but return to medical attention days or weeks later with vomiting, abdominal distention, and hematochezia. In particular, pancreatic pseudocysts and duodenal hematomas are characterized by late presentations. Handlebar injuries are the most common cause of pancreatic pseudocyst formation in children. A direct blow to the epigastrium by a small-diameter object such as a broom handle or edge of a shoe is the usual cause of duodenal hematomas.

PANCREATIC PSEUDOCYST
Symptoms
- Nonspecific abdominal pain
- Nausea and vomiting

Signs
- Classic triad of epigastric pain, palpable abdominal mass, and hyperamylasemia is rare in children

Workup
- Abdominal US ++.
- Abdominal CT with contrast recommended (acute pancreatic injuries may not be evident on the original CT scan) +++.
- Amylase ++.

Comments and Treatment Considerations
Diagnosis is often delayed because of nonspecific complaints and physical examination findings. The absence of hyperamylasemia does not preclude pancreatic injury. Also, the absolute value of amylase does not correlate with the degree of injury. Nonoperative treatment with nasogastric decompression and bowel rest is usually used for pancreatic pseudocysts in children. Surgical internal drainage is used if a pseudocyst persists >6 weeks.

DUODENAL HEMATOMA
Symptoms
- Nonspecific abdominal pain
- Nausea and vomiting (usually bilious)
- Gastric distention

Signs
- Midepigastric abdominal tenderness
- Abdominal distention

Workup
- Abdominal US +++ or UGI series ("coiled spring sign") +++.

Comments and Treatment Considerations
If the diagnosis of duodenal hematoma is made, injury to the pancreas must also be considered. Nonoperative management includes bowel rest, nasogastric decompression, and parenteral nutrition.

 GYNECOLOGIC DISEASE

ECTOPIC PREGNANCY
All women of childbearing age must be evaluated for the potential of pregnancy-related conditions. Because the classic triad of amenorrhea, abdominal pain, and abnormal bleeding is seen in only 70% of women with ectopic pregnancy, a pregnancy test is indicated to rule out pregnancy. Further evaluation for ectopic pregnancy is indicated (see Chapter 37, Vaginal Bleeding.)

OVARIAN TORSION
Ovarian torsion is a twisting of the ovary compromising ovarian blood supply, which may lead to ovarian ischemia if not rapidly diagnosed and treated.

Symptoms
- Sudden onset of severe unilateral or nonlocalized lower abdominal or pelvic pain
- Nausea or vomiting
- Low-grade fever
- Urinary symptoms

Signs
- Lower abdominal or pelvic pain tenderness +++++
- Adnexal mass +++++ (may need US to diagnose, especially in the prepubertal female)
- Peritoneal signs

Workup
- Pregnancy test.
- US is the imaging study of choice but does not have perfect sensitivity. Transvaginal US is particularly useful, but prepubertal and virginal girls may not tolerate a vaginal probe.
- Laparoscopy can be used for both diagnosis and treatment.

Comments and Treatment Considerations
In infants and children the ovaries are located higher in the abdomen. Ovarian torsion may be mistaken for appendicitis and care must be taken when making the diagnosis in adolescent girls. Usually, patients with torsion report a more sudden onset of pain than appendicitis. Other signs and symptoms can be identical.

PELVIC INFLAMMATORY DISEASE
Pelvic inflammatory disease (PID) is an infectious inflammation of the upper genital tract in females associated with multiple partners and nonbarrier contraceptive methods. Almost all first episodes of PID in adolescents are caused by chlamydial or gonococcal infections.

Symptoms
- Constant dull pelvic or bilateral lower quadrant pain +++++
- Abnormal vaginal discharge ++++
- Irregular vaginal bleeding ++
- Urinary symptoms ++

Signs
- Lower abdominal/pelvic tenderness ++++
- Adnexal tenderness ++++
- Cervical motion tenderness +++
- Abnormal vaginal discharge on examination
- Abnormal cervix on examination (erythematous, edematous, or friable) +++
- Temperature >38°C

Workup
- Pregnancy test.
- Cervical cultures for gonorrhea and chlamydia.
- Wet mount for clue cells and *Trichomonas*.
- Pelvic US to evaluate for tuboovarian abscess in select cases; approximately one third of patients with PID will have visible fallopian tubes and one fifth will have tuboovarian abscess.
- If measured, erythrocyte sedimentation rate (ESR) (>15 mm/hr) and C-reactive protein (CRP) are commonly elevated.

Comments and Treatment Considerations
Alternative diagnoses, such as ectopic pregnancy and appendicitis, should be considered. Because of the potential sequelae of untreated PID, the Centers for Disease Control and Prevention (CDC) recommends empiric use of antibiotics after the diagnosis is made. Ceftriaxone 250 mg IM × 1 and doxycycline 100 mg PO bid × 14 days with or without metronidazole 500 mg PO bid × 14 days are commonly used. Avoid the use of doxycycline in pregnancy and in children <8 years of age. Admission for IV antibiotics is recommended for any patient with PID whose diagnosis is uncertain, for patients with severe illness, and for patients who are pregnant, immunodeficient, or noncompliant.

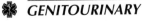

GENITOURINARY

TESTICULAR TORSION
Abdominal pain may be the only presenting symptom in males with testicular torsion. A complete genital examination should

be performed on all males with abdominal pain or testicular pain (see Chapter 31, Scrotal Pain or Swelling).

INCARCERATED HERNIA

Incarcerated inguinal hernia is a common cause of intestinal obstruction in childhood. It occurs more often in girls than in boys but usually involves the ovary rather than the intestine. Children may present with abdominal pain, irritability, and vomiting (see Chapter 31, Scrotal Pain or Swelling).

URINARY TRACT INFECTION

Children with urinary tract infection may have abdominal pain (see Chapter 18, Hematuria).

 ## CARDIAC DISEASE

Both myocarditis and pericarditis may present with abdominal pain, chest pain, dyspnea, and orthopnea (see Chapter 8, Chest Pain).

 ## LIVER/GALLBLADDER DISEASE

PANCREATITIS

Pancreatitis in younger patients is more unusual with a wider range of possible etiologies than in the older population, in which alcohol abuse and gallstones predominate. Most cases are idiopathic, but one third of pediatric cases are seen in patients with a systemic disease such as sepsis, hemolytic-uremic syndrome, systemic lupus erythematosus, or infection (e.g., mumps, coxsackie, salmonella, hemolytic streptococcus, and hepatitis A and B). Other less common causes are trauma (10%), structural defects including gallstones (10%), metabolic disease (10%), and drug induced (3%). No matter what the age of the patient, the presentation and evaluation are similar.

Symptoms

- Pain +++++ (epigastric ++, left upper quadrant pain ++, back pain ++)

- History of trauma
- Concurrent viral infection

Signs
- Abdominal tenderness ++++
- Vomiting ++++
- Low-grade fever ++
- Abdominal distention
- Guarding
- Dehydration (as a result of third spacing and possible hemorrhage)

Workup
- Lipase ++++ (tends to remain elevated for up to 14 days).
- Amylase ++++ (often returns to normal after 4 to 6 days).
- CT scan (contrast enhanced) ++++.
- US particularly useful for evaluating the biliary tract and following patients for complications such as pseudocyst formation.

Comments and Treatment Considerations

Children with pancreatitis are commonly acutely ill and require aggressive general supportive care.

Patients with acute pancreatitis require hospital admission for initial management. Most children require bowel rest for 1 to 2 days (range, 1 to 30), IV fluids or total parenteral nutrition for approximately 4 days (range 1 to 70), and hospitalization for an average of 15 days (range 3 to 90). Some children may require an NGT, but most will do well if left NPO until symptoms resolve. Antibiotics are not indicated unless treating a specific bacterial cause.

CT or US can be useful in the evaluation of complications, such as pseudocyst development, which occurs in approximately 10% of pediatric patients. Pancreatic necrosis and other complications commonly seen in older patients are rare in children.

CHOLANGITIS/CHOLELITHIASIS

The pain of biliary colic is generally acute in onset and colicky, often follows a meal, and is usually located in the right upper quadrant or epigastrium. Acute cholangitis should be suspected in the patient with right upper quadrant abdominal pain, fever, and jaundice (Charcot's triad). Severely ill patients may require biliary drainage and IV antibiotics (see Chapter 23, Jaundice).

HEPATITIS

Hepatitis usually causes variable constitutional symptoms such as right upper quadrant pain, anorexia, low-grade fever, nausea, vomiting, malaise, and fatigue. This is usually followed by scleral icterus, jaundice, and dark urine (see Chapter 23, Jaundice).

TUMOR

Abdominal tumors manifest either as discreet masses or as generalized enlargement but may be first noticed by a parent of a child complaining of a stomachache. Wilms' tumor and neuroblastoma are the most common malignant abdominal tumors in childhood.

WILMS' TUMOR
Symptoms
- Large flank mass in a well-appearing child
- Hypertension in 15% of cases
- Gross hematuria in <25% of patients

Signs
- Firm or soft abdominal mass
- Hypertension

Workup
- US is the preferred imaging study to initially localize the tumor.
- Abdominal x-ray may show a mass displacing the bowel but is not the study of choice.
- IV pyelogram (IVP) shows an intrarenal mass distorting the calyces.
- CT provides more anatomic detail.

Comments and Treatment Considerations

Children with presumed Wilms' tumor should be referred immediately to a pediatric surgeon. Disease-free survival after therapy approaches 90%.

NEUROBLASTOMA
Symptoms
- Midline or flank mass in an ill-appearing child
- Irritability
- Weight loss
- Pallor
- Bone pain

Signs
- Abdominal mass
- Periorbital metastases cause proptosis and "raccoon eyes" (periorbital ecchymosis)
- Cachexia
- Subcutaneous nodules
- Up to 3% of patients may have opsomyoclonus (myoclonic jerking and random eye movement) or a paraneoplastic syndrome

Workup
- US may show a suprarenal mass that displaces the kidney down and away from its normal axis.
- CBC looking for pancytopenia, which may occur with significant bone marrow involvement.
- CXR to identify any airway obstruction from large mediastinal masses.
- KUB may reveal a retroperitoneal mass, which may be calcified, displacing normal structures.
- Skeletal survey may show symmetric lytic lesions of the metastases of long bones.
- Bone scan looking for skeletal lesions.
- CT scan provides more anatomic detail.
- Bone marrow aspirate and biopsy looking for neuroblastoma cells and for possible staging.
- Serum ferritin and urinary catecholamines.

Comments and Treatment Considerations

Children diagnosed with neuroblastoma need referral to a pediatric oncologist for hospital admission and further evaluation. Approximately two thirds of patients have widespread metastases at the time of diagnosis. Opsoclonus and myoclonus (dancing eyes, dancing feet) are rare presenting symptoms of neuroblastoma. Prognosis is based on initial staging at diagnosis.

SYSTEMIC DISEASE

DIABETIC KETOACIDOSIS

Diabetic ketoacidosis (DKA) is a life-threatening complication seen in 20% to 40% of newly diagnosed diabetic patients. Abdominal pain may be one of the only presenting symptoms of ketoacidosis in children.

Symptoms
- Polyuria +++
- Polydipsia +++
- Abdominal pain
- Nausea and vomiting
- Weight loss

Signs
- Hyperpnea (Kussmaul's respirations) +++
- Dehydration
- Abdominal tenderness (some children may even have guarding and rigidity)
- Ketotic breath +++
- Change in mental status

Workup
- Venous blood gas (VBG), arterial blood gas (ABG), end-tidal CO_2 analysis to assess degree of acidosis.
- Serum glucose concentration.
- Electrolyte screening for abnormality and acidosis.
- CBC (WBC may be elevated).

- Urinalysis (UA) for glucose, protein, and ketones concentrations, as well as possible urinary tract infection.
- Baseline electrocardiogram (ECG) looking for cardiac arrhythmias associated with hyperkalemia or hypokalemia.

Comments and Treatment Considerations

For the severely dehydrated child, treatment should be directed toward the careful expansion of intravascular volume, as well as correction of the acidosis and potential shock (see Chapter 20, Hypotension/Shock). If shock is not present, hydration should be initiated with a bolus of 10 ml/kg of normal saline (NS) to begin to correct dehydration with the rest of the fluid replaced slowly over 24 to 48 hours, to minimize the potential for the development of cerebral edema. Ultimately, insulin will be required to arrest the ketotic process. For the patient with a serum pH < 7.3, blood glucose > 250 mg/dl, serum T_{CO_2} < 15 mEq/L, and ketonuria, the starting dose of regular insulin for continuous infusion is 0.1 unit/kg/hr and should be adjusted to a rate of glucose fall of 100 mg/dl/hr. Glucose-containing IV fluids need to be added when blood sugar levels approach 300 mg/dl. If any questions about management options exist, a pediatric endocrinologist should be consulted. All patients with DKA will need to be admitted to the hospital and intensive care monitoring should be strongly considered.

Patients with DKA will be depleted of total body potassium and will generally require early potassium repletion (despite normal or low normal serum potassium measurements), particularly while on insulin therapy, which further reduces serum potassium levels. Bicarbonate should be avoided. Ensure adequate urine output prior to instituting potassium-containing fluids. Consider repletion with a combination of potassium acetate and potassium phosphate because potassium chloride can contribute to hyperchloremic acidosis. To prevent significant hypokalemia, potassium levels must be followed carefully.

Treatment for the patient with new-onset diabetes without DKA should be discussed with a pediatric endocrinologist before beginning insulin therapy. These patients generally require admission or careful outpatient management for diabetic teaching.

❋ MISCELLANEOUS

PNEUMONIA

Lower lobe pneumonia may present with abdominal pain, fever, and respiratory distress and may be mistaken for appendicitis. The young child may have lethargy and a decreased appetite without any further symptoms (see Chapter 30, Respiratory Distress).

HENOCH-SCHÖNLEIN PURPURA

Abdominal pain usually precedes the rash and arthralgia of Henoch-Schönlein purpura (HSP) and may be the only presenting symptom. The pain is colicky and severe (see Chapter 6, Bleeding and Bruising).

STREPTOCOCCAL PHARYNGITIS

Many children with streptococcal pharyngitis will have abdominal pain. This diagnosis should be considered in any child with mild to moderate abdominal pain and throat complaints (see Chapter 26, Mouth and Throat Pain).

REFERENCES

Abi-Hanna A, Lake AM: Constipation and encopresis in childhood, *Pediatr Rev* 19:123-131, 1998.

Arkovitz MS, Johnson N, Garcia VF: Pancreatic trauma in children: mechanisms of injury, *J Trauma* 42:49-53, 1997.

Brodeur GM, Pritchard J, Berthold F, et al: Revisions of the international criteria for neuroblastoma diagnosis, staging and response to treatment, *J Clin Oncol* pp 1466-1477, 1993.

Centers for Disease Control and Prevention: Sexually transmitted diseases treatment guidelines 2002, *MMWR Morb Mortal Wkly Rep* 51 (RR-6):1-80, 2002.

Durbin DR, Liacouras CA: Gastrointestinal emergencies. In Fleisher GR et al., editors: *Textbook of pediatric emergency medicine*, Philadelphia, 2000, Lippincott Williams & Wilkins.

Eschenbach DA, Buchanan TM, Pollock HM, et al: Polymicrobial etiology of acute pelvic inflammatory disease, *N Engl J Med* 293: 166-171, 1975.

Fitzgerald JF: Constipation in children, *Pediatr Rev* 8:10299-10302, 1987.

Garcia Peña BM, Mandl KD, Kraus SJ, et al: Ultrasonography and limited computed tomography in the diagnosis and management of appendicitis in children, *JAMA* 282(11):1041-1046.

Garcia Peña BM, Taylor GA, Lund DP: Appendicitis in children. New insights into an age-old problem, *JAAPA* 13(1):65-67, 70, 73-76, 2000.

Green DM: Wilms' tumor, *Eur J Cancer* 33:409-418, 1997.

Gryboski JD: Peptic ulcer disease in children, *Med Clin North Am* 75(4):889-902, 1991.

Hale DE : Endocrine emergencies. In Fleisher GR et al., editors: *Textbook of pediatric emergency medicine*, Philadelphia, 2000, Lippincott Williams & Wilkins.

Harland RN: Diagnosis of appendicitis in childhood, *J R Coll Surg Edinb* 36:89-90, 1991.

Hogarty M, Lange B: Oncologic emergencies. In Fleisher GR et al., editors: *Textbook of pediatric emergency medicine*, Philadelphia, 2000, Lippincott Williams & Wilkins.

Holder WD: Intestinal obstruction, *Gastroenterol Clin North Am* 17:317, 1988.

Jaffe D, Wesson D: Emergency management if blunt trauma in children, *N Engl J Med* 324:1477-1482, 1991.

Judd RH: *Helicobacter pylori*, gastritis and ulcers in pediatrics, *Adv Pediatr* 39:283-306, 1992.

Kahn JG, Walker CG, Washington E, et al: Diagnosing pelvic inflammatory disease, *JAMA* 266:2594-2604, 1991.

Klekamp J, Churchwell KB: Diabetic ketoacidosis in children: initial clinical assessment and treatment, *Pediatr Ann* 25:387-393, 1996.

Long FR, Kramer SS, Markowitz RI: Intestinal malrotation in children: tutorial or radiographic diagnosis in difficult cases, *Radiology* 198:775, 1996.

Markowitz J, Ludwig S: Constipation. In Fleisher GR et al., editors: *Textbook of pediatric emergency medicine*, Philadelphia, 2000, Lippincott Williams & Wilkins.

Meyer JS, Harmon CM, Harty MP, et al: Ovarian torsion: clinical and imaging presentation in children, *J Pediatr Surg* 30:1433, 1995.

Paradise J: Pediatric and adolescent gynecology. In Fleisher GR et al., editors: *Textbook of pediatric emergency medicine*, Philadelphia, 2000, Lippincott Williams & Wilkins.

Powell OM, Othersen HB, Smith CD: Malrotation of the intestines in children: the effect of age on presentation and therapy, *J Pediatr Surg* 24:777-780, 1989.

Rosenbloom AL, Hamas R: Diabetic ketoacidosis (DKA): treatment guidelines, *Clin Pediatr* 35:261-266, 1996.

Saladino RA, Lund DP: Abdominal trauma. In Fleisher GR et al., editors: *Textbook of pediatric emergency medicine*, Philadelphia, 2000, Lippincott Williams & Wilkins.

Schnaufer L, Mahboubi S: Abdominal emergencies. In Fleisher GR et al., editors: *Textbook of pediatric emergency medicine*, Philadelphia, 2000, Lippincott Williams & Wilkins.

Schuh S, Wesson DE: Intussusception in children 2 years of age or older, *CMAJ* 136:269-272, 1987.

Spigland N, Brandt ML, Yazbeck S: Malrotation presenting beyond the neonatal period, *J Pediatr Surg* 25:1139-1142, 1990.

Weizman Z, Durie PR: Acute pancreatitis in childhood, *J Pediatr* 113: 24-29, 1988.

Young DG: Intussusception. In O'Neill JA, et al., editors: *Pediatric surgery*, St Louis, 1998, Mosby.

CHAPTER 2

Abuse/Rape

JOELI HETTLER

More than 3 million cases of child maltreatment are reported per year in the United States. Roughly 2 million cases are investigated and 1 million cases are substantiated. One needs to always maintain an index of suspicion for potential abuse, because an estimated 2000 to 5000 child fatalities occur per year as a result of maltreatment. Based on reports of all maltreatment cases from 1988, more than half (54%) suffer neglect, 23% suffer physical abuse, and 12% are sexually abused. Children younger than 5 years represent 88% of all cases reported and 77% of all fatalities.

Child abuse is legally defined by federal law as (1) any recent act or failure to act on the part of a parent or caretaker that results in death, serious physical or emotional harm, sexual abuse, or exploitation or (2) an act or failure to act that presents an imminent risk of serious harm. In addition, each state may have its own definition in addition to this minimal federal definition.

Health care providers play an important role in identifying suspected abuse. Any suspected abuse should be reported to child protective services when the suspected perpetrator is a caretaker (e.g., parent or baby-sitter). When the perpetrator is not a caretaker, suspected abuse should be reported to the police.

Certain patterns of injury are recognized as highly specific for abuse. In cases in which the observed injuries are not pathognomonic for abuse, a knowledgeable clinician and a high index of suspicion are required to make the diagnosis. Any child under 2 years of age who is suspected of being abused should have a skeletal survey (see skeletal trauma section).

There are historical features that would raise the concern of potential nonaccidental injury, such as the following:

- A delay in seeking medical care
- Evidence of trauma and no history of injury
- A history of injury that is not compatible with physical findings or the developmental level of the child
- A history of injury that changes over time

Although studies have demonstrated that child abuse can and does occur in almost any environment that a child is in, there are many risk factors that increase the potential for abuse, including the following:

- A child with special needs or physical deformity
- Prior involvement with child protective services
- Low-income family status
- A history of drug and alcohol abuse in the abuser
- A history of psychiatric disorders in the abuser
- Poor social support systems
- Social isolation of the child or the abuser
- Domestic violence in the home

ABUSIVE HEAD TRAUMA

Child abuse is responsible for up to 95% of serious head injuries in infants. Head injury is the most common cause of mortality among cases of abuse.

Symptoms (may be nonspecific)
- Excessive crying
- Poor feeding
- Vomiting
- Lethargy
- Seizures
- Apnea
- Unresponsiveness

Signs (may be absent)
- Bruising
- Full fontanelle
- Skull deformity

- Battle's sign
- Hemotympanum
- Neurologic abnormality
- Retinal hemorrhage (Fig. 2-1)

Workup
- Skull films.
- Head CT scan.
- Ophthalmologic examination.
- Head MRI scan.

Comments and Treatment Considerations
Certain types of head injuries are more typical of abuse. Skull fractures from abuse are likely to be bilateral, comminuted,

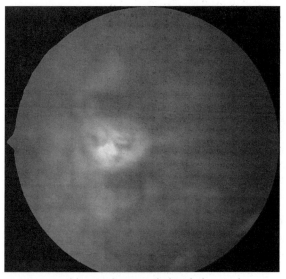

Fig. 2-1   Retinal hemorrhage in shaken baby syndrome. Visualization with the direct ophthalmoscope is not always possible. This child died of his injuries. (From Palay D, Krachmer J: *Ophthalmology for the primary care physician,* St. Louis, 1997, Mosby.)

depressed, involving nonparietal bone, or crossing suture lines (Fig. 2-2). Intracranial injuries are likely to present with subdural (Fig. 2-3) or subarachnoid hematoma, cerebral edema, or cortical injury.

Retinal hemorrhages after 4 weeks of age are highly associated with abuse. Retinal hemorrhages are most likely to be bilateral, involve many layers of the retina, and extend to the periphery of the retina.

A magnetic resonance imaging (MRI) scan may be more helpful than CT for dating intracranial injuries. All children whose symptoms are suggestive of abusive head trauma should have a dilated eye examination by an ophthalmologist.

SKELETAL TRAUMA

Many skeletal injuries from child abuse are discovered incidentally.

Symptoms
- Child not moving involved extremity
- Pain with movement or palpation of extremity

Signs
- Tenderness to palpation
- Redness
- Swelling
- Bruising of overlying skin
- Deformity

Workup
- Any child younger than 2 years who is suspected of being abused should have a complete skeletal survey. This includes the following views:
  - Anteroposterior (AP) and lateral chest.
  - AP humeri.
  - AP forearms.
  - Posteroanterior (PA) hands.
  - AP pelvis.

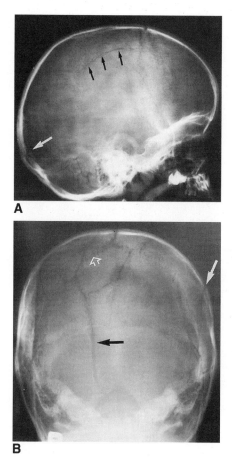

Fig. 2-2   Skull films of a 2-year-old abused child show multiple skull fractures in lateral and Towne's views. **A,** A linear left parietal fracture extending into the coronal suture (*black arrows* in **A**, *white arrow* in **B**). **B,** A complex parietooccipital fracture is present on the right, which is depressed (*white arrow* in **A**), crosses the lambdoid suture (*open white arrow* in **B**), and is diastatic (*black arrow* in **B**) as it extends inferiorly into the foramen magnum. (From Kleinman P: *Diagnostic imaging of child abuse,* 2nd ed, St. Louis, 1988, Mosby.)

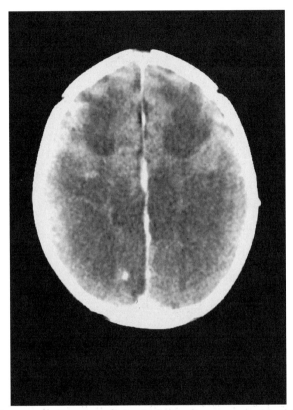

Fig. 2-3 Prominent subdural effusions are seen in this CT scan obtained during the tenth day of hospitalization of a shaken infant. The CT scan obtained on the day of admission failed to demonstrate these subdural hemorrhages. (From Grainger R, Allison D, et al.: *Grainger & Allison's diagnostic radiology*, 4th ed, Philadelphia, 2001, WB Saunders.)

- Lateral lumbar spine
- Lateral cervical spine
- AP femurs
- AP tibias
- AP feet
- AP and lateral skull
- Consider bone scan
- Consider MRI

Comments and Treatment Considerations

A "babygram" is not sufficient for identification of skeletal findings in abuse. All positive sites should be viewed in at least two projections. If abuse is strongly suspected and no fractures are found, a skeletal survey may be repeated in 2 weeks to evaluate for callus formation, evidence of a fracture not previously seen. Bone scan or MRI is also often helpful in identifying occult fractures or further defining questionable abnormalities on plain film.

Fractures may be further classified based on their specificity for abuse. Fractures that are specific to abuse include the following:
- Metaphyseal lesions (corner or bucket-handle fractures)
- Posterior rib fractures (especially in the first year of life)
- Scapular fractures
- Spinous process fractures
- Sternal fractures

Fractures with moderate specificity for abuse (high specificity when combined with head injury) include the following:
- The presence of multiple fractures (especially when they are bilateral or of different ages)
- Epiphyseal separations
- Vertebral body fractures and subluxations
- Digital fractures
- Complex skull fractures

Fractures that are common in abuse but have a low specificity for abuse include the following:
- Clavicular fractures
- Long bone shaft fractures
- Linear skull fractures

SOFT TISSUE INJURIES

Burns and bruises are common in cases of abuse. A careful and complete skin examination is essential in the evaluation when abuse is suspected. Certain soft tissue injuries have high specificity for abuse. All observed skin findings, including birthmarks and scars, should be documented with photography or careful description of size, color, location, and character of lesions.

BURNS

Features suggesting that burns are more likely to be due to abuse include the following:
- Delay in seeking care for burns or the mechanism is unexplained
- Contact burns (sharply demarcated edges, burn of uniform thickness) involving the dorsum of hands, buttocks, genitals, upper thigh or face, and neck
- When the burn is an imprint of a household item, such as iron or cigarette (this can happen unintentionally but is common in abuse)
- Scald burns (irregular margins, variable burn thickness, often extensive) in a stocking or glove distribution of the hands and feet (especially if bilateral) or of the genitalia (especially if there is central sparing present from contact with cooler bath base or if the flexor creases are spared)

BRUISES

Bruises are common in abuse but have a low specificity. Patterns of bruising more likely to be due to abuse include the following:
- Multiple bruises
- Bruises of varying ages as determined by color and stage of healing
- Bruising patterns that are in the shape of an object used to inflict injury such as a belt, buckle, stick, or cord (Fig. 2-4)
- Hand print (often a few finger-sized linear marks)
- Pinch marks (two opposing crescentic marks)
- Bite marks
- Ligature marks around extremities, neck, or genitals

Additionally, the location of bruises may be suggestive of nonaccidental injury, especially when they occur in areas related to punishment (e.g., buttocks, lower back, and outer thighs), areas not overlying a bony prominence (e.g., cheeks, calves, upper arms, and abdomen), other naturally protected areas of head and neck (e.g., external ear, posterior auricular area, lower jaw, and neck) or the digits.

OTHER SOFT TISSUE INJURIES

Other soft tissue injuries seen in abuse include traumatic alopecia, subungual hematomas, and frenulum lacerations.

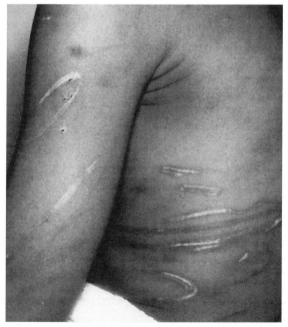

Fig. 2-4 Multiple scars produced by a prior whipping with a looped cord. (From Zitelli B, Davis H: *Atlas of pediatric physical diagnosis*, 4th ed, St. Louis, 2002, Mosby.)

Comments and Treatment Considerations

When significant bruising is present, blood dyscrasias must be ruled out. Prothrombin time (PT), partial thromboplastin time (PTT), and a platelet count are good initial screens.

 ## SEXUAL ABUSE

Sexual abuse is defined as contact or interaction between a child and an adult or older child when the child is being used for the sexual stimulation of that adult or older child or any sexual activity that a child cannot comprehend or give consent to or that violates the law.

Most sexual abuse occurs during preadolescence (ages 8 to 12 years) and girls are more likely to be abused than boys. Furthermore, boys are less likely to report abuse once it has occurred.

Risk factors include prior sexual abuse involving family members, poor parent-child relationships, poor relationships between parents, or the presence of a nonbiologically related male in the home.

Symptoms
- Disclosure of inappropriate sexual contact (sexual play involving another child of the same developmental age that includes mutual agreement to participate and does not result in injury is usually not considered "inappropriate")
- Behavioral changes
  - Sexual perpetration on others
  - Sexual acting out or promiscuity
  - School problems
  - Temper tantrums
  - Aggression
  - Sleep disturbances or nightmares
  - Appetite changes
  - Conduct disorders
  - Withdrawal
  - Self-injury
  - Substance use

- Medical complaints
  - Any complaint involving genital/rectal region
  - Abdominal pain
  - Headaches
  - Enuresis
  - Constipation/encopresis

Signs

In most cases of sexual abuse involving young children there are often no findings on examination.

Workup

Suspected sexual abuse is best evaluated by those experienced in interviewing and examining the sexually abused child. It is imperative to clearly document physical findings, and when possible, photographs should be obtained. Please see Fig. 2-5 for a diagram of normal female genitalia to aid in the description of findings.

In the many cases in which there are no physical findings of sexual abuse, successful prosecution is the result of a careful initial interview of the child by a person experienced in the conduct and documentation of such interviews. Pediatricians, social workers, law enforcement officers, and prosecutors must decide how to best coordinate the initial interview of the suspected sexual abuse victim in their community.

Physical examination

- A complete physical examination should include careful evaluation of the mouth and genital area.
- When a colposcope is not available, an otoscope provides additional light and magnification.
- Anal inspection should be performed in the lateral recumbent or supine position with the patient holding knees to chest. Gentle gluteal outward traction should be applied to evaluate presence of anal dilatation. Female genitalia should be examined first in the supine froglike position. Gentle outward and downward traction on the labia majora usually allows for sufficient visualization of vestibular structures. The knee-chest position often allows noninvasive visualization of the posterior hymen and cervix. In

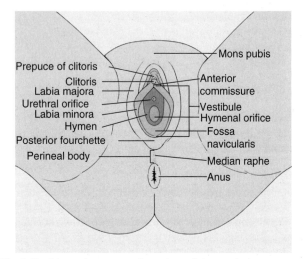

Fig. 2-5 Normal anatomy. Location of the genital structures of the prepubertal girl. (From Zitelli B, Davis H: *Atlas of pediatric physical diagnosis,* 4th ed, St. Louis, 2002, Mosby.)

estrogenized girls, a moist swab may be useful to separate hymenal folds for inspection.

Evidence collection

Evidence collection using an evidence collection ("rape") kit should be performed if the sexual contact occurred within 72 hours of the examination. Efforts should be made to collect linens and clothing worn during or just after the event.

Laboratory evaluation

- The CDC recommends screening for sexually transmitted diseases (STDs) in the following situations:
  - The suspected offender is at risk for having an STD.
  - The child has signs or symptoms of an STD.
  - STDs are especially prevalent in the community.
- Cultures (and not antigen-detection methods) should be used when screening for gonorrhea (GC) and chlamydia.

- In nonacute evaluations, careful examination without STD screening may be acceptable for an asymptomatic prepubertal child who lacks clear history or physical findings indicative of penetrating sexual abuse.
- Serologic testing for human immunodeficiency virus (HIV), syphilis, and hepatitis B (depending on immunization status) may be performed initially and 12 weeks after the assault. HIV testing should be repeated 6 months after the assault.

Comments and Treatment Considerations
Postexposure prophylaxis

Pregnancy prophylaxis with levonorgestrel (Plan B), 0.75-mg tablets, two tablets PO × 1 dose for postpubertal girls, should be offered if serum pregnancy test result is negative up to 5 days after the event. Chlamydia and GC prophylaxis should be given to postpubertal girls after sexual assault. Effective regimens include azithromycin 1 g PO × 1 dose plus cefixime 400 mg PO × 1 dose. If unavailable, cefixime may be replaced with ceftriaxone 125 mg IM × 1 dose. For patients older than 18 years, a fluoroquinolone such as ciprofloxacin 500 mg PO × 1 dose can be used in place of cefixime or ceftriaxone. Fluoroquinolones should not be used in patients who may have been exposed to *Neisseria gonorrhoeae* acquired in an area with known fluoroquinolone resistance. Metronidazole dosed at 2 g PO × 1 dose should also be considered for treatment of bacterial vaginosis. Prepubertal girls are at lower risk for ascending infection, so antimicrobial treatment should be based on the results of laboratory testing. In patients who have not been immunized, postexposure hepatitis B vaccination 0.5 ml IM should be initiated at the time of the evaluation. If the perpetrator is known to be positive for hepatitis B virus, give hepatitis B immune globulin 0.06 ml/kg (max 5 ml/dose) IM × 1 dose within 14 days of exposure in addition to initiating the vaccine.

Before offering postexposure antiviral therapy for HIV, one should consider the following:
- Likelihood of perpetrator being HIV infected
- Risk of transmission

- Vaginal/anal tears or bleeding
- Visible genital ulcers
- Time from assault
  - Prophylaxis most effective 1 to 2 hours after exposure
  - Prophylaxis has questionable efficacy if given more than 24-36 hours after exposure

Given the complexity of the various HIV prophylaxis regimens and resistance patterns, consultation with an expert in infection disease is warranted.

REFERENCES

Cahill LT, Kaminer RK, Johnson PG: Developmental, cognitive, and behavioral sequelae of child abuse, *Child Adolesc Psychiatr Clin N Am* 8(4):827-843, 1999.

Centers for Disease Control and Prevention: Discontinuation of cefixime tablets—United States, *MMWR Morb Mortal Wkly Rep* 51(46):1052, 2002.

Duhaime AC, Christian CW, Rorke LB, et al: Nonaccidental head injury in infants—the "shaken-baby syndrome," *N Engl J Med* 338(25):1822-1829, 1998.

Jain AM: Emergency department evaluation of child abuse, *Emerg Med Clin North Am* 17(3):575-593, 1999.

Kini N, Lazoritz S: Evaluation for possible physical or sexual abuse, *Pediatr Clin North Am* 45(1):205-219, 1998.

Nimkin K, Kleinman PK: Imaging of child abuse, *Radiol Clin North Am* 39(4):843-864, 2001.

Taketomo CK, et al, editors. *Pediatric dosage handbook, 2001-2002*, ed 8, Hudson, Ohio, 2001, Lexicomp.

Wissow LS: Child abuse and neglect, *N Engl J Med* 332(21):1425-1431, 1995.

CHAPTER 3

Altered Mental Status

DAVID GREENES

Altered mental status represents a spectrum of disability, from mild confusion to deep coma, and is a common reason for patients to seek emergency care. Initial evaluation and treatment are directed at rapidly identifying immediate threats to life and stabilization of the ABCs. This includes initial bedside check of oxygen saturation, glucose level, and cardiac monitor. The early provision of antibiotics in patients for whom a diagnosis of sepsis or meningitis is being considered is indicated.

The differential diagnosis for altered mental status is broad and includes several categories:

Primary brain insults
- Trauma (see Chapter 35, Trauma)
- Increased intracranial pressure (ICP) caused by tumor, meningitis, or ventriculoperitoneal (VP) shunt malfunction
- Cerebrovascular accident (CVA)
- Seizures (see Chapter 32, Seizures)
- Central nervous system (CNS) infections
- Toxic ingestions
- Carbon monoxide poisonings

Systemic illness leading to cerebral ischemia
- Hypoxia (see Chapter 30, Respiratory Distress)
- Hypotension (see Chapter 20, Hypotension/Shock)
- Hypoglycemia
- Hyperglycemia: DKA (see Chapter 1, Abdominal Pain)

Illness leading to generalized malaise and lethargy
- Intussusception
- Dehydration

Psychiatric disease

TRAUMA

Altered mental status is commonly seen in pediatric trauma (see Chapter 36, Trauma).

INCREASED INTRACRANIAL PRESSURE

Increased ICP may result from various causes including traumatic intracranial hematoma, cerebral contusion, spontaneous intracranial hemorrhage, cerebral edema, hydrocephalus, and brain tumor. Cerebral edema, in turn, may result from trauma, hypoxic-ischemic injury, infection, or metabolic disturbance (such as diabetic ketoacidosis).

Mild intracranial hypertension causes mild symptoms, such as headache and nausea. With more severe increases in ICP, neurologic deficits appear. Slowly advancing focal lesions may produce focal findings before generalized ones. Severe, generalized increased ICP causes the uncus of the temporal lobe to begin to herniate through the tentorial notch, causing compression of the adjacent brainstem structures. Without early reversal of this process, brainstem compression leads to progression of neurologic deterioration, cranial nerve dysfunction, and autonomic changes, culminating in death.

In general, the following symptoms and signs may occur as the disease process worsens, although individual cases may vary.

Symptoms
- Headache
- Nausea and vomiting
- Confusion/disorientation
- Lethargy

Signs
- Decorticate or decerebrate posturing
- Dilated and nonreactive ("blown") pupils
- Papilledema

- Hypertension, bradycardia, irregular respirations ("Cushing's triad") +
- Hemiparesis or other focal findings if mass or other slowly progressive process is present

Workup

- History directed toward identifying causes of intracranial hypertension: trauma, infection, metabolic disease, mass lesions.
- Focused neurologic examination: pupil reactivity and size, motor strength and tone, papilledema.
- Emergent head CT scan.
- Emergent neurosurgical consultation.
- Depending on the suspected diagnosis, additional workup may include the following:
  - Serum glucose and electrolytes
  - Blood culture
  - Further evaluation for associated medical illness or traumatic injury
- Deferral of lumbar puncture (LP) should be considered if there is concern of intracranial hypertension. Head CT and consultation with neurosurgery should be initiated. Antibiotics and other lifesaving therapies should not be withheld pending LP results if there will be a delay in LP performance.

Comments and Treatment Considerations

When intracranial hypertension is present, ABCs should be carefully evaluated and the airway managed as necessary. A mild degree of hyperventilation may be indicated (goal PCO_2 30 to 35 mm Hg). Therapeutic maneuvers include elevation of the head to promote venous drainage, restriction of hypotonic IV fluids, and endotracheal intubation to protect the airway. IV mannitol dosed at 0.5 to 1 g/kg given over 20 minutes should be initiated when tentorial herniation is suspected while awaiting surgical intervention. Neurosurgical interventions, if possible, can be lifesaving and should be pursued immediately.

BRAIN TUMOR

Brain tumors, especially if they involve the frontal lobe, may cause subtle changes in behavior or personality that occasionally persist for weeks before diagnosis. Depression of mental status can also occur secondary to intracranial hypertension if a posterior fossa tumor obstructs cerebrospinal fluid (CSF) outflow, thereby causing hydrocephalus.

Symptoms
- Headaches, especially in the morning +++
- Nausea and vomiting +++
- Ataxia ++
- Changes in behavior or school performance +
- Sleepiness +
- Irritability +

Signs
- Papilledema ++
- Focal neurologic deficits ++
- Bradycardia +
- Hypertension +

Workup

Head imaging (CT or MRI scans) should be pursued urgently whenever brain tumor is suspected and emergently in cases of suspected intracranial hypertension. Emergent neurosurgical consultation is indicated for patients with increased ICP. LP should not be performed in cases of suspected brain tumor, because cerebral herniation may result.

Comments and Treatment Considerations

Treatment of brain tumor includes surgical resection (when possible) and in some cases adjunct chemotherapy or radiation therapy. Emergency stabilization focuses on the ABCs of resuscitation and treatment for intracranial hypertension, if present. Emergent ventriculostomy may be lifesaving in patients with hydrocephalus and impending cerebral herniation. After stabilization the patient should be treated at a facility with neurooncology services.

SHUNT MALFUNCTION

Malfunction of VP shunts can result from mechanical disruptions of the shunt tubing or occlusion of the tubing with inflammatory or infectious material. Early symptoms may be very subtle. In some patients the only abnormality will be the parents' observation that the child "just doesn't look right" or is "acting a little different." As intracranial hypertension progresses, more obvious symptoms and signs will appear. If left untreated, cerebral herniation and irreversible brain injury or death may ensue.

Symptoms
- Headache ++++
- Change in behavior ++
- Lethargy ++
- Nausea and vomiting +++
- Fever (if simultaneous shunt infection) +
- Discomfort or swelling along the shunt track +
- Abdominal pain (if a CSF seroma is occluding outflow from the shunt) +

Signs
- Depressed mental status ++
- Pupillary asymmetry or lack of reactivity +
- Focal neurologic findings +
- Palpable discontinuity of the shunt or swelling around the shunt (in some patients) +
- Abnormal filling or emptying of the shunt reservoir with palpation (not reliable)
- Fever (in some cases of shunt infection)
- Abdominal tenderness or distention (in cases with abdominal CSF seroma)

Workup
In any child with a VP shunt and altered mental status, head CT scan, plain x-rays of the shunt ("shunt series"), and neurosurgical

consultation should be obtained without delay. In some patients, the neurosurgeon may aspirate fluid from the shunt to evaluate CSF pressure and cell counts. In some newer shunts, CSF pressure may be evaluated without aspiration.

Comments and Treatment Considerations

Intracranial hypertension can progress very quickly. In most cases a neurosurgeon will prefer to have the results of radiographic imaging before proceeding to surgery. However, if patients have signs of impending cerebral herniation, empiric bedside ventriculostomy or externalization of the shunt can be lifesaving.

CEREBROVASCULAR ACCIDENT

Cerebrovascular accidents (strokes) are rare in pediatrics but may occasionally lead to altered mental status. In most cases, however, focal neurologic findings will be evident at presentation when cerebrovascular accidents result from hemorrhage or ischemia.

Symptoms
- Sleepiness +
- Confusion ++
- Weakness +++
- Facial asymmetry +
- Abnormal speech +
- Headache (with hemorrhagic lesions) +

Signs
- Depressed mental status ++
- Focal neurologic findings ++++

Workup
- History directed at possible underlying causes: hypercoagulability, vasculitis, bleeding diatheses, sickle cell anemia, arterial dissection (traumatic or spontaneous).
- Careful neurologic examination.
- Emergent head CT scan.

- Emergent neurologic consultation.
- Further workup for underlying causes may be pursued semielectively.

Comments and Treatment Considerations

Thrombolytic therapy is increasingly being used in adults for acute thromboembolic stroke. To be effective, therapy must be initiated within 2 to 4 hours of symptom onset, ideally within 30 minutes. There is little published experience with thrombolytic therapy for pediatric stroke; therefore emergent neurologic consultation is indicated to consider all therapeutic possibilities. In some cases of hemorrhagic stroke, emergent neurosurgical intervention may be necessary.

 SEIZURES

Patients with altered mental status may be experiencing seizures or be in a postictal phase. Although many seizures have obvious generalized tonic-clonic activity, atonic or complex partial seizures may present with altered mental status as the sole abnormality. Some patients may have had an unwitnessed seizure before presentation with postictal lethargy as the only presenting finding (see Chapter 32, Seizures).

TEMPORAL LOBE EPILEPSY

Complex partial seizures involving the temporal lobe manifest as episodic impairment of consciousness, as episodic changes in affect or cognition, or as motor automatisms. In some cases it may be difficult to distinguish temporal lobe epilepsy from absence seizures, psychiatric illness, or toxic ingestion (see Chapter 32, Seizures).

 CENTRAL NERVOUS SYSTEM INFECTION

Infections of the CNS, either meningitis or encephalitis, may present with lethargy, confusion, or altered mental status. Bacterial meningitis is often a fulminating illness, which may be complicated by lethargy, seizures, coma, or stroke. Viral meningitis, in contrast, is generally mild and self-limited, causing minimal if any change in mental status. Infectious encephalitis may follow viral meningeal infection or may be the presenting manifestation of CNS viral infection. Cases may be mild and self-limited (as with varicella, Epstein-Barr virus, or influenza), but some cases (e.g., those caused by eastern equine encephalitis virus, West Nile virus, or herpes simplex virus [HSV]) may be quite severe, causing intractable seizures, coma, and long-term sequelae.

Symptoms
- Headache +++
- Lethargy ++
- Confusion +
- Photophobia
- Neck stiffness
- Seizures +
- Fever ++++
- Vomiting +++
- Rash (meningococcal disease, enteroviral meningitis)

Signs
- Irritability +++
- Nuchal rigidity +++
- Depressed mental status ++
- Delirium +
- Kernig's and/or Brudzinski's sign +
- Rash (petechiae/purpura with meningococcus, maculopapular with viral infections) +
- Signs of sepsis such as tachycardia, poor capillary refill, weak pulses, or hypotension (bacterial meningitis) +

Workup
- History including ill contacts, possible exposure to ticks or mosquitoes, and season of the year. Viral meningitis and arthropod-borne illnesses are more likely in the summer.
- Head CT scan if intracranial hypertension, focal neurologic findings, or seizures.

- LP with CSF for cell counts, chemistries, Gram stain, and culture. Latex agglutination studies for bacterial antigens may be helpful, especially if antibiotic therapy was initiated before CSF was obtained. CSF may also be sent for polymerase chain reaction testing for HSV.
  NOTE: LP is contraindicated if intracranial hypertension or uncontrolled bleeding diathesis is present.
- CBC count and blood culture.
- Electroencephalogram may be helpful in cases of encephalitis.

Comments and Treatment Considerations

Initial attention should be directed to the ABCs of resuscitation. IV access and simultaneous blood tests should be obtained immediately. IV boluses of isotonic fluids should be given to patients who are hypovolemic or in shock, taking into consideration that excess fluid may worsen cerebral edema.

In cases in which bacterial meningitis is a concern, steroids and antibiotics should be given immediately. Antibiotics may be delayed a few minutes while diagnostic specimens (CSF and blood cultures) are obtained, but prolonged delays should be avoided. Antibiotics should be given prior to LP or other tests if there will be a delay in performing these diagnostic procedures.

Ceftriaxone dosed at 100 mg/kg/day IV divided q12h (max 4 gm/day) with vancomycin dosed at 60 mg/kg/day IV divided q6h (max 3 gm/day) are good empiric choices. Recent studies suggest that steroids in the form of dexamethasone dosed at 0.15 mg/kg/dose IV (max 10 mg/dose) be considered in the patient with septic shock or meningitis if given concurrently or just before the first dose of antibiotics. For patients <30 days of age, give ampicillin to provide *Listeria* coverage (see Chapter 24, Fever).

For suspected HSV encephalitis, IV acyclovir (60 mg/kg/day divided q8h) should be initiated immediately.

❋ *TOXIC INGESTIONS*

Toxic ingestions are a leading consideration when evaluating patients with altered mental status. Toddlers and adolescents are the age-groups at highest risk. Some of the more common toxic ingestions to consider in a patient with altered mental status include ethanol, opiates, benzodiazepines, amphetamines and related "club drugs," antihistamines, antidepressants, clonidine, and salicylates (see Chapter 35, Toxic Ingestion, Approach To).

 ## CARBON MONOXIDE POISONING

Carbon monoxide poisoning may present with lethargy, confusion, or agitation, as a result of inadequate oxygen delivery to the brain. In addition to known exposures, it should be considered in particular during winter months when improperly ventilated heating systems may be in use (see Chapter 35, Toxic Ingestion, Approach To).

 ## HYPOXIA

Hypoxia requires immediate intervention to improve oxygenation and ensure adequate ventilation in parallel with rapid consideration of the cause. Hypoxia frequently results from respiratory illness (e.g., pneumonia, asthma, or anaphylaxis) but may occur with metabolic abnormalities such as sepsis, hematologic abnormalities, and toxic exposures (methemoglobinemia or carbon monoxide exposure), neurologic abnormalities (such as seizures or cerebral hematoma), or cyanotic heart disease. Patients who are hypoxic may exhibit either depressed mental status or agitation. Hypoxia-related agitation is sometimes initially mistaken for psychiatric illness. Unless preparing for definitive airway management, the physician should not use benzodiazepines and other anxiolytics as they may lead to further respiratory depression (see Chapter 30, Respiratory Distress).

 ## HYPOTENSION

Hypotension, with resultant hypoperfusion of the brain, may cause altered mental status. In most cases other historical features or physical findings indicating hypotension or shock will be evident. Occasionally, agitation, lethargy, or coma is the presenting manifestation of hypotension. Causes of hypotension include sepsis, anaphylaxis, acute blood loss, severe dehydration, toxic ingestions, adverse effects of medications, myocarditis, and spinal cord injury. Specific therapies addressing the cause of hypotension should be initiated without delay (see Chapter 20, Hypotension/Shock).

 METABOLIC DISEASE

HYPOGLYCEMIA

The leading cause of symptomatic hypoglycemia is an unintentional excess of exogenous insulin activity in a patient with diabetes mellitus. Other causes may include "ketotic hypoglycemia" (a syndrome of symptomatic hypoglycemia and ketosis in a young child after a prolonged fast), ethanol intoxication, ingestion of oral hypoglycemic agents, adrenal insufficiency, excess of endogenous insulin (with insulinoma or in infants born to diabetic mothers), and inborn errors of glycogenolysis, gluconeogenesis, or fatty acid oxidation.

Symptoms
- Lethargy +++
- Confusion +++
- Jitteriness +
- Diaphoresis +
- Seizures +

Signs
- Lethargy or confusion ++++
- Seizures +
- Diaphoresis +
- Jitteriness +

Workup

A bedside measure of serum glucose should be checked in all cases of altered mental status. If hypoglycemia is noted,

laboratory confirmation is desirable. In cases of hypoglycemia the following workup should be considered:
- Careful history, reviewing recent oral intake and use of insulin or other medications.
- History of illnesses, growth, and development.
- Urinalysis for ketones ± serum ketone screen.
- Serum electrolytes.
- Venous blood gas if appropriate, when hypoglycemia is not insulin related.
- Serum ammonia level if appropriate, when hypoglycemia is not insulin related.
- Serum ethanol level or comprehensive toxic screen (if indicated).
- Additional tests may include insulin and cortisol levels, serum lactate and pyruvate levels, serum amino acid levels, and urine organic acid levels. In many cases the clinician will opt simply to obtain a "critical sample" of several blood and urine specimens before therapy is initiated and hold for further testing pending consultation with a specialist.

Comments and Treatment Considerations

IV administration of dextrose 0.5 g/kg is appropriate initial therapy. The dose may be administered as D5W 10 ml/kg or D10W 5 ml/kg through a peripheral vein or D25W 2 ml/kg through a central line if possible. Depending on the cause of the hypoglycemia, ongoing dextrose infusions may be needed.

If IV access cannot be rapidly achieved, consider IM administration of glucagon dosed at 0.02 to 0.1 mg/kg (max 0.5 mg/dose) for patients ≤20 kg. Give 1 mg IM for patients >20 kg. The dose may be repeated × 1 and should be reconstituted with the provided diluent and may be repeated in 20 minutes if necessary. Glucagon tends to be more effective in patients with excess exogenous insulin. For alert cooperative patients with less severely altered mental status, oral administration of drinks with high sugar content (e.g., orange juice) may be helpful.

OTHER METABOLIC ABNORMALITIES

Electrolyte disturbances, such as hyponatremia, hypernatremia, and hypermagnesemia, may also cause lethargy. Previously undiagnosed inborn errors of metabolism may also present as depressed mental status. Inborn errors of metabolism usually are diagnosed within the first several weeks or months of life but occasionally may present later in childhood.

Specific clues indicating that altered mental status may be due to inborn errors of metabolism include the following symptoms and signs:

Symptoms
- Sleepiness +++
- Nausea and vomiting +++
- Deep or rapid breathing ++
- Unusual odors +

Signs
- Lethargy +++
- Emesis +++
- Tachypnea and/or Kussmaul's respirations ++
- Unusual odor +
- Hepatomegaly +
- Low weight ++
- Hypotonia +

Workup
- Medical history evaluating for growth failure, food aversions, developmental delay, frequent vomiting/lethargy.
- History evaluating for acute illness (vomiting, diarrhea, inadequate oral intake).
- Electrolytes, blood gases, urine for ketones, and blood ammonia levels as initial screen for metabolic illness.
- Other tests for metabolic illness may include blood lactate, pyruvate, and amino acid levels, as well as urine organic acid levels. The clinician may choose simply to obtain several blood tubes and a urine specimen, to be frozen and held pending consultation with a specialist in pediatric metabolism.

Comments and Treatment Considerations

If metabolic illness is suspected, laboratory specimens should be obtained before initiation of therapy. After stabilization of the ABCs, resuscitation should focus on correcting the metabolic defects. The vast majority of inborn errors of metabolism will present with an anion gap acidosis. The pathogenesis of the acidosis typically results from the accumulation of a substrate (e.g., ammonia, lactate, pyruvate, or other organic acids) caused by an enzyme deficiency. For most inborn errors of metabolism, it is appropriate to inhibit catabolism to halt further accumulation of the offending substrate by the administration of IV dextrose at a rate of 6 to 8 mg/kg/min (this is the rate of normal hepatic glucose production). One can achieve this rate of dextrose administration by giving a 10% dextrose solution at 1.0 to 1.5 times the maintenance fluid rate.

 INTUSSUSCEPTION

The diagnosis of intussusception should be considered in cases of altered mental status, especially for children 3 to 24 months of age. Usually other symptoms and signs of intussusception such as vomiting, intermittent abdominal pain, palpable abdominal mass, right-sided abdominal tenderness, or bloody stool are present. Occasionally, lethargy or depressed mental status may be the main presenting manifestation. In cases of altered mental status with no clear cause, rectal examination for occult blood and abdominal radiographs may be reasonable screening tests (see Chapter 1, Abdominal Pain).

 DEHYDRATION

Dehydration is a common cause of lethargy in children. It is, however, a diagnosis of exclusion once more serious causes such as infection have been considered. In most cases children will be less active but still easily aroused with a nonfocal neurologic status. Hypoglycemia and other metabolic disturbances (such as hyponatremia) may contribute to lethargy. Usually the history and physical examination will make dehydration obvious. However, especially for medically complex children with static encephalopathy or other chronic diseases, altered mental status may be the main presenting complaint (see Chapter 38, Vomiting).

 PSYCHIATRIC DISEASE

Acute psychiatric illness may lead to agitation, bizarre thinking (psychosis), or catatonia. In most cases there is a history of psychiatric illness, making the diagnosis easier. Rarely an acute change in mental status may be the presenting feature of psychiatric illness. This is a diagnosis of exclusion and it is imperative that presumed psychiatric patients receive a full medical evaluation.

Symptoms
- Disturbances in mood (sadness or mania) ++++
- Decreased appetite +
- Altered sleep patterns ++
- Increasing social isolation +++
- School failure +++
- Bizarre thinking or delusions ++
- Hallucinations (mainly auditory) ++
- Suicidal ideation ++

Signs
- Sad, manic, or flat affect ++++
- Lack of eye contact ++
- Incoherent speech ++
- Evidence of delusions or hallucinations on interview ++
- Catatonia +
- Absence of focal neurologic abnormalities ++++

Workup
- History of mental illness, school or social difficulties, recent stressors, family history of mental illness.

- History and physical examination to exclude other causes of altered mental status.
- History and physical examination directed at common comorbidities: substance abuse, child abuse or neglect, sexual abuse.
- Toxicologic screen of blood and/or urine.
- Psychiatric consultation.

Comments and Treatment Considerations

Patients with psychiatric illness and altered mental status may be dangerous to themselves or others. The patient should be kept in a safe room to minimize the possibility of harm to self and others. Patients who are psychotic, suicidal, or homicidal may need to be legally committed to inpatient therapy against their will. While pursuing psychiatric evaluation the clinician should be prepared for the need for chemical or physical restraint if less invasive measures are ineffective.

Medications to consider include lorazepam dosed at 0.05 to 0.1 mg/kg IM (max 4 mg/dose) or haloperidol dosed at 0.025 to 0.075 mg/kg IM (max 10 mg/dose). Some clinicians prefer to add diphenhydramine at 1 mg/kg/dose (max 50 mg/dose) IM when administering haloperidol to prevent dystonic reactions. The newer antipsychotic agents risperidone and ziprasidone may provide valuable alternatives. When giving any medication as a chemical restraint, the clinician must consider the patient's current medication regimen, to avoid several important potential drug interactions.

Potential drug-drug interactions include but are not limited to the following: haloperidol and clonidine (may result in hypotension), haloperidol and carbamazepine (decreased effectiveness of haloperidol), and haloperidol or chlorpromazine and lithium (increased incidence of neurotoxicity). If the patient has received a monoamine oxidase inhibitor (MAOI) within the prior 2 weeks, ensure that all potential interactions are reviewed before giving any medication. Meperidine, selective serotonin reuptake inhibitors, and tricyclic antidepressants are contraindicated with concurrent MAOI therapy. Droperidol should not be used in pediatric patients because of the risk of QT-interval prolongation. This adverse effect may potentially be exacerbated by antipsychotic medications that also prolong the QT interval.

REFERENCES

Aledo A, Heller G, Ren L, et al: Septicemia and septic shock in pediatric patients: 140 consecutive cases on a pediatric hematology-oncology service, *J Pediatr Hematol Oncol* 20:215-221, 1998.

Andrade R, Mathew V, Morgenstern MJ, et al: Hypoglycemic hemiplegic syndrome, *Ann Emerg Med* 13:529-531, 1984.

Andrews MM, Parent EM, Barry M, Parsonnet J: Recurrent nonmenstrual toxic shock syndrome: clinical manifestations, diagnosis, and treatment, *Clin Infect Dis* 32:1470-1479, 2001.

Berger MS, Edwards MS, LaMasters D, et al: Pediatric brain stem tumors: radiographic, pathological, and clinical correlations, *Neurosurgery* 12:298-302, 1983.

Bond GR: The poisoned child. Evolving concepts in care. *Emerg Med Clin North Am* 13:343-355, 1995.

Burton BK: Inborn errors of metabolism in infancy: a guide to diagnosis, *Pediatrics* 102(6):E69, 1998.

Cohen D, Flament M, Dubos PF, Basquin M: Case series: catatonic syndrome in young people, *J Am Acad Child Adolesc Psychiatr* 38:1040-1046, 1999.

Eick APT, Nakamura H, Reed MD: Drug-drug interactions in pediatric psychopharmacology, *Pediatr Clin North Am* 45(5):1233-1263, 1998.

Fullerton HJ, Johnston SC, Smith WS: Arterial dissection and stroke in children, *Neurology* 57(7):1155-1160, 2001.

Garton HJ, Kestle JR, Drake JM: Predicting shunt failure on the basis of clinical symptoms and signs in children, *J Neurosurg* 94:202-210, 2001.

Gordon GS, Wallace SJ, Neal JW: Intracranial tumors during the first two years of life: presenting features, *Arch Dis Child* 73(4):345-347, 1995.

Guerreiro C, Cendes F, Li LM, et al: Clinical patterns of patients with temporal lobe epilepsy and pure amygdalar atrophy, *Epilepsia* 40:453-461, 199X.

Halamandaris PV, Anderson TR: Children and adolescents in the psychiatric emergency setting, *Psychiatr Clin North Am* 22:865-874, 1999.

Harvey AS, Berkovic SF, Wrennall JA, Hopkins IJ: Temporal lobe epilepsy in childhood: clinical, EEG, and neuroimaging findings and syndrome classification in a cohort with new-onset seizures, *Neurology* 49:960-968, 1997.

Hasbun R, Abrahams J, Jekel J, Quagliarello VJ: Computed tomography of the head before lumbar puncture in adults with suspected meningitis, *N Engl J Med* 345:1727-1733, 2001.

Henriquez H, el Din A, Ozand PT, et al: Emergency presentations of patients with methylmalonic acidemia, propionic acidemia and branched chain amino acidemia (MSUD), *Brain Dev* 16(suppl):86-93, 1994.

Hoffman JR, Schriger DL, Votey SR, Luo JS: The empiric use of hypertonic dextrose in patients with altered mental status: a reappraisal, *Ann Emerg Med* 21:20-24, 1992.

Jozefowicz RF: Neurologic manifestations of pulmonary disease, *Neurol Clin* 7:605-616, 1989.

Kaplan SL: Clinical presentations, diagnosis, and prognostic factors of bacterial meningitis, *Infect Dis Clin North Am* 13:579-594, 1999.

Mahle WT, Forkey HC, Wernovsky G, Rhodes LA : Sepsis, septic shock, acute abdomen? The ability of cardiac disease to mimic other medical illness, *Pediatr Emerg Care* 12:317-324, 1996.

Osorio I, Arafah BM, Mayor C, Troster AI: Plasma glucose alone does not predict neurologic dysfunction in hypoglycemic nondiabetic subjects, *Ann Emerg Med* 33:291-298, 1999.

Perry HE, Shannon MW: Diagnosis and management of opioid- and benzodiazepine-induced comatose overdose in children, *Curr Opin Pediatr* 8:243-247, 1996.

Powers KS: Diagnosis and management of common toxic ingestions and inhalations, *Pediatr Ann* 29:330-342, 2000.

Rivkin MJ, Volpe JJ: Strokes in children, *Pediatr Rev* 17:265-277, 1996.

Rothrock SG, Green SM, Wren J, et al: Pediatric bacterial meningitis: is prior antibiotic therapy associated with an altered clinical presentation? *Ann Emerg Med* 21(2):146-152, 1992.

Ruiz-Contreras J, Urquia L, Bastero R : Persistent crying as predominant manifestation of sepsis in infants and newborns, *Pediatr Emerg Care* 15:113-115, 1999.

Theodore WH, Porter RJ, Penry JK: Complex partial seizures: clinical characteristics and differential diagnosis, *Neurology* 33:1115-1121, 1983.

Valentino TL, Conway EE Jr, Shiminski-Maher T, Siffert J: Pediatric brain tumors, *Pediatr Ann* 26:579-587, 1997.

Walsh-Kelly C, Nelson DB, Smith DS, et al: Clinical predictors of
    bacterial versus aseptic meningitis in childhood, *Ann Emerg Med*
    21:910-914, 1992.
Watkins L, Hayward R, Andar U, Harkness W: The diagnosis of blocked
    cerebrospinal fluid shunts: a prospective study of referral to a
    pediatric neurosurgical unit, *Childs Nerv Syst* 10:87-90, 1994.

CHAPTER 4

Apnea

SUSAN B. TORREY

The management of a child who is apneic on arrival to the ED requires emergent application of the ABCs of pediatric resuscitation. When the event has resolved before arrival, the ED physician must determine whether the child was truly apneic, whether the event is likely to recur, and whether there is an underlying cause that requires immediate treatment. The term *apnea* refers to a ≥20-second pause in breathing or <20 seconds if associated with significant bradycardia, cyanosis, or pallor. Although apnea can occur as a manifestation of significant disease throughout childhood, in pediatrics the term is commonly applied to infants only. An older patient with "apnea" is considered to be in respiratory failure.

The frequency of apnea demonstrates an inverse relationship to gestational age at birth. Infants born at less than 32 weeks of gestation have a >50% probability of exhibiting significant apnea, whereas apnea in a full-term or older infant is considered abnormal and requires evaluation.

The initial approach to the patient who may have had an apneic episode should include a complete history and physical examination. The history should be obtained from firsthand observers as objectively as possible. Questions such as "What did the baby look like?" "What color was he?" and "Was she awake?" may be useful. A thorough physical examination including rectal temperature, pulse oximetry, and lung, heart, and neurologic examinations should be performed.

APPARENT LIFE-THREATENING EVENT (ALTE)

Symptoms
- Cyanosis or pallor
- Unresponsive to caretaker
- Loss of tone or posture
- Required resuscitation
- Occurred while infant was in a car seat, bouncy chair, or swing

Signs
- Physical examination, including rectal temperature and pulse oximetry, is usually unremarkable
- Signs of an underlying etiology of the event, such as respiratory distress (pneumonia), fever (sepsis), or abnormal neurologic examination findings (trauma/abuse)
- Signs of inflicted injury

Workup
The workup is directed toward identifying the cause of the event and is guided by the history and physical examination. A history that is inconsistent with the physical examination findings or a delay in seeking treatment suggests the possibility of inflicted injury (see Chapter 2, Abuse/Rape). If a significant event has occurred but there are no defining elements in the history or physical examination, the following studies should be considered (see Chapter 3, Altered Mental Status):
- CBC, electrolytes (including Ca, Mg, and Po_4), and UA, which might indicate possible infection or metabolic abnormalities associated with a possible seizure.
- CXR to identify lower airway disease or an abnormal cardiac silhouette.
- Electrocardiogram (ECG) may suggest a rhythm disturbance or congenital heart disease.
- Consider head CT.
- Consider sepsis evaluation.

Comments and Treatment Considerations

Admission and observation with heart rate, respiratory rate, and pulse oximetry monitoring are suggested for all patients who have had a significant event. If there is clinical evidence of recurrent apnea and/or gastroesophageal reflux (GER), a pneumogram with or without a pH probe may provide useful information.

 ## SUDDEN INFANT DEATH SYNDROME

Sudden infant death syndrome (SIDS) is the unexpected death of a healthy infant for whom no cause is found at autopsy. Some investigators believe that a death scene investigation should be included to exclude factors such as smothering or inflicted injury. Associated factors are multiple, including socioeconomic status, ethnic origin, maternal drug use, and discharge from a neonatal intensive care unit. A decline in the incidence of SIDS has been observed coincident with the American Academy of Pediatrics recommendation in 1992 to position infants supine during sleep, the "Back to Sleep" campaign.

 ## ABUSE

Apnea or recurrent ALTE can be a manifestation of inflicted injury. It is important to consider this possibility while taking care not to alienate the caretakers and ensuring the child's safety. A social service evaluation and admission to the hospital for observation may be necessary (see Chapter 2, Abuse/Rape).

 ## INFANT BOTULISM

If apnea has occurred as a result of botulinum toxin, the infant will require intensive respiratory and nutritional support. The patient should be stabilized and transferred to a pediatric intensive care unit (see Chapter 39, Weakness/Fatigue).

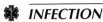 INFECTION

Almost any infection can cause an infant to become apneic. Infants with bacterial sepsis and meningitis presenting with apnea are usually moribund on arrival to the ED. Both respiratory syncytial virus (RSV) and pertussis are notable viral illnesses that may cause apnea in young infants. Suspicion for RSV and pertussis should be heightened when presented with a premature infant who has not received RSV immune globulin (Synagis or RespiGam) or an infant who has not completed the diphtheria and tetanus toxoids and acellular pertussis vaccine (DTaP) series. Older infants with RSV who have been apneic are usually ill appearing on arrival with obvious signs of lower airway disease. However, premature infants and neonates can develop apnea early in the course of their RSV illness with only a history of rhinorrhea. Infants with pertussis often appear well on initial evaluation. There is a history of rhinorrhea and apnea occurring with paroxysmal cough. It is important to observe the infant during a coughing spell to make the diagnosis. A generalized approach to ruling out an infectious cause is necessary in the otherwise stable infant, as there may be only subtle clues from the history or physical examination.

Symptoms
- Rhinorrhea
- Cough
- Lethargy or irritability

Signs
- Fever or hypothermia
- Hypoxia
- Rales or wheezes

Workup
- CBC to look for signs of leukocytosis (consistent with possible bacterial infection), lymphocytosis (consistent with pertussis), or anemia (indicative of decreased oxygen-carrying capability).

- Blood culture in all febrile infants younger than 3 months, in all infants who have not completed three doses of pneumococcal vaccination (Prevnar), or in those in whom sepsis is a concern.
- Urine for culture and UA (specimen obtained by bladder catheterization).
- Consider CSF analysis for cell count, gram stain, glucose, protein, and culture.
- CXR.
- Consider nasal swab for pertussis.

Comments and Treatment Considerations

If the child is unstable, cultures of blood and urine should be obtained and antibiotics given before a lumbar puncture is performed.

RSV usually occurs in winter months. It is prudent to consider hospital admission for any infant younger than 6 weeks with RSV and signs of lower airway disease. Infants discharged from the ED should have daily follow-up with the primary care provider.

Infants with pertussis should be admitted to the hospital to ensure that they are not becoming apneic with coughing. Recommended therapy includes erythromycin base dosed at 40 mg/kg/day (max 2 g/day estolate or base and 3.2 g/day ethylsuccinate) PO divided q6h for 14 days. Secondary to gastrointestinal intolerance and concerns of an increased incidence of pyloric stenosis in infants younger than 6 weeks receiving erythromycin, azithromycin has been successfully used to treat pertussis. Azithromycin should be dosed at 10 mg/kg/day (max 500 mg/dose) PO every day for 5 days. Household members and close contacts should also be prophylactically treated (see Chapter 14, Fever, and Chapter 30, Respiratory Distress).

Consider admission based on age, symptoms, and suspected diagnosis.

 GASTROESOPHAGEAL REFLUX DISEASE

Apnea can be the first manifestation of GERD. With close observation, laryngospasm (including choking, loss of voice, and an anxious appearance) may be noted to precede the apneic event. Historical clinical evidence may not be available from the parents and these children may need to be admitted for observation by experienced nursing staff looking for signs of GERD (see Chapter 38, Vomiting).

APNEA OF PREMATURITY

Apnea occurs frequently in premature infants. It is usually not seen in full-term infants unless the child is actually premature and the estimated gestational age was incorrect. The frequency with which apnea occurs increases with degree of prematurity. Infants with apnea of prematurity have usually had an extensive evaluation in the neonatal intensive care unit and are often discharged with instruction to use a monitor and a respiratory stimulant, usually theophylline or caffeine. Factors such as anemia, hypoglycemia, and hypoxemia can worsen apnea and other diagnoses such as sepsis should be considered. An increased frequency of apneic episodes can occur in an infant who has outgrown his or her stimulant dose.

Symptoms
- Apnea
- History of respiratory stimulant medication

Signs
- Physical examination consistent with prematurity

Workup
- CBC to identify anemia.
- Glucose to exclude hypoglycemia.
- Pulse oximetry to identify hypoxemia.
- Consider blood, urine, and CSF evaluations for possible infection.
- Pneumogram if diagnosis is in question.

Comments and Treatment Considerations
If signs of concurrent infectious disease exist, further care is dictated based on pertinent features of history, physical

examination, and laboratory study results. These patients should be admitted for observation when respiratory stimulant medication is introduced or adjusted. Pneumograms may be helpful in making the diagnosis and for determining the characteristics of the immature breathing pattern.

 ## SEIZURE

Apnea (usually without bradycardia) may be a manifestation of seizure activity in small infants. A neurologic evaluation is warranted if seizure activity is suspected (see Chapter 32, Seizures).

 ## BREATH-HOLDING SPELL

Breath-holding spells are involuntary and most children outgrow them.

Symptoms
- Child who has been interrupted during favorite activity or reprimanded
- Child first holds breath then turns blue and finally becomes apneic
- A history of similar episodes in the past

Workup
- ECG to rule out prolonged QT syndrome or a conduction abnormality.

Comments and Treatment Considerations
Some breath-holding spells are associated with conduction disturbances such as prolonged QT syndrome. Pediatric cardiology referral is recommended for any patient with abnormal ECG findings.

REFERENCES
Anas N et al: The association of apnea and respiratory syncytial virus infection in infants, *J Pediatr* 101:65-68.

Bass J, Mehta KA: Oxygen desaturation of selected term infants in car seats, *Pediatrics* 96:288-290, 1995.

Davies F, Gupta R: Apparent life threatening events in infants presenting to an emergency department, *Emerg Med J* 19:11-16, 2002.

DiMario FJ: Breath holding spells in childhood, *Am J Dis Child* 146:125-131, 1998.

Orenstein SR: An overview of reflux-associated disorders in infants: apnea, laryngospasm, and aspiration, *Am J Med* 111;8:60-63, 2001.

Southall DP, Plunkett CB, Banks MW, et al: Covert video recordings of life-threatening child abuse: lessons for child protection, *Pediatrics* 100:735-760, 1997.

Task Force on Infant Positioning: Positioning and sudden infant death syndrome (SIDS): update, *Pediatrics* 98:1216-1218, 1996.

CHAPTER 5

Bites

JACQUELINE BRYNGIL CORBOY

Bites and envenomations are responsible for great morbidity and mortality worldwide. In the United States, mammalian bites account for approximately 1% of ED visits in the pediatric population both for management of wound complications and for postexposure prophylaxis. Approximately 85% of these visits are the result of dog bites in the 5- to 14-year-old age-group. Though rare in the United States, rabies prevention and prophylaxis are important when dealing with certain mammalian exposures, as rabies remains a universally fatal disease. Envenomations, most commonly from hymenopteran and spiders in the United States, also account for a small percentage of ED visits per year.

 MAMMALIAN BITES (Table 5-1)

Comments and Treatment Considerations
Evaluation by x-ray to rule out fractures
- For bites to head or face in infants
- Evaluation of hand bites
- Consider for long bones if bite inflicted by large mammal

Local care
- Copious irrigation (100 ml/cm estimate) and debridement helps to prevent most infectious complications; however, human and cat bites have a high infection rate.

Table 5-1 Types of Bites

Types	Incidence Among Bites	Infection Rate	Flora	Other Infectious Risks	Rabies Risk
Human	2%–3%	High	*Streptococcus viridans, Staphylococcus aureus, Bacteroides, Peptostreptococcus, Eikenella corrodens*	Hepatitis B and C virus, syphilis, HIV	None
Dog	90%	Moderate	*S. aureus, Pasteurella multocida,* coagulase-negative staphylococci, enterics	None	High
Cat	5%–10%	High	*S. aureus, P. multocida,* coagulase-negative staphylococci, enterics	*Bartonella henselae* (upper extremity cat scratches)	Present but low
Bat	Low	Unknown	Staphylococci and streptococci	None	High

Continued

Table 5-1 Types of Bites—Cont'd

Types	Incidence Among Bites	Infection Rate	Flora	Other Infectious Risks	Rabies Risk
Rodent	Low	Low	Staphylococci and streptococci	*Streptobacillus moniliformis, Spirillum minus* (ratbite fever)	None
Lagomorph (rabbits, skunks, raccoons)	Low	Low	Staphylococci and streptococci	*Francisella tularensis* (tularemia)	High

Suturing

To suture or not to suture depends on location, age of wound, and effectiveness of local debridement. Most facial wounds can be safely sutured after copious irrigation because the blood supply is good.

High-risk wounds include the following:

- Any human or cat bite
- Hand bites are particularly high risk and should be left open
- Puncture wounds
- Wounds open >12 hours

ANTIBIOTIC TREATMENT ISSUES

Antibiotics should be administered for all human, all cat, and most dog bites. Parenteral antibiotics should be considered for almost all hand bites or severe wounds (i.e., deep tissue injury). No single antibiotic is perfect for all bites. However, in patients with mammalian bites who are not allergic to penicillin derivatives, ampicillin-sulbactam (Unasyn) is the current parenteral drug of choice and amoxicillin-clavulanate (Augmentin) is the current oral drug of choice. It should be noted that cephalexin (Keflex), usually a good choice for skin infections, is generally not effective for mammalian bites.

Parenteral Antibiotics

- **Ampicillin-Sulbactam (Unasyn)**

Infants/children: 100-200 mg ampicillin component/kg/day IV divided q6h (max 2 g ampicillin/dose)

Adults: 1-2 g ampicillin component IV q6h (max 12 g ampicillin/day)

- **Cefoxitin (Mefoxin)**

Infants/children: 80-160 mg/kg/day IV divided q4-6h (max 12 g/day)

Adults: 2 g IV q8h (max 12 g/day)

- **Ticarcillin-Clavulanate (Timentin)**

Infants/children: 200-300 mg ticarcillin component/kg/day IV divided q4-6h (max 24 g ticarcillin/day)

Adult: 3.1 g (3 g ticarcillin) IV q6h (max 24 g ticarcillin/day)

- **Piperacillin-Tazobactam (Zosyn)**

Infants/children: 240-400 mg piperacillin component/kg/day IV divided q6-8h (max 18 g piperacillin/day)

Adults: 3.375 g (3 g piperacillin) IV q6h or 4.5 g (4 g piperacillin) IV q8h (max 18 g piperacillin/day)

Oral Antibiotic Choices

- **Amoxicillin-Clavulanate (Augmentin)**

Infants younger than 3 months: 30 mg amoxicillin component/kg/day PO divided q12h

Children <40 kg: 20-40 mg amoxicillin component/kg/day PO divided q8h (max 500 mg amoxicillin/dose)

Adults: 500 mg PO q8h or 875 mg PO bid
    OR

- **If allergic to penicillin**

Infants/children:

Dog or human bite: clindamycin 30 mg/kg/day PO divided q6-8h plus trimethoprim-sulfamethoxazole 6-10 mg trimethoprim/kg/day PO divided bid

Cat bite: doxycycline 5 mg/kg/day PO divided q12h (max 100 mg/dose). Use with caution in children younger than 8 years; consultation with pediatric infectious disease specialist is recommended.

Adolescents older than 16 years and adults:

Dog or human bite: clindamycin 300 mg PO qid plus ciprofloxacin 250-750 mg PO bid or clindamycin 300 mg PO qid plus trimethoprim-sulfamethoxazole one DS tab PO bid

Cat bite: doxycycline 100 mg PO q12h

TETANUS PROPHYLAXIS ISSUES

Tetanus immunization should be given if last immunization was more than 5 years ago, history is indeterminate, or immunization schedule is not complete. Tetanus immunoglobulin should be given for all patients who have not received at least three primary immunizations. See Tables 5-2 and 5-3 for wound classification and prophylaxis recommendations.

Table 5-2 Wound Classification

Clinical Features	Tetanus Prone	Non–Tetanus Prone
Age of wound	>6 hr	≤6 hr
Configuration	Stellate or avulsion	Linear
Depth	>1 cm	≤1 cm
Mechanism of injury	Missile, crush, burn, frostbite	Sharp surface
Devitalized tissue	Present	Absent
Contaminants (dirt, saliva, etc.)	Present	Absent

Table 5-3 Prophylaxis Recommendations

No. of Primary Immunizations	Years Since Last Booster	Type of Wound	Recommendations*
≤2	Irrelevant	Non–tetanus prone	DTaP/DT or Td
		Tetanus prone	DTaP/DT or Td + TIG†
3	10	Low risk	DT, Td
		Tetanus prone	DT, Td
3	5-10	Low risk	No treatment
		Tetanus prone	DT, Td
3	<5	Low risk	No treatment
		Tetanus prone	No treatment

*DTaP or DT should be used in all children who have not completed their primary immunization schedule or in whom immunization status is unknown and are 7 years or younger. Td should be used in children older than 7 years.

†Human TIG 250 to 500 units/dose intramuscularly × 1 at the site opposite to Td administration.

RABIES PROPHYLAXIS ISSUES

Rabies is a viral infection affecting the central nervous system, causing an encephalomyelitis that is always fatal. Prophylaxis with rabies vaccine and immunoglobulin should be provided for all patients with potential risk (Table 5-4).

Table 5-4 Rabies Prophylaxis Guidelines

Animal Type	Evaluation and Disposition of Animal	Postexposure Prophylaxis Recommendations
Dogs, cats, ferrets	Healthy and available for 10-day observation period	Do not begin prophylaxis unless animal develops clinical symptoms
	Rabid or suspected rabid	If animal has symptoms, vaccinate immediately with
	Escaped	RIG and HDCV; consult public health officials
Skunks, raccoons, foxes, carnivores, bats	Regarded as rabid unless proven otherwise by negative laboratory test results	Vaccination with RIG and HDCV
Livestock, small rodents, lagomorphs, large rodents, and other mammals	Consider individually	Consult public health officials; these bites rarely require postexposure prophylaxis

HDCV, Human diploid cell rabies vaccine; *RIG*, Rabies immune globulin.

Postexposure Prophylaxis Regimen

- **Rabies immune globulin (RIG)**

    RIG provides rapid passive immunity lasting approximately 21 days. Do not use RIG in patients who have previously received human diploid cell rabies vaccine (HDCV).

    Day 0: RIG 20 units/kg/dose IM × 1. Give half the dose infiltrated into wound(s), give the remaining half of dose IM in deltoid opposite HDCV site in older children and adults. May administer in midlateral aspect of thigh in infants and small children.

- **Rabies vaccine (HDCV)**

    HDCV induces active immune response and production of antibodies to the rabies virus. Response develops in 7 to 10 days and persists for approximately 2 years.

    Day 0: HDCV 1 ml IM in deltoid opposite RIG site in older children and adults. May administer in midlateral aspect of thigh in infants and small children.

    Days 3, 7, 14, and 28: HDCV 1 ml IM in deltoid. May administer in midlateral aspect of thigh in infants and small children.

 SNAKE ENVENOMATIONS

PIT VIPERS (CROTALIDAE) ENVENOMATION

Includes rattlesnake, water moccasin (cottonmouth), and copperhead snakes, which are responsible for 99% of venomous snakebites in the United States. Most signs and symptoms develop within 6 hours.

Symptoms

Report of a bite by a snake with a triangular head, pits between nostrils, elliptical and vertical pupils, wide-spaced curved fangs, and a single row of ventral tail scales.

Signs

- Pain, edema, hemorrhage, ecchymosis +++
- Anxiety, diaphoresis, weakness ++++

- Nausea/vomiting ++++
- Paresthesias ++++
- Tachycardia, muscle fasciculations ++
- Local pain with the potential for compartment syndrome in extremities
- Convulsions, paralysis, pulmonary edema, respiratory failure, hypotension, and shock ++ within 2 to 6 hours in severe envenomations

Workup

- CBC to detect thrombocytopenia, which should be repeated in 6 hours.
- PT/PTT to detect elevation of coagulation parameters, which should be repeated in 6 hours.
- Type and crossmatch.
- Electrolytes to detect hemoconcentration.
- Fibrin and fibrin split products may be increased.
- Creatine phosphokinase (CPK) may be increased.
- UA to detect proteinuria and hematuria.

Comments and Treatment Considerations

Management of ABCs as indicated. Systemic symptoms are caused by the intravascular depletion that results from increased venous capacitance, third spacing, and hemorrhagic losses. Immediate therapy should include splinting and positioning of the affected extremity below the level of the heart. The incision, suction, and constriction band technique is only recommended for pit viper strikes. Incision and suction should be considered only if within 5 to 10 minutes of the snake strike and used in conjunction with a constriction band of at least 2 cm wide placed 5 to 10 cm proximal to the wound that is loose enough to ensure arterial flow (able to place one finger width beneath band) but that restricts lymphatic and venous flow. Use of a constriction band can also be considered if transport will be significantly delayed. Ice application is contraindicated.

Determination of severity of envenomation (mild, moderate, or severe) is based on age and size of victim, depth of fang penetration, and size of snake (if known). Consult your local poison control experts. Once at a treatment facility (*not* in the field!) and if <12 hours since the snakebite, consider antivenin therapy. Benefits of antivenin are greatest when administered within 4 hours of the bite. Efficacy after 12 hours is controversial.

Currently two types of antivenin are available, the antivenin (crotalidae) polyvalent by Wyeth and crotalidae polyvalent immune Fab (CroFab) by Savage Laboratories. The Wyeth antivenin is made from horse serum and is extremely antigenic; skin testing is *mandatory* before administration. A 1:10 dilution test vial is supplied in the kit. Inject 0.02 to 0.03 ml intradermally (*not* subcutaneously) and check for positive reaction (erythema, spreading) within 30 minutes. A delayed serum sickness will develop in 4 to 21 days in up to 75% of patients given pit viper antivenin.

CroFab is prepared from affinity-purified, sheep-derived Fab fragments and is less antigenic than the Wyeth product. Skin testing before infusion is not necessary. CroFab should not be used in patients allergic to papaya or papain unless the benefit outweighs the risk and appropriate measures are taken to treat anaphylaxis if it occurs.

Doses of both antivenin products are based on degree of envenomation (see Tables 5-5 and 5-6) and children commonly require larger doses than adults. Snake species covered by the Wyeth product include North and South American crotalus, rattlesnake, copperhead, cottonmouth, tropical moccasin, fer-de-lance, and bushmaster. CroFab can be used for envenomations by North American crotalids, western diamondback rattlesnake, eastern diamondback rattlesnake, Mojave rattlesnake, cottonmouth, and water moccasin.

Supportive care, local wound care, tetanus prophylaxis, and antibiotic coverage for *Clostridium*, *Pseudomonas*, *Proteus*, *Micrococcus*, *Enterobacter*, *Staphylococcus*, *Streptococcus*, *Corynebacterium*, and *Citrobacter* should be provided. All snakebites are considered a risk factor for tetanus and prophylaxis should be provided (see the previous section on mammalian bites for further information on tetanus prophylaxis). Antibiotic recommendations include the following.

Table 5-5 Pit Viper Antivenin Guidelines for Wyeth Antivenin

Degree of Envenomation	Symptoms	Antivenin Determination
No envenomation	Fang marks, no local or systemic reaction	No antivenin
Minimal envenomation	Fang marks, local swelling and pain, no systemic reaction	0 or 5 vials*
Moderate envenomation	Fang marks with swelling that progresses beyond bites; systemic symptoms including nausea, vomiting, paresthesias or blood pressure changes; laboratory findings of mild coagulopathy	10-20 vials*
Severe envenomation	Fang marks with severe swelling of extremity, subcutaneous ecchymosis; severe systemic symptoms; severe laboratory pathology with coagulopathy, thrombocytopenia, proteinuria and hematuria	20 or more vials*

*Vials should be diluted per package directions. The amount is determined by symptomatic improvement when antivenin is administered at a rate of 1 ml/min; one may increase the rate if no adverse reaction is noted. Urine output should be monitored in children.

Table 5-6 Pit Viper Antivenin Guidelines for Crofab

Degree of Envenomation	Symptoms	Antivenin Determination
No envenomation	Fang marks, no local or systemic reaction	No antivenin
Minimal envenomation	Fang marks, local swelling and pain, no systemic reaction	4-6 vials*
Moderate envenomation	Fang marks with swelling that progresses beyond bites; systemic symptoms including nausea, vomiting, paresthesias or blood pressure changes; laboratory findings of mild coagulopathy	As above, repeat dose as needed until envenomation syndrome is controlled*
Severe envenomation	Fang marks with severe swelling of extremity, subcutaneous ecchymosis; severe systemic symptoms; severe laboratory pathology with coagulopathy, thrombocytopenia, proteinuria and hematuria	As above, repeat dose as needed until envenomation syndrome is controlled, may require maintenance dosing*

*Vials should be diluted per package directions. The amount is determined by symptomatic improvement when antivenin is administered at an initial rate of 25-50 ml/hr; increase to 250 ml/hr if no adverse response. Initial dose is four to six vials. Repeat initial dose as needed at 1-hour intervals until envenomation syndrome is controlled. Maintenance dosing of two vials q6h for 18 hours may be required.

Antibiotic Choices

- **Cefuroxime (Ceftin)***

Infants/children: suspension 20-30 mg/kg/day PO divided bid
   (max 500 mg/day) or 75-150 mg/kg/day IV divided q6-8h
   (max 6 g/day)

Adults: tablets 250-500 mg PO bid or 750-1500 mg IV q8h

- **Ceftriaxone (Rocephin)**

Infants/children: 50-75 mg/kg/day IV/IM divided q12-24h
   (max 4 g/day)

Adults: 1-2 g IV/IM q24h (max 4 g/day)

CORAL SNAKE (ELAPIDAE) ENVENOMATION

Known for its characteristic appearance of multiple red, yellow
(or white), and black bands, the mnemonic "red on yellow, kill
a fellow; red on black, venom lack" is often recited to distinguish this highly venomous snake from its nonvenomous
cousins.

Coral snakes are responsible for less than 1% of envenomations
in the United States and are found in Arizona, New Mexico, and
states east of the Mississippi River excluding the northeast. Fewer
than 40% of bites lead to symptoms of envenomation.

Symptoms

- Report of a bite by a snake with a blunt head, no pits, round
  pupils, small round fangs, ventral caudal scales with red,
  black, and yellow bands as described above

Signs

- Develop within 90 minutes, progress to severe over 5 to 12
  hours affecting neurologic and respiratory systems
- Very little pain or swelling (edema in <50%)
- Limb weakness ++
- Paresthesias +++
- Nausea ++
- Malaise
- Muscle fasciculations +
- Impaired swallow and cranial nerve dysfunction
- Respiratory failure +

---

*Cefuroxime suspension and tablets are not bioequivalent or interchangeable.

Comments and Treatment Considerations

Management of ABCs as indicated. Local measures such as constriction bands, suction, and drainage do not retard absorption of coral snake venom and are not recommended. Antivenin is available only for eastern and Texas coral snakes. Consider antivenin therapy in consultation with your local poisoning control experts. Note that Wyeth antivenin must be used in coral snake envenomations.

Wyeth antivenin is made from horse serum and is highly antigenic, requiring skin testing before administration. All bites require early treatment with four to six vials to prevent neurologic dysfunction. Follow directions in the kit for administration. See the earlier section on mammalian bites for further information on tetanus prophylaxis. See section on pit vipers for antibiotic recommendations.

SPIDER ENVENOMATIONS

BROWN RECLUSE (*LOXOSCELES RECLUSA*)

The brown recluse is found primarily in southern and midwestern states, indoors and outdoors, and is sometimes called a *fiddle-back spider*.

Symptoms
- History of a bite by a spider that is small (1.0 to 1.5 cm) with a brown violin-shaped marking on the back (Fig. 5-1).

Signs
- Local findings
  - 2 to 8 hours: mild to moderate pain at site
  - 6 to 20 hours: erythema and central blistering at bite site
  - 24 hours: subcutaneous discoloration lasting 3 to 4 days, growing between 10 and 15 cm
  - 72 hours: central pustules burst, revealing necrotic crater
- Systemic symptoms more common in children, developing within 24 to 48 hours; fever, chills, malaise, weakness, nausea, vomiting, joint pain, rash, and renal failure secondary to hemolysis

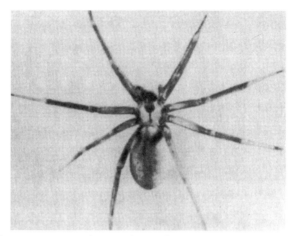

Fig. 5-1 Brown recluse spider. Violin-shaped mark on the cephalothorax. (From Goddard J: *Physicians' guide to arthropods of medical importance,* 2nd ed, Boca Raton, 1996, CRC Press.)

Workup

- For systemic symptoms, CBC with platelets, BUN and SCr, and UA to monitor hemolysis.

Comments and Treatment Considerations

Supportive care as indicated. Initially only local care is needed, but occasionally debridement and grafting is required if a large necrotic area develops. Dapsone therapy is controversial in children and should be used only in adults (50 mg PO every day) because it may result in methemoglobinemia and hypersensitivity reactions in pediatric patients < 16 years. Dapsone is contraindicated in patients with glucose-6-phosphate dehydrogenase (G6PD) deficiency.

BLACK WIDOW (*LATRODECTUS MACTANS*)

The black widow spider bite yields the highest fatality rate among spider bites in the United States.

Symptoms

- History of a bite from a female black widow spider that has a shiny black body with a red hourglass on the abdomen and is 2.0 to 2.5 cm long (Fig. 5-2). Males are not harmful because they are only one fourth of the female size and their fangs are not long enough to penetrate human skin.

Signs

- Usually no local signs are associated with this spider bite
- Nausea and vomiting +++
- Abdominal pain +++ and muscle rigidity +++ occur 1 to 8 hours after bite.
- Hypertension ++

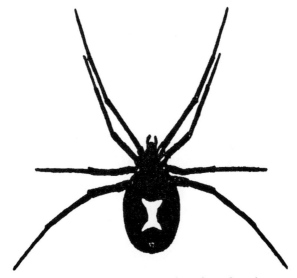

Fig. 5-2 Black widow spider. Hourglass-shaped mark is visible on the abdomen. (From Goddard J: *Physicians' guide to arthropods of medical importance,* 2nd ed, Boca Raton, 1996, CRC Press.)

- Respiratory distress
- Chills
- Urinary retention
- Priapism

Comments and Treatment Considerations

Supportive care as indicated. Consultation with local poison center. *Latrodectus* antivenin 2.5 ml is recommended for all confirmed bite victims weighing ≤40kg; suggested in all individuals younger than 16 years or those who exhibit systemic complications of respiratory distress or hypotension. Sensitivity testing to horse serum is recommended before use. In severe cases, the antivenin should be given by IV infusion in normal saline (NS) over 15 minutes. IM injection can be used in less severe cases. Calcium gluconate for muscle cramping dosed at 50 mg/kg/dose (suggested max 4 g/day) slow IV push via central line or peripheral line in large vessel has traditionally been used. Recently calcium gluconate has been shown to be beneficial only for 4% of cases. Muscle relaxants such as diazepam have been advocated by some authors but are not clearly efficacious. Pain control with narcotics such as morphine sulfate is usually effective. Hospital admission is required for all pediatric and pregnant patients with systemic signs and symptoms.

 HYMENOPTERA ENVENOMATIONS

Hymenoptera envenomations are responsible for 50% of all deaths from venomous bites and stings worldwide. This category includes insects with barbed stingers such as bees, hornets, yellow jackets, and nonbarbed stingers such as wasps (which can inflict multiple stings at one time). Most severe reactions are due to allergic responses. See Table 5-7 for types of reactions and recommended therapy. All patients in groups II through IV should carry EpiPen. Patients should receive teaching and a prescripton for EpiPen Jr (0.15 mg) if <30 kg and EpiPen Adult (0.3 mg) if >30 kg at discharge.

Table 5-7 Types of Hymenoptera Reactions and Treatment Considerations

Type	Signs/Symptoms	Treatment Considerations
Group I	Local erythema, puncture mark	Ice and local wound care
Group II	Local or generalized urticaria without respiratory symptoms	1. Diphenhydramine 1-1.25 mg/kg/dose (max 50 mg/dose) PO q6h for 48-72 hr 2. Ice and local wound care
Group III	Generalized urticaria with systemic reactions such as wheezing, angioedema, nausea/vomiting	1. Epinephrine (1:1000) 0.01 ml/kg (max 0.5 ml/dose) IM × 1 dose; or epinephrine (1:10,000) 0.01 ml/kg IV; may repeat every 15-20 min as needed 2. Diphenhydramine 1-1.25 mg/kg/dose (max 50 mg/dose) IV/PO q6h for 48-72 hr 3. Ranitidine 2 mg/kg/dose (max 150 mg/dose) PO bid or 1 mg/kg/dose (max 50 mg/dose) IV q8h 4. Prednisone 1 mg/kg/day PO daily or methylprednisolone 2 mg/kg/day IV bolus then 2-4 mg/kg/day IV divided q6h or hydrocortisone 4-8 mg/kg (max 250 mg/dose) IV bolus and then 2 mg/kg/dose IV q6h 5. Consider admission for 24-hr observation

Continued

Table 5-7 Types of Hymenoptera Reactions and Treatment Considerations—Cont'd

Type	Signs/Symptoms	Treatment Considerations
Group IV	Severe systemic reactions with laryngospasm, laryngoedema, hypotension and shock[*]	1. Manage ABCs, intubate if necessary 2. Epinephrine (1:1000) 0.01 ml/kg (max 0.5 ml/dose) IM × 1 dose; or epinephrine (1:10,000) 0.01 ml/kg IV; may repeat every 15-20 min as needed 3. Diphenhydramine 1-1.25 mg/kg/dose (max 50 mg/dose) IV/IM q6h for 48-72 hr 4. Ranitidine 1 mg/kg/dose (max 50 mg/dose) IV q8h 5. Albuterol inhalation (0.5%) 0.03 ml/kg/dose (max 1 ml) via nebulizer and/or aminophylline 6 mg/kg load IV over 30 min for wheezing 6. Methylprednisolone 2 mg/kg IV bolus then 2-4 mg/kg/day IV divided q6h or hydrocortisone 4-8 mg/kg (max 250 mg/dose) IV bolus and then 2 mg/kg/dose IV q6h 7. NaCl (0.9%) 20-ml/kg IV bolus for hypotension; consider further doses of epinephrine IV and if resistant via infusion, 0.1-1 mcg/kg/min 8. Admit to intensive care unit for monitoring

[*]See Chapter 29, Rash, for further recommendations for the treatment of anaphylaxis.

REFERENCES

Auerbach PS: *Wilderness medicine: management of wilderness and environmental emergencies*, 3rd ed, St. Louis, 1995, Mosby–Year Book.

Centers for Disease Control and Prevention: Human rabies prevention—United States, 1999. Recommendations of the Advisory Committee on Immunization Practices (ACIP), *MMWR Morb Mortal Wkly Rep* 48(RR-1):1-21, 1999.

Dart RC, McNally J: Efficacy, safety, and use of snake antivenoms in the United States, *Ann Emerg Med* 37(2):181-188, 2001.

Hodge D III, Tecklenburg FW: Bites and stings. In Fleisher GR, Ludwig S, editors: *Textbook of pediatric emergency medicine*, 4th ed, Philadelphia, 2000, Lippincott Williams & Wilkins.

Gilbert DN: *The Sanford guide to antimicrobial therapy*, Hyde park, Vermont, 31st ed, 2001, Antimicrobial Therapy, Inc.

Rosen P: *Emergency medicine: concepts and clinical practice*, 4th ed, St. Louis, 1998, Mosby–Year Book.

Taketomo CK, Hodding JH, Kraus DM: *Pediatric dosage handbook*, 8th ed, Cleveland, 2001/2002, Lexicomp.

CHAPTER 6

Bleeding and Bruising

ALEXANDRA EPEE-BOUNYA

To many parents a child with unexplained bruising or bleeding is cause for great concern. Normal toddler behavior resulting in minor injuries must be differentiated from nonaccidental trauma and an entire spectrum of bleeding disorders. Several very serious conditions can present with bleeding or bruising. The patient must be quickly stabilized and treated, appropriate subspecialists consulted, and the family kept informed. In most cases a careful history, physical examination, and a few simple tests are enough to differentiate between life-threatening and minor conditions.

 ## INFECTIONS

Petechiae and purpura can be the symptoms of life-threatening infections such as staphylococcal, streptococcal, *Haemophilus influenzae,* or gram-negative sepsis; meningococcemia; or Rocky Mountain spotted fever. A high degree of suspicion must be present on the part of the clinician, as prompt diagnosis and administration of antibiotics may save the patient's life (see Chapter 14, Fever; Chapter 19, Hypertension; and Chapter 29, Rash).

 ## LEUKEMIA

Leukemia is the most common form of childhood malignancy. The yearly incidence is 4 cases per 100,000 children. Leukemias are classified according to their onset (chronic vs. acute), the morphology of the abnormal cells, and the markers on their surface. Most cases of childhood leukemia are acute; 75% are lymphoblastic. The cause of leukemia is unknown, but there are some high-risk populations such as children with Down syndrome, children already treated for malignancy, and those affected by certain syndromes (e.g., Peutz-Jeghers syndrome).

Symptoms
- Pallor +++
- Fatigue +++
- Spontaneous bruising +++
- Epistaxis
- Oozing from gums
- Bone pain ++++
- Joint pain ++
- Irritability ++
- Weight loss +++

Signs
- Petechiae, ecchymoses ++++
- Adenopathy
- Hepatosplenomegaly ++
- Mediastinal mass
- Chloromas (localized masses of leukemic cells that can develop at any site, including the skin; may precede the leukemic infiltration of the bone marrow)
- Fever +++
- Testicular mass

Workup
- CBC with manual differential and smear to identify any abnormalities such as:
  - Blasts ++++.
  - Anemia +++.
  - Thrombocytopenia +++.
  - Leukopenia +++.
- PT and PTT.
- CXR to rule out mediastinal mass.

- Electrolytes, blood urea nitrogen, creatinine, uric acid, calcium, and phosphorus to assess for tumor lysis syndrome.
- Liver function tests, lactate dehydrogenase.
- Blood type and screen (to facilitate further crossmatch if the patient is anemic).
- Blood culture if febrile.
- Bone marrow aspirate or biopsy for definitive diagnosis.

Comments and Treatment Considerations

Except in rare cases definitive diagnostic workup and management of a newly diagnosed leukemic patient is done by a pediatric oncology team. Immediate management considerations should be discussed in the emergent setting with a pediatric oncologist and may include the need to begin alkalinization of the urine, blood transfusion, and/or empiric antibiotics.

Alkalinization of the urine should be considered if the white blood cell (WBC) count is greatly elevated, if the electrolytes suggest tumor lysis, or if a mediastinal mass or hepatosplenomegaly is present. A continuous infusion of D5W with sodium bicarbonate 75 mEq/L administered at 1.5 to 2 times the maintenance rate should be initiated. Additionally, consider the use of allopurinol or rasburicase therapy to reduce the concentration of uric acid.

If the patient is symptomatic from anemia (or has a hemoglobin <8 g/dl), a packed red blood cell transfusion should be given very slowly. All blood products should be irradiated and cytomegalovirus negative secondary to the potential need for future bone marrow transplantation (see Chapter 28, Pallor).

Treatment with broad-spectrum antibiotics (ensure *Pseudomonas* coverage) should be instituted if the patient is febrile or has evidence of a bacterial infection. Corticosteroids are usually not indicated and should not be given without consultation with a pediatric oncologist.

✳ HEMOPHILIA AND DISORDERS OF COAGULATION

Bleeding in patients with hemophilia can have very serious consequences. Any bleeding must be evaluated and corrected rapidly.

Hemophilia A (factor VIII deficiency) and hemophilia B (factor IX deficiency) are the most common inherited bleeding disorders. The severity of the bleeding episodes is related to the quantity of factor present (<1% is severe, 1% to 5% is moderate, and >5% is mild). Patients with von Willebrand's disease tend to have minimal significant clinical bleeding. Many patients who were treated with factor concentrate in the early 1980s are now HIV positive. Persistent bleeding in a patient not previously diagnosed with hemophilia requires a high index of suspicion and consultation with a pediatric hematologist.

Symptoms

- History of excessive bruising once ambulation starts (in toddlers) or of large hematoma formation with minor trauma ++
- Joint pain
- Joint swelling
- Bruising
- Abdominal pain
- Prolonged bleeding from circumcision site ++
- Headache/lethargy

Signs

- Hemarthroses ++
- Muscle bleeding ++
- Subcutaneous bleeding +++
- Oral mucosa bleeding
- Melena
- Hematuria

Workup

- For known hemophilic patients, CBC and reticulocyte count.
- If you suspect a disorder of coagulation in a patient not previously diagnosed, obtain a CBC with differential, platelets, PT, and PTT. After consultation with a pediatric hematologist, consider obtaining factor levels and bleeding time. If possible, laboratory specimens should be drawn before giving any factor or blood products.
- Have a low threshold for neuro-imaging a patient with known coagulopathy sustaining even a mild head injury to

confirm the presence or absence of an intracranial hemorrhage.

Comments and Treatment Considerations

The severity of the hemophilia and the type of injury dictate treatment. There is clear clinical evidence of bleeding in 90% of patients with hemophilia by 1 year of age. Factor replacement is the mainstay of therapy for all serious hemorrhages. Most known pediatric hemophiliacs will have a pediatric hematologist and a plan for emergency therapy. Many patients are known to respond well to specific factor types and doses.

Consider consultation with a pediatric hematologist before instituting care. Cryoprecipitate enriched for factor VIII (5 to 10 units/mg of protein) may be used in cases of significant active bleeding. Cryoprecipitate contains 80 to 120 units of factor VIII per unit and the dose volume is calculated from the desired factor VIII correction. However, secondary to concerns about viral transmission, recombinant factor is more commonly used. Two formulas are routinely used to determine the number of units of factor concentrate required to achieve a particular level of correction.

Recombinant factor VIII: (weight in kg) $\times$ (desired level of correction in %) $\times$ (0.5) = no. of units

Recombinant factor IX: (weight in kg) $\times$ (desired level of correction in %) $\times$ (1.2) = no. of units

The degree of correction required depends on the severity of the disease and the extent of the injury or bleeding.

Site of Bleeding	Desired Level of Correction (%)
Joint or simple hematoma	20-40
Simple dental extraction	50
Major soft tissue bleed	80-100
Head injury	100+
Major surgery	100+

Some children require additional doses of factor in 12 to 14 hours based on severity of disease and bleeding site. Desmopressin (DDAVP) at a dose of 0.3 mcg/kg/dose given either SC or via IV infusion over 30 minutes may be useful in a subset of patients. Adjuvant antifibrinolytic therapy with either aminocaproic acid dosed at 100 mg/kg/dose (max 5 g/dose) IV/PO q6h or tranexamic acid dosed at 25 mg/kg/dose (max 1.5 g/dose) PO q8h or 10 mg/kg/dose (max 1 g/dose) IV q8h may be useful, particularly for oral bleeding. Dry topical thrombin may be useful for oral mucosa bleeding. There are some children with hemophilia and known antibodies (inhibitors) to the missing factor. These children are very difficult to clinically manage and their hematologist should be consulted.

 THROMBOCYTOPENIA

Thrombocytopenia may be due to decreased platelet survival, decreased platelet production, or platelet sequestration. The most common form of thrombocytopenia in children is immune thrombocytopenic purpura (ITP). This condition is due to increased platelet destruction. Disseminated intravascular coagulation and hemolytic uremic syndrome are also associated with decreased platelet survival. Leukemias and neuroblastomas are common causes of decrease platelet production, secondary to bone marrow suppression. Platelet sequestration occurs when an enlarged spleen removes platelets from the circulation. This can result from numerous causes including storage disorders and portal hypertension.

DISSEMINATED INTRAVASCULAR COAGULATION
See Chapter 20, Hypotension.

HEMOLYTIC UREMIC SYNDROME
See Chapter 10, Diarrhea.

IMMUNE THROMBOCYTOPENIC PURPURA
ITP most commonly occurs in children 2 to 6 years of age. When one is faced with a child with purpura, a detailed history including surgeries, dental extractions, and trauma is crucial. The results of the blood tests and the clinical status of the patient will guide further management. The cause of ITP is unknown,

but its onset is often temporally related to an antecedent non-specific viral infection. ITP may occur in association with HIV, mononucleosis, CMV, rubeola, mumps, or varicella. The differential includes aplastic anemia and acute leukemia. A bone marrow biopsy is sometimes performed to rule out other causes. Normal megakaryocytes are found in ITP.

Symptoms
- History of mild viral illness (up to 6 weeks prior) followed by acute onset of bruising and bleeding

Signs
- Acute onset of petechiae and ecchymoses (Fig. 6-1) +++
- Mucosal bleeding +
- Epistaxis +

Workup
- CBC with differential is usually notable for thrombocytopenia only; anemia is unusual unless large blood loss has occurred.
- PT and PTT are usually normal.
- Platelet count is usually <20,000.
- Antinuclear antibody (as a screening test for collagen disorders).

Comments and Treatment Considerations
ITP has an excellent prognosis, even when no specific treatment is administered. Only those patients with significant bleeding or platelet counts <10,000 are routinely treated. Children should be protected from potential trauma until the platelet count normalizes, which usually occurs spontaneously within 3 months.

Before the initiation of any therapy a pediatric hematologist should be consulted. Platelet transfusions are indicated only in the management of life-threatening intracranial hemorrhages (a rare complication in <1% of patients). Randomized controlled trials have demonstrated that therapy with IV immune globulin (IVIG) shortens the duration of severe thrombocytopenia. A single dose of 1 g/kg has been shown to be effective. Severe or recalcitrant cases may require a second dose of IVIG at 1 g/kg on day 2 and may even require maintenance IVIG doses every

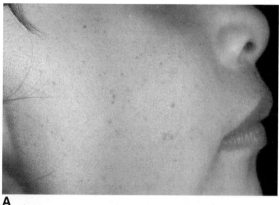

A

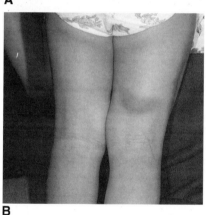

B

Fig. 6-1 A, Petechiae over face. **B,** Petechiae and ecchymoses over lower extremity in this 2-year-old girl, who had normal values of white blood cells, differential, and hemoglobulin. Her platelet count was 13,000 cells/mm³. Interestingly, she had received the varicella vaccine 3 weeks before the onset of purpura. Purpura is most prominent over the legs and typically is asymmetric in acute immune thrombocytopenic purpura. In Henoch-Schönlein purpura, purpuric lesions are symmetrically distributed over the lower extremities. (From Shah B, Laude T: *Atlas of pediatric clinical diagnosis,* Philadelphia, 2000, WB Saunders.)

3 to 6 weeks. The rate of IVIG administration is brand specific, so confirm appropriate infusion rate with the blood bank or pharmacy. $Rh_o(D)$ immune globulin (WinRho) can be used in patients who have a rhesus-positive blood type. Anemia should be expected in patients receiving $Rh_o(D)$ immune globulin secondary to the destruction of Rh-positive red blood cells. Dosing is dependent on hemoglobin level and should be given by IV infusion only. Steroids, such as prednisone at a dose of 2-8 mg/kg/day PO divided q6h, have been shown to sometimes decrease the severity and duration of the initial phase, but their use should be discussed with a consultant hematologist. Adjuvant therapy for acute severe bleeding may include antifibrinolytic treatment with aminocaproic acid dosed at 50 to 100 mg/kg/dose (max 5 g/dose) IV/PO q6h.

 ## PHYSICAL ABUSE

Physical abuse is the most often reported form of child abuse. The skin is the most commonly injured organ. All active children will sustain bruises, but pediatricians must have a low threshold for suspicion of child abuse when evaluating patients with any kind of nonspecific skin injury, especially those involving areas rarely exposed to trauma (e.g., back of legs and back). Nonconcerning trauma is usually located in areas that are exposed (e.g., shins and elbows). Inconsistent histories and inappropriate affects are also red flags (see Chapter 2, Abuse/Rape).

 ## HENOCH-SCHÖNLEIN PURPURA

Henoch-Schönlein purpura (HSP) is an immunologically mediated inflammatory disorder of unknown etiology that manifests itself as a diffuse vasculitis causing skin, gastrointestinal, renal, or joint symptomatology. Symptoms are thought to be related to those systems affected by an increased capillary permeability caused by the underlying vasculitis.

The characteristic rash of HSP can be very troubling to families. Despite its appearance, which may resemble coagulopathy or abuse, HSP is usually a fairly benign disease.

Symptoms

- History of an antecedent upper respiratory tract infection. Exposure to other viruses, bacteria, drugs, foods, insect bites, immunizations, cold, or chemicals have also been implicated in pathogenesis
- Malaise and low-grade fever
- Age 3 to 10 years (but can occur in younger and older patients)
- Abdominal pain (most often described as colicky) ++++; gross or occult rectal bleeding may occur
- Joint pain (most commonly knees and ankles but may be wrists and elbows) +++/++++
- Angioedema, especially of the hands and feet

Signs

- The rash usually begins as erythematous macules and papules becoming hemorrhagic and then purpuric. In its classic form the rash is palpable and tends to have a symmetric distribution over the buttocks and extensor surfaces of the lower extremities. The upper extremities, trunk, and face may also be less commonly involved (Fig. 6-2)
- Painful, warm, swollen joints (most commonly knees, ankles, and feet but may be wrists and elbows)
- Gastrointestinal tract bleeding may occur, with complications of intussusception, obstruction, or infarction with bowel perforation
- Seizures, paresis, and coma
- Respiratory involvement and testicular hemorrhage and/or torsion are less commonly seen

Workup

- Diagnosis is predominantly clinical and based on the constellation of rash, arthritis, gastrointestinal, and/or renal

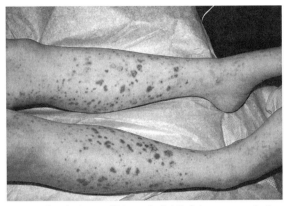

Fig. 6-2 Skin lesions of Henoch-Schönlein purpura in its typical symmetric distribution on the lower extremities. (See Color Insert.) (From Shah B, Laude T: *Atlas of pediatric clinical diagnosis*, Philadelphia, 2000, WB Saunders.)

symptoms; however, diagnosis may be difficult if joint and abdominal symptoms begin before the rash is evident.

- Urinalysis should be performed for evidence of nephritis. Renal involvement occurs in 25% of children younger than 2 years and 50% of children older than 2 years, manifesting as a nephritis with gross or microscopic hematuria with or without casts and proteinuria.
- Erythrocyte sedimentation rate may be elevated.
- WBC count may be increased with an eosinophilia.
- Coagulation study results are normal.
- Stool for occult or gross blood.
- Serum complement titers are normal or elevated.
- Serum levels of immunoglobulin A (IgA) are elevated +++.
- Cultures, particularly of the throat, are indicated.

Comments and Treatment Considerations

Prognosis is excellent for most patients, particularly young children who usually have milder symptoms of a shorter duration with fewer renal and gastrointestinal manifestations. Serial urinalyses should be performed until the results are normal for a few months. Approximately 5% of patients with nephritis will develop advanced glomerular disease leading to renal failure. Although no specific therapy for the underlying process exists, systemic steroids such as prednisone dosed at 1 to 2 mg/kg/day may be beneficial in reducing severe abdominal and CNS manifestations. Cytotoxic agents and anticoagulants have been used in cases of severe nephritis but remain controversial.

REFERENCES

Aysun S, Topcu M, Gunay M, Topaloglu H: Neurologic features as initial presentations of childhood malignancies, *Pediatr Neurol* 10(1):40-43, 1994.

Bevan JA, Maloney KW, Hillery CA, et al: Bleeding disorders: a common cause of menorrhagia in adolescents, *J Pediatr* 138(6):856-861, 2001.

Bickert B, Kwiatkowski JL: Coagulation disorders. In DiPiro JT, editor: *Pharmacotherapy: a pathophysiologic approach*, 5th ed, New York, 2002, McGraw-Hill.

Cabral DA, Tucker LB: Malignancies in children who initially present with rheumatic complaints, *J Pediatr* 134(1):53-57, 1999.

Conway JH, Hilgartner MW: Initial presentations of pediatric hemophiliacs, *Arch Pediatr Adolesc Med* 148(6):589-594, 1994.

Ljung R, Petrini P, Nilsson IM: Diagnostic symptoms of severe and moderate haemophilia A and B. A survey of 140 cases, *Acta Paediatr Scand* 79(2):196-200, 1990.

Ma SK, Chan GC, Ha SY, et al: Clinical presentation, hematologic features and treatment outcomes of childhood acute lymphoblastic leukemia: a review of 73 cases in Hong Kong, *Hematol Oncol* 15(3):141-149, 1997.

Minhas HI, Giangrande PL: Presentation of severe haemophilia—a role for accident and emergency doctors? *Emerg Med J* 18(4):246-249, 2001.

Parkin JD, Smith IL, O'Neill AI, et al: Mild bleeding disorders. A clinical and laboratory study, *Med J Aust* 156(9):614-617, 1992.

Taketomo CK, Hodding JH, Kraus DM: *Pediatric dosage handbook*, 8th ed, Cleveland, 2001/2002, Lexicomp Inc.

Tarantino MD: Acute immune (idiopathic) thrombocytopenic purpura in childhood, *Blood Rev* 16(1):19-21, 2002.

Thiam D, Diop S, Berrada S, et al: Presenting features at diagnosis and complications of hemophilia in Dakar: apropos of 25 cases, *Hematol Cell Ther* 39(1):1-4, 1997.

Venkateswaran L, Wilimas JA, Jones DJ, Nuss R: Mild hemophilia in children: prevalence, complications, and treatment, *J Pediatr Hematol Oncol* 20(1):32-35, 1998.

Young G, Toretsky JA, Campbell AB, Eskenazi AE: Recognition of common childhood malignancies, *Am Fam Physician* 61(7): 2144-2154, 2000.

CHAPTER 7

Burns

MICHELLE M. CARLO

Approximately 30,000 children are hospitalized with burns each year. Unintentional burns are more common in children younger than 4 years and adolescents. When treating patients with burns, the clinician must consider the mechanism and etiology, as well as the risk for inhalation injury. Immediate attention must be paid to early signs of impending or potential airway compromise. Intentional burns comprise approximately 10% of child abuse injuries (see Chapter 2, Abuse/Rape). Associated traumatic injuries should not be overlooked.

Emergent transfer to a burn center should be considered in children with thermal burns covering full-thickness >10% body surface area (BSA) or partial-thickness >20% BSA. Patients with serious burns to the hands, feet, face, and genitalia or burns across joints should also be transferred emergently. Electrical and chemical burns are special considerations that are discussed separately.

 ## INHALATION INJURY

Smoke exposure or close contact with intense heat can have life-threatening consequences secondary to inflammation and edema of the upper airways and lungs. Swelling of the upper airways can quickly become obstructive and may result in devastating consequences. Empiric intubation for airway protection may be indicated. Carbon monoxide (CO) exposure should be considered for patients involved in fires in enclosed areas, with motor engine exhaust exposure, with exposure to fumes produced by malfunctioning or inappropriate indoor heaters, or with unexplainable nausea, headache, or altered mental status (see Chapter 33, Syncope, and Chapter 35, Toxic Ingestion, Approach To). Cyanide exposure is rare in pediatrics but should be considered if the child is involved in a fire or other environmental disaster (see Chapter 35, Toxic Ingestion, Approach To).

Symptoms
- Shortness of breath
- Sore throat
- Drooling
- Brassy cough
- Facial burns
- Hoarseness

Signs
- Stridor
- Singed facial hair
- Sooty sputum
- Airway erythema

Workup
Do not postpone immediate airway management to obtain laboratory or radiographic studies.
- Pulse oximetry may be normal in the patient with asphyxiant exposure to CO or other toxins.
- CXR.
- Consider CO and cyanide levels.

Comments and Treatment Considerations
Support the ABCs with particular attention to the need for prophylactic intubation in any patient with burns to the face, singed facial hairs, hoarseness, or soot in nares or oropharynx. Delaying intubation may result in edema and difficulty in securing the airway. Additionally, a smaller sized endotracheal tube may be necessary to stabilize an edematous airway. Radiographic evidence of inhalational injury may not manifest for 24 to 36 hours. Patients with suspected injury should be observed for at least 24 hours. Severely ill patients will require ICU admission and management. Associated burns and trauma should be managed appropriately.

THERMAL INJURY

When evaluating a patient with thermal injuries, the clinician must examine the wound closely to estimate accurately both the extent and the depth of the burn, which will determine treatment and disposition. Attention should be paid to fluid balance, thermoregulation, and pain control when managing significant burns. Determine BSA involvement by using the "rule of nines" (Fig. 7-1). In children, the surface of the child's hand approximates 1% of BSA.

FIRST-DEGREE BURNS

First-degree burns involve the superficial epidermal layer only and usually heal in 1 week without scarring.

Signs
- Pain
- Redness
- Dry
- Sensation intact
- No sloughing
- No blisters
- Blanching

SECOND-DEGREE BURNS

Second-degree partial-thickness burns are subdivided into superficial (involving the papillary layer) or deep (involving the reticular layer). Superficial burns usually heal in 2 to 3 weeks and do not leave major scars. Deep burns may be difficult to differentiate from third-degree burns and may require longer than 3 weeks for healing. They may be associated with scar formation.

Signs
Superficial
- Very painful
- Thin-walled blisters
- Tender to touch
- Pink or mottled color

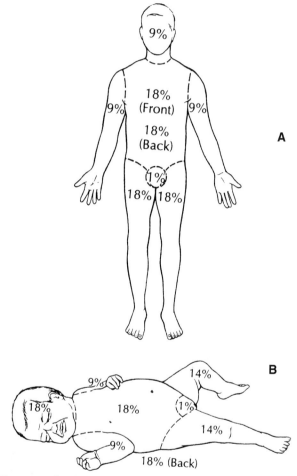

Fig. 7-1 Rule of nines. **A,** Adult. **B,** Infant. (From Rosen P, Barkin RM, Hockberger RS, et al (eds): *Emergency medicine: concepts and clinical practice,* 4th ed, St. Louis, 1998, Mosby.)

- Blanches
- Moist
- Sensation intact

Deep

- Extremely painful
- Thick-walled blisters
- Dark red or yellow skin
- Nonblanching
- Mostly dry skin
- Sensation to pressure intact
- Poor capillary refill

THIRD-DEGREE BURNS

Third-degree burns or full-thickness burns involve loss of all skin components. This type of burn usually requires grafting.

Symptoms and Signs

- White
- Leathery
- Firm
- Dry
- Sensation to deep pressure only

Workup

- UA for hemoglobinuria or myoglobinuria.
- Consider CO and cyanide levels as indicated.

Comments and Treatment Considerations

Immediately remove any hot clothing to prevent further injury and cover burns with wet gauze or bed sheets until adequate pain relief can be provided. Severely burned children will require support of the ABCs with careful attention to possible inhalation injury (see previous section), pain relief, and fluid resuscitation. Morphine sulfate 0.1 mg/kg/dose (max 15 mg/dose) IM, IV, or SC q2-4h prn should be given for pain control, with the initial dose given as soon as possible, certainly before cleaning and debridement.

Fluid shifts become significant at >20% BSA involvement. Initial fluid management should consist of normal saline or Ringer's lactate. Half of the calculated requirements should be given in the first 8 hours and the rest over the next 24 hours. The Parkland formula can be used to estimate fluid needs:

$$3 \times \text{wt (kg)} \times \% \text{ total BSA burn} + \text{standard maintenance fluids}$$

For example, for a 10-kg child with 20% total BSA burns, use the following:

$$3 \times 10 \times 20 = 600 \text{ ml/day} + 960 \text{ ml/day maintenance fluid}$$
$$= 1560 \text{ ml/day}$$

Consider emergent escharotomy if circumferential burns of chest or extremity are present. Mineral oil can be used to remove tar. Do not unroof any intact blisters unless very large or in areas prone to breaking. Blister fluid should not be aspirated. Burns may be covered with topical antibiotics such as silver sulfadiazine (Silvadene) or bacitracin. Topical antibiotic use is controversial and many suggest simple sterile dressings with sterile Vaseline jelly. Initial use of systemic antibiotics is not indicated unless evidence of infection is present. If the hands or feet are involved, each finger or toe should be dressed individually and placed in position of function. Daily dressing changes are required, with a wound recheck in 24 to 48 hours. Patients require tetanus prophylaxis and tetanus immune globulin if immunization status is unknown (see Chapter 5, Bites).

If there is evidence of rhabdomyolysis on UA, ensure hydration is sufficient to produce a urine output of at least 2 ml/kg/hr and consider alkalinization of urine (see the section on malignancy for information on how to alkalinize urine in Chapter 6, Bleeding and Bruising). Monitor patients for the development of hyperkalemia. Ileus is common with >15% to 20% BSA burns and usual resolves within 72 hours.

Transfer of the patient to a burn center should be considered in children with thermal burns covering full-thickness >10% BSA or partial-thickness >20% BSA or those with serious burns to the hands, feet, face, genitalia, or burns across joints. Patients with first-degree burns or small areas of second- or third-degree burns may be managed as outpatients as long as adequate follow-up can be arranged. Intermediate cases may be initially managed as inpatients.

For mild pain after debridement, ibuprofen 10 mg/kg/dose (max 800 mg/dose) PO q6h or acetaminophen 15 mg/kg/dose (max 1000 mg/dose, 4000 mg/day) PO q4-6h can be used with oral narcotics such as oxycodone 0.15 mg/kg/dose (initial max 10 mg/dose) PO q4h or codeine 0.5 to 1 mg/kg/dose PO q4-6h for mild to moderate pain. The combination of acetaminophen and codeine elixir (acetaminophen 120 mg and codeine 12 mg/5 ml) dosed at 0.5 to 1 mg/kg/dose of the codeine component PO q4-6h prn is another option. Pain medication should be given 1 hour before follow-up visits where the need for repeated debridement or painful dressing changes is expected. Inpatients may benefit from patient-controlled analgesia use.

 ## ELECTRICAL INJURY

A number of factors determine the effect of electrical activity on the body and include resistance, type of current (alternating current or direct current), frequency, intensity, duration, and current pathway. Tissue injury is inversely proportional to resistance, with wet skin or mucosa providing low resistance. Alternating current at low voltage is able to induce tetanic muscle contractions and is more dangerous than direct current. High-voltage injury is more dangerous than low-voltage injury and may cause "locking on" and deep tissue injury. Current pathway is complex and is affected by multiple factors; however, low-voltage current tends to follow the path of least resistance and high-voltage current follows a more direct course to ground. Tissues or organs in the pathway are those at greatest risk of injury. If the heart is in the pathway, ventricular fibrillation may ensue.

In children, electrical injuries usually arise from household currents and children are rarely exposed to high-voltage shock (>1000 V) with the possible exception of lightning strikes. Common sources of pediatric injury develop from a child chewing on an extension cord or placing an object into an outlet.

Signs and Symptoms
- Entrance/exit wounds (may not always be present, especially if low voltage)
- Superficial burns to fingers or mouth

Workup
- ECG.
- Consider UA for hemoglobinuria or myoglobinuria with baseline BUN and SCr clearance.
- For severe electrocutions obtain a CBC and CPK level.

Comments and Treatment Considerations
Patients who are acutely ill after significant electrical trauma require support of the ABCs with special attention to treating arrhythmias per standard protocols (see Chapter 34, Tachycardia). Further management of injuries should be undertaken as outlined earlier in the section on thermal injury, including the need for significant fluid support, management of mucosal wounds, and close observation for evidence of rhabdomyolysis. Fluid needs are difficult to assess because of large third-space shifts; however, indicators of adequate resuscitation include peripheral perfusion and urine output. Patients with severe symptoms should be transferred and managed at a burn center.

Injuries to the corner of the mouth from biting a cord can be minimal or quite extensive. In severe cases the early involvement of a plastic surgeon is recommended. Rarely, prophylactic intubation may be necessary to prevent airway compromise that may result from progressive swelling, which commonly occurs over the first few hours. A child with significant oral wounds may require hospitalization for IV/nasogastric hydration while the wound heals. At 2 to 3 weeks copious bleeding can ensue from the labial artery from eschar separation and families should be forewarned. Oral injuries have become less common as manufacturers have increased the thickness of electrical cord plastic insulation.

Children who have sustained minor household electrical injuries and are asymptomatic usually do not require laboratory evaluation, cardiac evaluation, or hospitalization.

CHEMICAL INJURIES

Chemical injuries can arise from many products, some of which are available at home. The most important aspect of care is to remove the offending agent and all clothing and to proceed with decontamination via copious irrigation. Health care providers need to protect themselves by wearing the appropriate gear while caring for patients with chemical injuries. Alkali burns are usually worse than acidic injury secondary to deeper skin penetration. After irrigation, epidermal injuries are treated the same as outlined earlier for thermal injury.

Chemical injuries to the eye are discussed in Chapter 12, Eye Pain and Redness. Caustic ingestions are discussed in the following section.

CAUSTIC INGESTIONS

The most common agents involved in caustic ingestions are household products such as drain, toilet, and oven cleaners; detergents; disc batteries; lye; and ammonia. Initial care is centered on the protection of the airway, because this type of injury can result in significant edema and potential obstruction.

Alkali ingestions can result in significant damage to the oropharynx and esophagus. Acidic ingestions tend to inflict greater damage to the gastric mucosa. Remember not to induce emesis in patients with possible caustic ingestions because of the risk of reexposure of the mucosa to the offending agent.

Symptoms
- Pain
- Vomiting (hematemesis particularly concerning)
- Retrosternal burning

Signs
- Drooling
- Oropharyngeal burns (if present are concerning, but their absence has no prognostic value for lower injury)
- Erythema
- Stridor

- Hoarseness
- Dyspnea
- Abdominal pain

Workup

- Determine the pH level of the product; pH < 2.0 or >12.5 particularly concerning for deeper injury.
- Obtain CXR looking for evidence of mediastinal air (suggesting esophageal perforation and risk of mediastinitis) and aspiration pneumonia. Consider abdominal radiographs looking for free air in particularly ill patients.
- CBC, electrolytes, and type and cross.

Comments and Treatment Considerations

Initial management is directed to the ABCs, with specific concern for protection of the airway given the risk for progressive edema and potential obstruction. Emesis should not be induced. Prophylactic intubation may be lifesaving and should be strongly considered in any patient with evidence of significant injury such as drooling, stridor, or vomiting. Toxicology, gastroenterology, and/or surgical consultation is indicated for symptomatic patients. If the patient is in stable condition, elective endoscopy can be scheduled within 24 hours.

If no serious injury is suspected, CXR findings are normal, and patient is able to drink, the patient may be discharged home with close follow-up.

REFERENCES

Hansbrough JF, Hansbrough W: Pediatric burns, *Pediatr Rev* 20(4):117-124, 1999.

Joffee MD: Burns. In Fleisher GR, Ludwig S, editors: *Textbook of pediatric emergency medicine*, 4th ed, Philadelphia, 2000, Lippincott Williams & Wilkins.

Morgan ED, Bledsoe SC, Barker J: Ambulatory management of burns, *Am Fam Physician* 62(9), 2000.

Nichols et al, editors: *Golden hour: the handbook of pediatric advanced life support*, St Louis, 1996, Mosby.

Schonwald S: *Medical toxicology: a synopsis and study guide*, New York, 2001, Lippincott Williams & Wilkins.

Stranger G, editor: *APLS: The pediatric emergency medicine course*, 3rd ed, Dallas, 2000, American College of Emergency Physicians.

Viccellio P, editor: *Emergency toxicology*, 2nd ed, New York, 1998, Lippincott–Raven Press.

CHAPTER 8

Chest Pain

SARITA A. CHUNG

Chest pain is a common presenting symptom in the pediatric population. Unlike adult patients, children who have chest pain are unlikely to have cardiac disease and/or a life-threatening cause. Etiologies of chest pain in children include idiopathic (12% to 85%), musculoskeletal (15% to 31%), pulmonary (12% to 21%), psychiatric (5% to 17%), gastrointestinal (4% to 7%), cardiac (4% to 6%), and other (4% to 21%).

 TRAUMA

Tension pneumothorax must be emergently diagnosed and treated to prevent cardiopulmonary collapse (see Chapter 30, Respiratory Distress).

 MYOCARDIAL INFARCTION

Myocardial infarction (MI) is rare in the general pediatric population, so few data are available to aid in the diagnosis and therapy for children presenting with MI. There are subgroups in the pediatric population that are at increased risk of myocardial ischemia or MI such as children with a history of Kawasaki disease, cardiomyopathy, congenital heart disease, myocarditis, or collagen vascular disease. Children who have familial hypercholesterolemia, familial combined hyperlipidemia, hypoalphalipoproteinemia, and hypobetalipoproteinemia can develop premature coronary artery disease and have an MI before age 20 years. Cocaine ingestion should be considered a possible cause of cardiac ischemia in adolescents being evaluated for chest pain.

Most of the data describing the signs and symptoms of pediatric MIs come from patients with a history of Kawasaki disease. One should be careful not to extrapolate adult MI data to the pediatric population. Signs and symptoms are commonly more subtle and the ECG findings (as noted later in this chapter) are different in children versus adults with MI. Arrhythmias, particularly ventricular tachycardia, are a risk factor for MI. Ventricular hypertrophy is also a risk factor.

Symptoms
- Chest pain
- Poor feeding
- Dyspnea
- Vomiting
- Colic
- Irritability
- Anxiety
- Arrhythmia (in children signs of arrhythmias can present as abdominal pain, palpitations, syncope, or easy fatigability)

Signs
- Friction rub
- Gallop
- Dilated jugular veins
- Shock
- Cyanosis
- Diaphoresis
- Tachypnea
- Rales
- Arrhythmias

Workup
- 12-Lead ECG: Normal characteristics of ECG are different depending on the age of the child. Pediatric ECG changes in MI are new Q waves (>35 ms), notched Q waves, ST-segment elevation (>2 mm), and a prolonged corrected QT interval (Fig. 8-1).
- CXR may be helpful for identifying other causes of chest pain, such as pneumonia or pneumothorax.

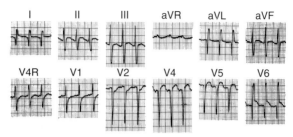

Fig. 8-1 Tracing from a 2-month-old infant who has an anomalous origin of the left coronary artery from the pulmonary artery. An abnormally deep and wide Q wave (0.04 seconds) is seen in leads I, aV_L, and V_6, and a QS pattern seen in leads V_2 through V_6 is characteristic of anterolateral myocardial infarction. (From Park M, Troxler RG: *Pediatric cardiology for practitioners,* 4th ed, St. Louis, 2002, Mosby.)

- Serum creatine kinase (CK), specifically CK (MB); isoenzyme elevation indicates ischemic cardiac muscle.
- Cardiac troponin I may be elevated before visible ECG changes consistent with ischemia or infarction.

Comments and Treatment Considerations

Very few data exist for the management of pediatric MI. Emergent cardiology consultation is recommended and further diagnostic testing such as cardiac catheterization is usually necessary to confirm the diagnosis. Most treatment options are extrapolated from adult experience. Oxygen, aspirin, and morphine for pain support may be initiated before cardiology consultation; however, a pediatric cardiologist should dictate any further medical therapy, including the initiation of thrombolytic therapy.

CONGENITAL HEART DISEASE

Patients with a history of corrected or uncorrected congenital heart disease are at particular risk for multiple cardiac issues later in life. Any patient with a history of congenital heart disease and chest pain should have an emergent ECG performed and consultation with their cardiologist (see Chapter 9, Cyanosis).

 ## PULMONARY EMBOLISM

Pulmonary embolism (PE) is rare in children but should be considered in a number of scenarios, particularly in a patient exhibiting significant hypoxia without other obvious causes of respiratory distress. The diagnosis should be considered in female adolescents who are taking oral contraceptives or who have had a recent abortion; children with hypercoagulable states such as antiphospholipid antibody syndrome, antithrombin III deficiency, lupus anticoagulants, protein C, and protein S deficiencies; children with central vascular access; and children with a history of trauma, congenital heart disease, prolonged immobilization, or surgery.

In general, PE is rare in healthy patients and is a difficult diagnosis to make unless the embolism is large. Frequency data for signs and symptoms (as indicated below) are derived from adult and adolescent patients. Younger patients often present with subtle symptoms and delayed diagnosis is common.

Signs
- Apprehension +++
- Chest pain, often pleuritic +++
- Dyspnea ++++
- Fever +++
- Palpitations
- Cough +++

Symptoms
- Tachypnea ++++
- Hypoxemia ++++
- Hemoptysis +++

Workup
- Ventilation/perfusion (V/Q) scan and/or spiral CT scan may identify an area of concern (Fig. 8-2).

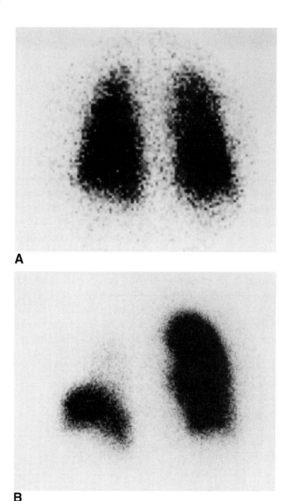

Fig. 8-2 Ventilation/perfusion scans from a patient with pulmonary embolism. **A,** Posterior view of the ventilation scan shows normal xenon-133 distribution in both lungs. **B,** Posterior view of the perfusion scan demonstrates markedly decreased perfusion of the left upper lobe with smaller filling defects of the right lung. (From Taussig L, Landau L: *Pediatric respiratory medicine,* St. Louis, 1999, Mosby.)

- ECG changes are nonspecific, but an $S_1Q_3T_3$ pattern ++ or ST-segment/T-wave changes +++ are suggestive.
- CXR findings are usually nonspecific, but an infiltrate with an elevated ipsilateral hemidiaphragm is suggestive.
- Consider lupus anticoagulants, protein C, and protein S levels.
- Pulmonary angiography is considered the gold standard for confirmation of diagnosis. Reliability diminishes with time after acute PE.

Comments and Treatment Considerations

Emergent hematology consultation is recommended. Initial management includes supplemental oxygen and heparinization. Heparin is commonly dosed at 75 to 100 units/kg IV bolus followed by 20 to 25 units/kg/hr as a continuous infusion. Dose should be adjusted based on heparin levels or activated partial thromboplastin time (aPTT). Enoxaparin, a low-molecular-weight heparin, may be considered in place of unfractionated heparin and is generally dosed at 1.5 mg/kg/dose SC q12h if the patient is younger than 2 months and 1 mg/kg/dose SC q12h if older than 2 months. Enoxaparin dosing is adjusted based on anti–factor Xa levels. Consider thrombolytic agents for severe distress with evidence of acute pulmonary arterial hypertension by echocardiography. Surgical thrombectomy is indicated if medical treatment is unsuccessful. Long-term oral anticoagulation may be necessary.

 TUMORS

Mediastinal tumors can present with chest pain. Included in the differential are Hodgkin's disease, T-cell lymphoma, thymoma, thymolipoma, teratoma, germ cell tumor, liposarcoma, and neuroblastoma.

Signs
- Chest pain
- Cough
- Dyspnea

- Hemoptysis
- Hoarseness
- Inspiratory stridor

Symptoms
- Cyanosis
- Retractions
- Tachypnea
- Wheeze

Workup
- Supplemental oxygen.
- CXR as initial radiographic evaluation of mass and airway compromise.
- Chest CT or magnetic resonance imaging to better delineate mass.

Comments and Treatment Considerations

Provide supplemental oxygen. Avoid intubation in the emergency department whenever possible. Intubation medications or general anesthetics can eliminate the negative thoracic pressure caused by the expansion of the chest wall and result in respiratory deterioration. Admission to the hospital with surgical or oncologic consultation is usually necessary for respiratory support and further diagnostic evaluation.

 ACUTE CHEST SYNDROME

Children with sickle cell disease may present with chest pain as a symptom of acute chest syndrome. This is a potentially life-threatening condition and a leading cause of death in patients with sickle cell disease. During evaluation of a patient with sickle cell disease for possible acute chest syndrome, one must remember that pulse oximetry may not reflect true Pao_2 in the presence of abnormal hemoglobin.

Symptoms
- Cough ++++
- Chest pain +++

- Shortness of breath ++
- Chills ++

Signs
- Dullness to percussion
- Fever ++++
- Wheezing ++
- Hemoptysis +
- Rales +
- Tachypnea (more common in younger patients)

Workup
- CXR to demonstrate the presence of new infiltrate. Upper lobe infiltrates ++++ are more common than lower lobe infiltrates ++.
- CBC and reticulocyte count to evaluate degree of anemia.
- Consider blood cultures if the child is febrile.
- Type and cross for later need for transfusion.
- Pulse oximetry (caution is warranted because the pulse oximetry reading may not correlate to the actual oxygenation).
- Arterial blood gas for measurement of true Pao_2.

Comments and Treatment Considerations:
Patients with sickle cell disease and symptoms suggestive of acute chest syndrome require hospital admission because the disease may be rapidly progressive. Significant respiratory distress requiring intubation and ventilatory support may develop. Initial therapy includes supplemental oxygen, early empiric broad-spectrum antibiotics such as ceftriaxone 50 mg/kg IV × 1 (max 2 g/dose), analgesia, and hydration. Consultation with a pediatric hematologist is recommended, particularly in the more severe case that may require simple blood or exchange transfusion.

 ## MYOCARDITIS

Myocarditis can be caused by a number of processes including infectious, bacterial, viral, rickettsial, fungal, or parasitic organisms; collagen vascular disease, systemic lupus erythematosus, or juvenile rheumatoid arthritis; and hypersensitivity drug reactions. Of the viral etiologies, coxsackie and echoviruses predominate. Clinically, the disease is difficult to diagnose because signs and symptoms are not pathognomonic and are often subtle. Frequently the cause of myocarditis is not identified.

Symptoms
- Chest pain
- Dyspnea
- Easy fatigability
- General malaise
- Fever
- Vomiting
- Lightheadedness
- Shortness of breath

Signs
- Tachypnea
- New onset of congestive heart failure (rales, hepatomegaly, jugular venous distention, pulmonary edema)
- Resting sinus tachycardia
- Arrhythmias
- Gallop rhythms
- Indistinct heart sounds
- Cardiovascular collapse

Workup
- ECG: variable findings but can show generalized low-voltage, left ventricular hypertrophy, ST-segment changes, and T-wave flattening.
- CXR may show cardiomegaly (late finding).
- Echocardiogram may show ventricular dysfunction, decreased cardiac function.
- ESR or CK (specifically CK MB) may be elevated.
- White blood cell count may be elevated.

Comments and Treatment Considerations
Treatment of myocarditis remains supportive and symptomatic. Options to consider are digoxin for inotropic support and

diuretics for afterload reduction. The angiotensin-converting enzyme inhibitor captopril has been shown to be beneficial in coxsackie myocarditis. Immunosuppression may be harmful and steroids should be avoided. Cardiology consultation is strongly recommended.

 PERICARDITIS

Acute pericarditis, or inflammation of the pericardium, can be caused by infection, collagen vascular disease, cardiac surgery, or rheumatic fever.

Symptoms
- Chest pain exacerbated by breathing, coughing, or motion; pain is usually decreased in the sitting position
- Fever
- Dyspnea

Signs
- Pericardial friction rub
- Tachycardia (out of proportion to fever)
- Distant heart sounds
- Pulsus paradoxus may be present (a decrease in systolic blood pressure of >10 mm Hg when compared from inspiration to expiration)

Workup
- ECG may show diffuse ST-segment elevation in all leads and/or PR-segment depression.
- Echocardiography to determine the presence and amount of intrapericardial fluid.
- CXR may show enlarged pericardium.

Comments and Treatment Considerations
Treat the underlying cause if due to infection. Symptomatic support includes rest, analgesia, and antiinflammatory drugs. Consider consultation with a pediatric cardiologist.

PNEUMONIA AND PULMONARY ASPIRATION

Pneumonia commonly causes chest pain in children (see Chapter 30, Respiratory Distress).

 ## GASTROINTESTINAL

Gastrointestinal pain can manifest itself as chest pain, particularly when caused by gastroesophageal reflux. Symptoms include a worsening of pain after eating or a metallic taste in the mouth with vertical radiation of pain along the sternum (see Chapter 1, Abdominal Pain).

 ## MUSCULOSKELETAL

Musculoskeletal complaints are common in children as a result of straining of the chest wall muscles while exercising or heavy lifting. Direct impact to the chest can lead to contusions, fractures, and/or more severe injuries.

Symptoms
- Tenderness to palpation of the specific muscle group, costochondral junction, or bone
- No history of cardiac disease

Signs
- Chest pain may be exacerbated with movement
- No history of palpitations

Workup
- CXR may be useful to rule out pneumothorax resulting from trauma; routine x-rays for rib fractures not indicated unless performed as part of an evaluation for abuse.

Comments and Treatment Considerations
Supportive care is usually all that is necessary, providing rest and nonsteroidal antiinflammatory analgesics such as ibuprofen

dosed at 10 mg/kg/dose (max 800 mg/dose) PO q6-8h prn for pain.

REFERENCES

Beck C: Incidence and risk factors of catheter-related deep vein thrombosis in a pediatric intensive care unit: a prospective study, *J Pediatr* 133:237-241, 1998.

Bor I: Myocardial infarction and ischemic heart disease in infants and children, *Arch Dis Child* 44:268-281, 1969.

Allen HD, Gutgesell HP, Clark EB, et al: *Moss and Adams: heart disease in infants, children and adolescents*, 5th ed, Baltimore, 1995, Williams & Wilkins.

Emre U, Miller S, Gutierez M, et al: Effect of transfusion in acute chest syndrome of sickle cell disease, *J Pediatr* 127:901-904, 1995.

Hoffman RS, Hollander JE: Evaluation of patients with chest pain after cocaine use, *Crit Care Clin* 13(4):809-828, 1997.

Kocis K: Chest pain in pediatrics, *Pediatr Clin North Am* 46:189-203, 1999.

Manco-Johnson MJ: Combined thrombolytic and anticoagulant therapy for venous thrombosis in children, *J Pediatr* 136:2000.

Monagle P, Michelson AD, Bovill E, Andrew M: Antithrombotic therapy in children, *Chest* 119(1 suppl):344S-370S, 2001.

Nuss R: Childhood thrombosis, *Pediatrics* 96:291-294, 1995.

Patterson MD, Ruddy RM: Pain-chest. In Fleisher GR, Ludwig S, editors: *Textbook of pediatric emergency medicine*, 4th ed, Philadelphia, 2000, Lippincott Williams & Wilkins.

Quinn C, Buchanan G: The acute chest syndrome of sickle cell disease, *J Pediatr* 135:205-216, 1999.

Reich J, Campbell R: Myocardial infarction in children, *Am J Emerg Med* 16:296-303, 1998.

Sharma GVRK, Schoolman M, Sasahara AA, et al: Pulmonary thromboembolism, *JAMA* 249(21):2945-2950, 1983.

Selbst SM: Pediatric chest pain: a prospective study, *Pediatrics* 82:319-323, 1988.

Selbst SM: Consultation with the specialist: chest pain in children, *Pediatr Rev* 185:169-173, 1997.

Siberry GK, Iannone R: *The Harriet Lane Handbook*, St Louis, 2000, Mosby.

Sprinkle RH, Smith S, Cole T, Buchanan GR: Acute chest syndrome in children with sickle cell disease: a retrospective analysis of 100 hospitalized cases, *Am J Pediatr Hematol Oncol* 8(2):105-110, 1986.

Strollo DC, Rosado-de-Christenson ML, Jett JR: Primary mediastinal tumors. Part 1: Tumors of the anterior mediastinum, *Chest* 112:511-522, 1997.

Towbin JA: Myocardial infarction in infants and children. In Garson A, Bricker JT, McNamara DG, editors: *The science and practice of pediatric cardiology*, vol 3, Philadelphia, 1990, Lea & Febiger.

von Scheven E, Athreya BH, Rose CD, et al: Clinical characteristics of antiphospholipid antibody syndrome in children, *J Pediatr* 129:339-345, 1996.

Wright EC, Vichinsky EP, Styles LA, et al, and the Cooperative Study of Sickle Cell Disease: Acute chest syndrome in sickle cell disease: clinical presentation and course, *Blood* 89(5):1787-1792, 1997.

Zavaras-Angelidou KA, Weinhouse E, Nelson DB: Review of 180 episodes of chest pain in 134 children, *Pediatr Emerg Care* 8(4):189-193, 1992.

CHAPTER 9

Cyanosis

ANNE M. STACK

Cyanosis is a bluish-purple discoloration of the tissues, most easily appreciated on the lips, nail beds, earlobes, mucous membranes, and locations where the skin is thin. It may be made more or less apparent by lighting conditions and skin pigmentation. Cyanosis in an acutely ill patient may indicate respiratory failure, shock, and/or cardiopulmonary failure; however, in other individuals it may represent a chronic illness of little immediate concern.

There are three factors that ultimately determine the occurrence of cyanosis: the total amount of hemoglobin (Hb) in the blood (anemia), the degree of Hb oxygen saturation/qualitative changes in the Hb molecule (lung disease, toxins), and the state of the circulation (shunt). Cyanosis is evident when the reduced or deoxygenated Hb level in the blood exceeds 5 g/100 ml or when oxygen saturation approaches 85%.

The state of the circulation plays an important role in the presence and degree of cyanosis via several mechanisms. First, if a left-right shunt is present, cyanosis can present. A shunt is defined as a mechanism by which blood that has not traveled through the ventilated alveolar capillary bed mixes with arterial blood. Factors that slow blood flow, such as poor perfusion states and cold temperature, favor the unloading of oxygen and thus increase the amount of unsaturated Hb in the tissue capillaries, also contributing to cyanosis. A third contribution from the circulation concerns ventilation/perfusion mismatch within the lung. In healthy subjects this depression is only a few millimeters of mercury; however, in patients with diseased lungs, the contribution of ventilation/perfusion inequality to lowering of blood Po_2 can be significant.

The most common causes of cyanosis are cardiac and respiratory diseases, but many other conditions can also cause a patient to appear blue.

Only the following etiologies of cyanosis are discussed in this chapter because many etiologies are covered elsewhere (see Chapter 20, Hypotension/Shock; Chapter 28, Pallor; Chapter 30, Respiratory Distress; and Chapter 34, Tachycardia).

Vascular	
Cardiac	Congenital heart disease, congestive heart failure (CHF), cardiogenic shock
Pulmonary	Edema, hypertension, embolism, hemorrhage
Peripheral	Cold exposure, acrocyanosis
Neurologic	Hypoventilation, central nervous system (CNS) depression or malfunction
Hematologic	Methemoglobinemia, polycythemia
Dermatologic	Blue dye, pigmentary lesions, amiodarone

 ## RESPIRATORY ETIOLOGIES

A cyanotic or "blue" patient with signs and symptoms of respiratory distress demands immediate attention to the ABCs of resuscitation (see Chapter 30, Respiratory Distress).

 ## VASCULAR ETIOLOGIES

CYANOTIC CONGENITAL HEART DISEASE

One of the most common causes of cyanosis in children is congenital heart disease. The most common of these conditions include tetralogy of Fallot, transposition of the great vessels, truncus arteriosus, and pulmonary atresia. In each of these conditions cyanosis is caused by an intracardiac *shunt*. Although most newborns with cyanotic congenital heart disease are diagnosed while still in the newborn nursery, sometimes such newborns will initially present to the pediatrician or emergency department (ED) in the first few days or weeks of life. One condition particularly prone to such late presentation is tetralogy of Fallot, specifically in those infants who have patent ductus arteriosus–dependent pulmonary blood flow. As the ductus closes, profound cyanosis ensues. Rarely, an infant with mild tetralogy of Fallot (or "pink tet") may come to the ED with intermittent cyanosis during a "tet spell," which is a 15- to 30-minute self-limited episode of cyanosis caused by increased right-to-left shunting and decreased pulmonary blood flow.

Symptoms
- Poor feeding +++
- Lethargy ++
- Poor weight gain +++
- Diaphoresis ++

Signs
- Cyanosis
- ± Murmur
- ± Respiratory distress

Workup
- Echocardiography.
- ECG, which may show abnormal axis and forces for age.
- CXR, which may show increased heart size, right-sided aortic arch, or abnormal pulmonary blood flow based on etiology. The classic CXR findings of tetralogy of Fallot with pulmonary stenosis include a "boot-shaped" heart (Fig. 9-1) and the CXR finding of transposition of the great arteries is an "egg-on-a-string" heart (Fig. 9-2).
- Four-extremity blood pressures may show a decrease of 20 mm Hg in lower extremities relative to upper extremities in a patient with coarctation of the aorta.
- ABG, which may show diminished PaO_2 and/or metabolic acidosis.
- Cardiac monitor and continuous pulse oximetry.

Comments and Treatment Considerations
Cardiology consultation and echocardiography are necessary for definitive diagnosis. Consider alprostadil (also called *prostaglandin E_1* [PGE_1]) 0.05 to 0.1 mcg/kg/min continuous

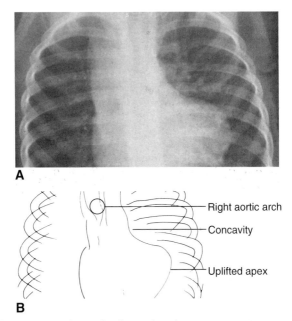

A

B

Right aortic arch

Concavity

Uplifted apex

Fig. 9-1 Tetralogy of Fallot with pulmonary stenosis produces this "boot-shaped" heart. Because of right ventricular hypertrophy, the apex is tilted upward and the small right ventricular infundibulum and small main pulmonary artery cause the concavity in the left upper border of the heart. Right aortic arch is present. (From Zitelli B, Davis H: *Atlas of pediatric physical diagnosis*, 4th ed, St. Louis, 2002, Mosby.)

infusion to keep the ductus arteriosus open. The usual dose ranges from 0.01 to 0.4 mcg/kg/min. Use the lowest effective rate to minimize side effects of bradycardia and hypotension. Alprostadil (PGE₁) is contraindicated in patients with total anomalous venous return. Prepare for possible intubation before initiating infusion secondary to PGE-induced respiratory distress and apnea. Other supportive measures consist of oxygen, IV fluid, keeping the patient NPO, and possible dopamine infusion.

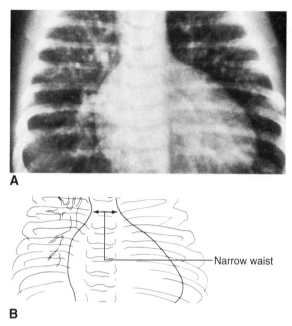

Fig. 9-2 "Egg-on-a-string" heart shadow resulting from trans-position of the great arteries. The main pulmonary artery is posterior and slightly to the left of the aorta, contributing to the narrow waist (the "string"). (From Zitelli B, Davis H: *Atlas of pediatric physical diagnosis,* 4th ed, St. Louis, 2002, Mosby.)

CONGESTIVE HEART FAILURE
CHF is caused by dysfunction of either or both right and left car-diac ventricles and may cause cyanosis (see Chapter 11, Edema).

CARDIOGENIC SHOCK
Cardiogenic shock is an uncommon cause of shock in the gen-eral pediatric population. It occurs when myocardial contractil-ity is so impaired the heart is incapable of delivering adequate cardiac output. More common causes of hypoperfusion such as sepsis should be considered before a diagnosis of cardiogenic shock is made.

Common Causes of Cardiogenic Shock
Direct Myocardial Damage
- Viral myocarditis
- Arrhythmia
- Drug ingestions
- Postoperative complications
- Metabolic derangements
- Congenital heart disease

Mechanical Obstruction to Cardiac Output
- Tamponade
- Tension pneumothorax

Cardiogenic shock can be distinguished from other forms of shock by associated signs of CHF, including: rales, gallop rhythm, hepatomegaly, and jugular venous congestion. Initial therapy in the ED is directed toward the ABCs of resuscitation and reversing or halting further tissue injury (see Chapter 20, Hypotension/Shock).

PULMONARY VASCULAR ABNORMALITIES
Several pulmonary vascular abnormalities can lead to cyanosis. These include pulmonary edema, primary pulmonary hypertension of the newborn (PPHN), pulmonary hypertension, pulmonary embolism (PE), and pulmonary hemorrhage. In pulmonary hypertension, high pulmonary pressures cause blood to be shunted away from the lungs, resulting in hypoxia. PE and pulmonary hemorrhage, though rare in children, also impair lung perfusion and must be considered (see Chapter 8, Chest Pain and Chapter 30, Respiratory Distress).

PERIPHERAL CAUSES OF CYANOSIS
Low perfusion states may lead to local cyanosis, particularly of the hands, face, and lips.

Cold Exposure
Moderate cold exposure slows transit time for RBCs across capillary beds, leading to greater unloading of oxygen to the tissues and local blueness.

Acrocyanosis

Blueness of the hands and feet with preserved pinkness in the mucous membranes and elsewhere, defined as *acrocyanosis*, is seen commonly in newborns and is related to variable perfusion in the extremities. It is seen in well-appearing babies and resolves within the first few days of life but may reappear when the infant is cold, such as after a bath.

 ## NEUROLOGIC ETIOLOGIES

Neurologic conditions can lead to Hb desaturation and cyanosis. Patients either hypoventilate because of CNS depression or inhibition of normal respiration from other neurologic causes. These may include CNS lesions, neuromuscular disease, toxins, seizure, or breath-holding spells (see Chapter 4, Apnea; Chapter 30, Respiratory Distress; Chapter 32, Seizures; and Chapter 35, Toxic Ingestion, Approach To).

 ## HEMATOLOGIC ETIOLOGIES

METHEMOGLOBINEMIA

When heme iron is oxidized to the ferric state from its normal ferrous state, it is called *methemoglobin* and it is incapable of binding O_2. Therefore, hemoglobin will remain deoxygenated. Methemoglobin itself is a brownish-purple color. Methemoglobinemia may be a congenital or acquired condition. Congenital methemoglobinemia is caused by either Hb variants designated M hemoglobins or deficiency of NADH-dependent Hb reductase. The acquired form is more common and occurs when RBCs are exposed to oxidant chemicals (nitrates, nitrites, aniline dyes, and naphthalene) or drugs (dapsone, phenazopyridine, and benzocaine, among others). Young infants with gastroenteritis, oxidant toxin exposure, or exposure to certain drugs are particularly susceptible to the development of methemoglobinemia as a result of immature enzyme systems required to reduce Hb.

Symptoms

Symptoms are caused by decreased blood oxygen content and cellular hypoxia and depend on the concentration of methemoglobin.

At 10% to 30% of total hemoglobin:
- Only cyanosis occurs

At 30% to 50% of total hemoglobin:
- Headache
- Dizziness
- Nausea
- Fatigue
- Dyspnea

At >50% total hemoglobin:
- Confusion
- Seizure
- Stupor
- Coma

Signs

- Tachycardia +++
- "Slate gray" cyanosis

Workup

The diagnosis should be strongly considered when oxygen fails to ameliorate the cyanosis.

- A rapid screening test is to place a drop of blood on filter paper, wave in the air for 30 to 60 seconds—normal blood appears red, methemoglobinemia blood appears reddish-brown.
- Pulse oximetry may be normal despite cyanosis.
- ABG analysis shows a normal Pao_2.
- Methemoglobin level.

Comments and Treatment Considerations

Treatment depends on the severity of the methemoglobinemia. One should determine the oxidant stress and remove the causative agent. If symptoms are mild, no treatment is necessary. If symptoms are severe, methylene blue should be given, dosed at 1 to 2 mg/kg/dose undiluted via direct IV administration over 5 minutes. The dose may be repeated if symptoms are still present 1 hour later. Total dose should not exceed 4 mg/kg in an infant and 7 mg/kg in an older child. Of note, methylene blue will not be effective in a patient with G6PD deficiency. Admit to hospital for further management.

POLYCYTHEMIA

Polycythemia occurs when the total amount of Hb in the blood is increased in relation to blood volume. Hb values >2 standard deviations above normal should be considered polycythemia. There is substantial contribution to the overall appearance of the patient from the increased RBC mass and the patient may appear ruddy. The relative increase in the amount of unsaturated Hb in the polycythemic patient will add a blue hue to the skin. The etiology of the polycythemia is irrelevant to its initial management but includes delayed clamping of the umbilical cord or twin-to-twin transfusion in a newborn, primary or secondary causes of increased RBCs, high-altitude living, chronic hypoxia, or an Hb abnormality. Signs and symptoms are related to the underlying cause of the increase in RBC mass.

Symptoms
- Patients may be asymptomatic
- Headache ++
- Weakness ++
- Dizziness ++

Signs
- Generally ruddy appearance to skin
- Periphery and lips may appear bluish
- May have liver or spleen enlargement

Workup
- CBC to assess Hb and hematocrit.
- Consider ABG.
- Search for the underlying cause.

Comments and Treatment Considerations
Treatment is directed at elimination or correction of the primary or underlying cause. Treatment consists of phlebotomy to keep

the hematocrit <60% if it is not possible to eliminate the underlying condition.

 # DERMATOLOGIC ETIOLOGIES

BLUE DYE
A benign yet sometimes perplexing presentation of localized blue discoloration may be related to blue dye of clothing. A careful history and swipe with an alcohol wipe will usually reveal the cause of the apparent cyanosis.

PIGMENTARY LESIONS
Large pigmentary lesions can be confused with cyanosis, especially when uncharacteristically large or in unusual locations.

AMIODARONE
Chronic treatment with the antiarrhythmic medication amiodarone can produce a characteristic slate blue color of the skin. The discoloration may occur secondary to amiodarone accumulation in the lysosomes. Usually the reaction is cosmetic and may not completely resolve despite discontinuation of the drug.

REFERENCES
Elias SS, Patel NM, Cheigh NH: Drug-induced skin disorders. In DiPiro JT, et al, editors: *Pharmacotherapy: a pathophysiologic approach*, 5th ed, New York, 2002, McGraw-Hill.

Grant JB, Saltzman AR: Respiratory functions of the lung. In Baum GL, Wolinsky, editors: *Textbook of pulmonary diseases*, 5th ed, Boston, 1994, Little Brown and Company.

Stack A: Cyanosis. In Fleisher GR, Ludwig S, editors: *Textbook of pediatric emergency medicine*, 4th ed, Philadelphia, 2000, Lippincott Williams & Wilkins.

West JB: Pulmonary gas exchange. In West JB, editor: *Physiologic basis of medical practice*, 12th ed, Baltimore, 1990, Williams & Wilkins.

CHAPTER 10

Diarrhea

LAURA A. DRUBACH

Most episodes of diarrhea in children are acute, self-limited, and transient. However, there are severe and life-threatening syndromes in which diarrhea is the initial presenting symptom. Acute diarrhea in younger children and infants tends to have a higher morbidity. These patients have smaller fluid reserves and can quickly become significantly dehydrated. The most common causes of diarrhea in the pediatric population are infectious (viral and bacterial) and diarrhea secondary to antibiotic treatment (especially amoxicillin-clavulanate). Causes of chronic diarrhea are not covered. See Chapter 16, Gastrointestinal Bleeding, for a discussion of bloody diarrhea.

HEMOLYTIC UREMIC SYNDROME

Hemolytic uremic syndrome (HUS) is a clinical syndrome characterized by acute renal failure, microangiopathic hemolytic anemia, and thrombocytopenia. The pathogenesis of HUS is due to endothelial cell damage, which gives rise to microthrombi resulting in a consumptive thrombocytopenia and red blood cell fragmentation. HUS is the most common cause of acute renal failure in children, with two distinct presentations: associated with diarrhea and not associated with diarrhea.

The diarrhea-associated form has a peak seasonal incidence in summer and fall and both sexes are equally affected. The most common causative infectious agents are *Escherichia coli* serotype O157:H7 (with the production of verotoxins or Shiga-like toxins) and *Shigella*. Diarrhea-associated forms usually have a favorable prognosis.

The non–diarrhea-associated form has a worse prognosis. It has a genetic predisposition, does not have a seasonal variation, and is not associated with verotoxins or Shiga-like toxins. This form has been linked to *Streptococcus pneumoniae* infections.

Symptoms
- A history of diarrhea, which may be bloody, 2 to 7 days before the onset of renal failure is present ++++
- Abdominal cramps ++
- Weakness +++
- Lethargy ++
- Seizures, irritability, lethargy ++
- Fever is rare

Signs
- Pallor ++++
- Reduced urine output ++++
- Hypertension +++
- Edema ++
- Easy bruising ++
- Petechiae ++

Workup
- CBC shows microangiopathic hemolytic anemia and thrombocytopenia.
- Blood smear with schistocytes, burr cells, and helmet cells.
- UA can show hematuria, proteinuria, and presence of hyaline casts.
- Liver function test results may show elevated bilirubin and lactate dehydrogenase (LDH) levels.
- Electrolytes show markedly elevated BUN and creatinine.
- PT, PTT, D-dimer, and fibrinogen levels are within the normal range.
- Stool analysis for the presence of the antigen for *E. coli* O157:H7.
- Stool culture.

Comments and Treatment Considerations
The diagnosis is based on signs of acute renal failure associated with thrombocytopenia and anemia. Approximately 85% of

children with the diarrheal form recover completely with supportive therapy.

Treatment is primarily supportive, with attention to the control of hypertension, fluid and electrolyte imbalances, azotemia, and other complications. Antibiotics and antidiarrheal agents are contraindicated in children with *E. coli* O157:H7 infection because they may actually increase the risk of HUS; however, *Shigella* infections should be treated with antibiotics to shorten the duration of diarrhea and eradicate organisms from feces. Peritoneal dialysis or hemodialysis is necessary in selected cases. Plasmapheresis has been used for the nondiarrheal form of HUS. A pediatric nephrologist should be consulted in any case exhibiting renal failure.

HIRSCHSPRUNG'S DISEASE

Hirschsprung's disease is a congenital aganglionosis of the distal bowel. The pathogenesis of this condition is a lack of normal motility in the aganglionic portion of the bowel, with subsequent dilation of the more proximal bowel. The areas most commonly involved are the rectosigmoid (80%), entire colon (10%), and small bowel (10%). It is more common in males (4:1).

Hirschsprung's disease–associated enterocolitis is a very severe complication of Hirschsprung's disease that presents with explosive diarrhea. It is caused by ulcerations in the intestinal mucosa proximal to the aganglionic portion. Mild cases may be confused with gastroenteritis.

Hirschsprung's disease may be associated with other entities such as Down syndrome, Laurence-Moon-Bardet-Biedl syndrome, Waardenburg's syndrome, ventricular septal defect, Meckel's diverticulum, and cryptorchidism.

Symptoms
- In the neonate, Hirschsprung's disease can present as symptoms of complete obstruction with bilious emesis, abdominal distention, and failure to pass meconium
- Chronic constipation is the usual presentation in the older child

- Alternating episodes of diarrhea and constipation
- Explosive and/or bloody stools
- Failure to thrive

Signs

- Palpable abdominal feces with no palpable stool in the vault on rectal examination with a constricted anus
- Abdominal distention
- Older children may be pale and malnourished, with hypoproteinemia and edema resulting from a protein-losing enteropathy (less common)
- Encopresis is very rare in Hirschsprung's disease in contrast with functional constipation, in which encopresis is common
- Enterocolitis can occur with colonic distention and severe dehydration, abdominal pain, fever, sepsis, intestinal necrosis, and perforation

Workup

- CBC in cases of suspected enterocolitis may show leukocytosis.
- Radiography of the abdomen shows dilated loops of bowel with lack of air in the rectal ampulla on the erect view.
- Barium enema shows narrow bowel that expands into a dilated segment.
- Anal manometry shows abnormal lack of sphincter relaxation after distention of a balloon placed in the rectal ampulla.
- Definitive diagnosis is made by rectal biopsy, showing absence of ganglion cells in the submucosa.

Comments and Treatment Considerations

In cases of obstruction, initial treatment should include hydration and gastric decompression with an NG tube. In cases of enterocolitis, antibiotics may be necessary and should include anaerobic and gram-negative coverage. The definitive treatment of Hirschsprung's disease is surgical.

PSEUDOMEMBRANOUS COLITIS

Pseudomembranous colitis develops as a result of overgrowth of *Clostridium difficile* and the production of at least two toxins (A and B) that are cytotoxic. *C. difficile* is normally present in the bowel of 2% to 3% of healthy adults and 20% to 40% of healthy children. Overgrowth of this pathogen occurs as a result of disruption of the normal intestinal flora after antibiotic therapy. Symptoms can develop from the first day of antibiotic treatment up to 3 weeks after treatment (average 5 days) and range from mild to copious bloody diarrhea, resulting in dehydration.

Antibiotics commonly associated with pseudomembranous colitis include ampicillin, amoxicillin, clindamycin, and cephalosporins; however, all antibiotics have the potential for causing this disease. Infection from external sources can occur and outbreaks with cross-infection have been reported.

Symptoms

There are a wide variety of symptoms, ranging from only mild nonbloody diarrhea to hemorrhagic colitis, tenesmus, and severe abdominal pain. Diarrhea is always present.

Signs

- Various degrees of dehydration are often present
- Fever
- Examination varies according to severity of disease, from normal abdominal examination findings to signs of peritonitis, sepsis, and shock

Workup

- The diagnosis is usually made with enzyme immunoassay of the stool. This test is rapid, inexpensive, and highly specific. Sensitivity ranges from 78% to 85% for one sample and increases as multiple samples are analyzed.
- The most sensitive and specific test is a tissue culture assay for the cytotoxicity of toxin B (+++++). This test is seldom used because it takes up to 3 days to complete.

- Leukocytosis.
- Electrolytes in severe cases may show abnormalities resulting from dehydration.
- Abdominal x-ray study results may show ileus and dilated colon. Thickened and edematous colonic mucosa will appear as "thumbprinting" on x-ray of the abdomen.
- Colonoscopy shows characteristic yellow plaques over the colonic mucosa. This procedure is not necessary for the diagnosis and is reserved for special situations.

Comments and Treatment Considerations

Treatment consists of correction of dehydration and electrolyte abnormalities. Discontinuation of the causative antibiotic is essential. The use of antimicrobials should be reserved for patients who do not improve 48 hours after discontinuation of antibiotic or who are exhibiting significant symptomatology. First-line therapy includes metronidazole dosed at 30 mg/kg/day (max 2 g/day) PO or IV divided q6h for 7 to 10 days. Patients requiring IV metronidazole therapy should be admitted to the hospital. If metronidazole is not effective, then vancomycin dosed at 40 mg/kg/day (max 2 g/day) PO divided q6h for 7 to 10 days may be substituted. Vancomycin is effective only against *C. difficile* when given orally and is not recommended as first-line therapy in the hope to minimize the development of vancomycin-resistant organisms. Toxic megacolon is a complication of pseudomembranous colitis. It can result in bowel perforation and sepsis.

Barium enema is contraindicated in pseudomembranous colitis secondary to the risk of perforation. Drugs that decrease intestinal motility such as antidiarrheal agents should not be given.

 INTUSSUSCEPTION

Intussusception is the most common cause of bowel obstruction in infants. A prodromal diarrheal illness is common, followed by the onset of colicky abdominal pain, vomiting, and apparent lethargy between episodes of irritability (see Chapter 1, Abdominal Pain).

INFLAMMATORY BOWEL DISEASE

Common presenting symptoms of inflammatory bowel disease include abdominal pain, diarrhea with or without blood, fever, joint pain, anemia, hypoproteinemia, and weight loss. Toxic megacolon is a life-threatening complication of inflammatory bowel disease (see Chapter 16, Gastrointestinal Bleeding).

GASTROENTERITIS

Gastroenteritis is one of the most common causes of diarrhea in the pediatric age-group. Associated symptoms include nausea, vomiting, fever, and abdominal pain (see Chapter 38, Vomiting).

REFERENCES

Bartlett J: *Clostridium difficile* infection: pathophysiology and diagnosis, *Semin Gastrointest Dis* 8:12-21, 1997.

Coran AG, Teitelbaum DH: Recent advances in the management of Hirschsprung's disease, *Am J Surg* 180(5):382-387, 2000.

Fekety R: Guidelines for the diagnosis and management of *Clostridium difficile*–associated diarrhea and colitis, *Am J Gastroenterol* 92:739-750, 1997.

Mylonakis E, Ryan ET, Calderwood SB: *Clostridium difficile*–associated diarrhea: a review, *Arch Intern Med* 161(4):525-533, 2001.

Reding R, de Ville de Goyet J, Gosseye S : Hirschsprung's disease: a 20-year experience, *J Pediatr Surg* 32(8):1221-1225, 1997.

Remuzzi G, Ruggenenti P: The hemolytic uremic syndrome, *Kidney Int* 66:554-557, 1998.

Rondeau R, Peraldi MN: *Escherichia coli* and the hemolytic uremic syndrome, *N Engl J Med* 335:660-662, 1996.

Ryan ET, Ecker JL, Christakis NA, et al: Hirschsprung's disease: associated abnormalities and demography, *J Pediatr Surg* 27(1):76-81, 1992.

Siegler RL: Management of hemolytic-uremic syndrome, *J Pediatr* 112(6):1014-1020, 1988.

Wong CS, Jelacic S, Habeeb RL: The risk of the hemolytic-uremic syndrome after antibiotic treatment of *Escherichia coli* O157:H7 infections, *N Engl J Med* 342(26), 2000.

CHAPTER 11

Edema

SUJIT SHARMA

Edema is a common complaint in the emergency department. Symptoms and signs may be localized to a specific anatomic area or may be generalized. Although the specific etiologies of edema are numerous, one of the following pathophysiologic mechanisms is always involved: increased venous or lymphatic hydrostatic pressure, decreased intravascular oncotic pressure, or increased vascular permeability. Localized edema is almost always infectious or inflammatory/allergic in nature. This chapter focuses on life-threatening conditions associated with generalized edema.

 ## *HEREDITARY ANGIONEUROTIC EDEMA*

Hereditary angioneurotic edema (HAE) is an autosomal dominant disorder in which a mutation occurs in the gene that produces C1 inhibitor. This results in inadequate production of C1 inhibitor (85% of cases) or a functional abnormality in the protein. Edema in this disease is due to increased vascular permeability. Affected individuals usually become symptomatic in the second decade of life. The most common trigger is mechanical trauma (even minor trauma).

Symptoms
- Generalized or localized swelling
- Difficulty breathing or "throat feels like it is closing up"
- Nausea, vomiting, severe abdominal pain

Signs
- Generalized or localized subcutaneous or submucosal edema; edema is usually nonpitting and nonpruritic (Fig. 11-1)
- Respiratory distress
- Stridor
- Abdominal tenderness mimicking acute surgical abdomen

Workup
- Serum studies of C1 inhibitor levels and function.

Comments and Treatment Considerations
HAE is a rare disease with similar presentation to allergic reactions, although swellings are usually painful rather than pruritic and skin lesions are typically lacking. It is inherited in an autosomal dominant pattern so the family history is usually positive. Because allergic reactions are much more common, treatment is generally directed to this as a presumptive cause in patients without previous episodes or known positive family history (see Chapter 5, Bites, and Chapter 29, Rashes). One

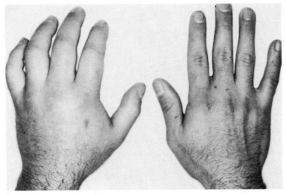

Fig. 11-1 Angioedema of the left hand in a patient with hereditary angioedema. (From Middleton E: *Allergy: principles and practice,* 5th ed, St. Louis, 1998, Mosby.)

should have a high index of suspicion for HAE in cases of supposed allergic reactions that are unresponsive to antihistamines, corticosteroids, and epinephrine.

Acute laryngeal edema is a life-threatening emergency that can occur in these patients. Investigational C1 inhibitor concentrate dosed at 25 units/kg intravenously may help alleviate this edema within 30 to 90 minutes. If C1 inhibitor is not readily available, surgical airway management may be necessary. For long-term therapy, danazol and tranexamic acid may provide treatment options.

 ## NEPHROTIC SYNDROME

Nephrotic syndrome is defined as edema associated with heavy proteinuria (>40 mg/m^2/hr in a 24-hour urine), hypoproteinemia (serum albumin <3 g/dl), and hyperlipidemia. Generalized edema in this condition is therefore a result of decreased oncotic pressure. Primary glomerular dysfunction is the most common cause of nephrotic syndrome, usually manifesting as minimal change disease or "nil disease" (76%), followed by various forms of glomerulosclerosis and glomerulonephritis. Nephrotic syndrome can also be a secondary result of other systemic diseases.

Symptoms
- Generalized or localized edema +++++
- Oliguria
- GI complaints: nausea, vomiting, abdominal pain (secondary to edema of the mucosal lining of the GI tract or peritonitis)
- Respiratory distress (secondary to a combination of hydrothorax and diaphragm elevation from ascites)
- Age younger than 6 years ++++
- History of atopy +++

Signs
- Periorbital/facial edema early in the disease (Fig. 11-2)
- Generalized/dependent pitting edema later in the disease +++++ (Fig. 11-3)

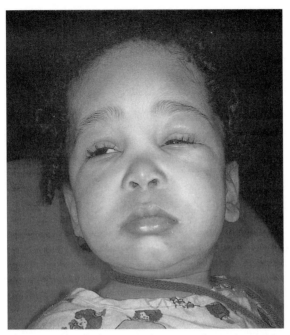

Fig. 11-2 Minimal change nephrotic syndrome in an 18-month-old child with periorbital and facial edema (picture taken right after he awoke in the morning). (From Shah B, Laude T: *Atlas of pediatric clinical diagnosis,* Philadelphia, 2000, WB Saunders.)

- Tachycardia and hypotension in cases of severe intravascular volume depletion
- Hypertension in cases in which significant glomerulonephritis is the cause of the nephrotic syndrome ++
- Abdominal distention, dullness to percussion, and fluid wave when ascites present
- Tachypnea, diminished breath sounds, and dullness to percussion when pleural effusion present
- Abdominal tenderness

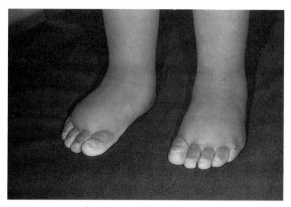

Fig. 11-3 Minimal change nephrotic syndrome in an 18-month-old child with edema of the feet. (From Shah B, Laude T: *Atlas of pediatric clinical diagnosis,* St. Louis, 2000, WB Saunders.)

Workup

- Serum albumin and total protein levels will be low.
- Serum cholesterol level will be elevated.
- UA with large protein. If present, 24-hour collection for quantification.
- Urine microscopy for RBCs ++ and casts (if nephritis present). Casts may be missed if there is a delay in microscopy.
- Serum electrolytes, BUN, calcium, and uric acid (ensure no evidence of renal failure).
- CBC may show hemoconcentration.
- Other serum studies: immunoglobulins, C3 complement, antinuclear antibody, DNA binding.
- Also consider sickle cell screening, hepatitis B surface antigen, HIV screening.

Comments and Treatment Considerations

Diagnosis of nephrotic syndrome can be made fairly rapidly on the basis of clinical and laboratory findings. The most pressing concern for a patient presenting de novo is intravascular volume status. For a patient who is severely depleted or in shock, small boluses of normal saline are warranted but need to be given very carefully. For the hemodynamically stable patient, low-sodium fluids can be attempted orally. The decision to administer diuretics or albumin for the child who is symptomatic from significant hypoproteinemia and edema is best made in consultation with a nephrologist.

Approximately 90% of patients with minimal change disease respond to corticosteroid therapy, although most will have a chronic relapsing course (60% to 80%). Initial therapy often consists of prednisone dosed at 2 mg/kg/day (max 80 mg/day) PO divided daily qd-tid until the urine is clear of protein for 4 to 6 weeks. Maintenance dosing follows with prednisone at 2 mg/kg/dose (max 80 mg/dose) PO daily and is gradually tapered over 4 to 6 weeks. Six-week courses tend to produce longer remission than 4-week regimens but will likely result in a higher incidence of side effects. Approximately 80% of these patients will eventually recover. Those who do not respond to steroids or have unusual courses will require renal biopsy. A small subset of patients will develop chronic renal failure. Infection and hypercoagulability occur more frequently in patients with nephrotic syndrome who are receiving steroid therapy.

 ## CONGESTIVE HEART FAILURE

Congestive heart failure (CHF) is a syndrome in which cardiac output cannot keep up with metabolic demands. Congenital or acquired conditions that lead to CHF include disorders of the heart (e.g., septal defects and aortic stenosis), disorders of the pericardium (e.g., pericarditis), or extracardiac disorders (e.g., severe anemia and hypertension). Regardless of the etiology of CHF, one or more of the following physiologic determinants of cardiac output are affected: preload, afterload, contractility, or heart rate. Edema in CHF is due to increased venous hydrostatic pressure. However, peripheral edema is uncommon in young infants because of increased venous capacitance.

Symptoms
- Respiratory distress
- Growth failure
- Fatigue
- Dyspnea on exertion
- Feeding difficulty

Signs
- Tachypnea, wheezing, rales, or rhonchi
- Tachycardia
- Cardiac ausculatory abnormalities include murmurs, S_3 or S_4
- Pulsus alternans
- Hepatomegaly
- Jugular venous distention
- Cool, moist extremities
- Generalized pallor

Workup
- CXR to evaluate for increased heart size.
- ECG to assess ventricular changes, such as ventricular enlargement indicated by increased R wave in left precordial leads, as well as to exclude arrhythmia.
- Electrolytes, CBC (expect to find dilutional hyponatremia, hypochloremia, and lowered hematocrit).
- Blood gas analysis (assess degree of metabolic acidosis if present).
- Echocardiography to assess structure, function, and presence of pericardial fluid accumulation.
- Creatine phosphokinase may be elevated if perfusion abnormalities or myocarditis is suspected.

Comments and Treatment Considerations
Supportive care for CHF includes elevation of the head and chest while providing supplemental oxygen and establishing IV access. More specific therapy aimed at correcting cardiac output depends on the etiology. Therapies may include reduction of preload with diuretics, improvement contractility with inotropes, and reduction of afterload with angiotensin-converting enzyme inhibitors. Rhythm abnormalities, such as supraventricular

tachycardia, should be treated immediately (see Chapter 34, Tachycardia). Consider cardiac consultation.

 PROTEIN MALNUTRITION

Though usually a disease found in underdeveloped nations, protein malnutrition (known as *kwashiorkor* in its advanced stages) does occur even in industrialized nations. When it does occur in countries such as the United States, it is most likely due to nutritional ignorance on the part of the caregiver or neglect. Overall appearance of the child may be misleading secondary to the development of edema.

Symptoms
- Lethargy, apathy, or irritability (earlier in the disease)
- Generalized edema
- Inadequate growth
- Recurrent infections
- Hair loss
- Anorexia
- Vomiting and persistent diarrhea

Signs
- Generalized pitting edema, which led to the term "sugar baby"
- Apathy
- Loss of muscle tone
- Flabbiness of subcutaneous tissue
- Hepatomegaly
- Dermatitis or dyspigmentation
- Hair is thin and sparse with loss of elasticity, may show bands of hypopigmentation

Workup
- Serum albumin and total protein levels should be decreased.
- Serum glucose and electrolytes (including calcium, magnesium, and phosphorus), which will commonly show abnormalities in glucose, potassium, and magnesium.

- BUN and SCr (look for evidence of renal failure).
- CBC (normocytic anemia).
- UA (ketonuria present early in disease but then disappears).

Comments and Treatment Considerations

In the acute setting the most life-threatening complications of severe protein malnutrition are dehydration, renal failure, or infection. Once these issues have been addressed, enteral feedings should be introduced gradually. Extreme caution should be taken to avoid refeeding syndrome. A nutrition service consultation is warranted to assist with appropriate electrolyte supplementation (especially phosphorous). In addition, a social service consultation is recommended for evaluation of possible neglect in cases in which poverty is not the clear cause.

REFERENCES

Barnes LA, Curran JS: Nutrition. In Nelson WE, Behrman RE, Kliegman RM, Arvin AM, editors: *Nelson textbook of pediatrics*, 15th ed, Philadelphia, 1998, WB Saunders.

Carvalho NF, Kenney RD, Carrington PH, Hall DE: Severe nutritional deficiencies in toddlers resulting from health food milk alternatives, *Pediatrics* 107:e46, 2001.

Chase HP, Kumar V, Caldwell RT, O'Brein D: Kwashiorkor in the United States, *Pediatrics* 66:972-976, 1980.

Chesney RW: The idiopathic nephrotic syndrome, *Opin Pediatr* 11:158, 1998.

Cicardi M, Agostini A: Hereditary angioedema, *N Engl J Med* 334:1666-1667, 1996.

Cicardi M, Bergamaschini L, Marasini B, et al : Hereditary angioedema, an appraisal of 104 cases, *Am J Med Sci* 284:2-9, 1982.

Cronan K, Norman ME: Renal and electrolyte emergencies. In Fleisher GR, Ludwig S, editors: *Textbook of pediatric emergency medicine*, 4th ed, Philadelphia, 2000, Lippincott Williams & Wilkins.

Gewitz MH, Vetter VL: Cardiac emergencies. In Fleisher GR, Ludwig S, editors: *Textbook of pediatric emergency medicine*, 4th ed, Philadelphia, 2000, Lippincott Williams & Wilkins.

Hogg RJ, et al: Evaluation and management of proteinuria and nephrotic syndrome in children: recommendations from a pediatric nephrology panel established at the National Kidney Foundation Conference on Proteinuria, Albuminuria, Risk, Assessment, Detection, and Elimination (PARADE), *Pediatrics* 105(6):1242-1249, 2000.

Orth SR, Ritz E: The nephrotic syndrome, *N Engl J Med* 338(17):1202-1211, 1998.

Rudloph CD et al, editors: *Rudloph's pediatrics*, 21st ed, New York, 2003, McGraw-Hill.

Shaddy RE: Optimizing treatment for chronic congestive heart failure in children, *Crit Care Med* 29(10 suppl):S237-S240, 2001.

CHAPTER 12

Eye Pain and Redness

ATIMA C. DELANEY

Eye complaints must be thoroughly addressed to prevent the devastating consequence of permanent vision loss. Most cases will be uncomplicated bacterial or viral conjunctivitis or a minor corneal abrasion, but vision-threatening etiologies must be ruled out. A ruptured globe is the most emergent of the ocular injuries, but chemical burns, foreign bodies, infections, and corneal abrasions must be identified and properly managed. Newborn infants often present with conjunctivitis or excess tearing and are discussed at the end of this section.

It may be a challenge to adequately examine the eye of a child. If a chemical burn is suspected, immediate irrigation should begin (after testing for ocular pH level, if immediately available) even before completing the full examination. Visual acuity should at least be attempted in all verbal children with any complaint relating to the eye. Lid eversion should be performed to rule out foreign body, and slit-lamp and funduscopic examination should be performed as indicated. If sufficient concern exists and a child cannot cooperate with the examination, an ophthalmologist should be consulted and the child may need to be sedated.

RUPTURED GLOBE

Ruptured globe is caused by a laceration or a puncture of the cornea or sclera. This may occur after trauma by a projectile sharp implement or blunt trauma. In the older adolescent or young adult the chiseling and hammering of metal on metal is often associated with metal fragments that cause globe perforation. Because any pressure on the eyeball may cause extrusion of intraocular contents through the ruptured site, a ruptured globe must be recognized early and no pressure should be applied to the globe during examination. The ruptured globe may present with a surprisingly normal-appearing eye. Except in the most severe lacerations, the intraocular tissue will plug the wound so that intraocular pressure is preserved and the shape of the eyeball remains intact.

Symptoms
- Eye pain
- Decreased visual acuity
- Possible systemic symptoms including agitation and nausea/vomiting

Signs
- Iris or choroid plugs the wound (blue, brown, or black material on the surface of sclera) (Fig. 12-1)
- Teardrop pupil with narrowest segment pointing toward the ruptured site (see Fig. 12-1)
- Hyphema may be present (Fig. 12-2)
- May have remarkably normal appearance
- 360 degrees of subconjunctival hemorrhage or chemosis may obscure the underlying scleral rupture

Workup
- Immediate ophthalmology consultation is needed when the diagnosis is confirmed, strongly suspected, or when evaluation findings do not rule out the diagnosis.
- Orbital x-ray to rule out metallic foreign body, if suspected.
- MRI or CT scanning may be useful to help localize the ruptured site, detect intraocular foreign bodies, and evaluate for other potential injuries to surrounding bony structure. MRI scans should never be obtained if a metal foreign body is present or suspected.
- Fluorescein streaming on slit-lamp examination.

Comments and Treatment Considerations
A ruptured globe should be protected by a hard plastic or metal protective eye shield until evaluated by an ophthalmologist. If a

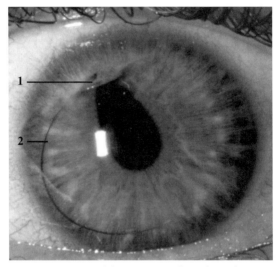

Fig. 12-1 Acute corneal laceration with prolapsed iris (*1*) and resultant peaked pupil. An eyelash (*2*) has entered the anterior chamber. (From Palay D, Krachmer J: *Ophthalmology for the primary care physician*, St. Louis, 1997, Mosby.)

ruptured globe is not seen clearly on examination but is suspected (based on high-risk history, severe lid swelling, or extreme resistance to examination), the patient should be given an eye shield and seen by an ophthalmologist immediately.

The eye shield should fit entirely over the bony orbit and completely encase the eye without putting pressure on the eyeball when taped to the face. Eye patches that may apply pressure to the globe are contraindicated to avoid any further extrusion of vitreous. When ophthalmic supplies are not available, a disposable Styrofoam coffee cup can be cut about 1 inch from its base and used for the same purpose.

Crying, vomiting, screaming, and the Valsalva maneuver should be avoided since they can result in extrusion of intraocular contents through the rupture. Mild sedation and an antiemetic may be indicated. A broad-spectrum antibiotic with gram-positive and gram-negative coverage should be given. Possible choices include cefoxitin 100 to 160 mg/kg/day (max

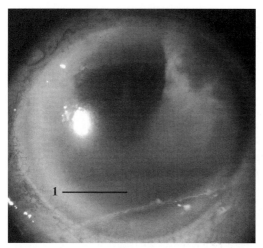

Fig. 12-2 Hyphemas layer with time, much like a hematocrit in a test tube. Here, a 30% hyphema (*1*) is noted. (From Palay D, Krachmer J: *Ophthalmology for the primary care physician*, St. Louis, 1997, Mosby.)

12 g/day) IV divided q6-8h or piperacillin-tazobactam 300 mg/kg/day piperacillin component (max 18 g of piperacillin per day) IV divided q6-8h. Tetanus status should be confirmed and appropriate treatment given based on immunization history (see Chapter 5, Bites, for tetanus prophylaxis).

 ## ANTERIOR UVEITIS, IRITIS, AND HYPOPYON

The hallmark of acute anterior uveitis, also called *iritis*, is the presence of inflammatory cells and proteinaceous flare in the anterior chamber of the eye. If the inflammation is severe, leukocytes in the anterior chamber settle and form a hypopyon, or white layer of cells usually visible on direct visualization. Anterior uveitis and iritis can be caused by a number of systemic and local processes including viral, fungal, or bacterial infection, juvenile rheumatoid arthritis, ulcerative colitis, ankylosing spondylitis, Reiter's syndrome, leukemia, lymphoma, and trauma. Approximately 5% to 10% of cases will present in children younger than 16 years. Children are at risk of delayed diagnosis and increased permanent sequelae.

Symptoms
- Photophobia +++++
- Unilateral gradual onset of eye pain
- Red eye without discharge
- Blurred vision (common)
- Excessive tearing
- Other symptoms of primary medical condition

Signs
- Perilimbal injection
- Consensual photophobia, pain in the involved eye when light is shined in the uninvolved eye ++++
- Miosis may be present
- Cornea may be normal

Workup
- Slit-lamp examination showing cells and flare (WBCs and RBCs in the anterior chamber) are the hallmark signs. In a hypopyon, the WBCs will layer in the bottom of the chamber.
- Posterior synechia (i.e., iris adherent to the lens) may be seen.
- Intraocular pressure may be low.
- Evaluation for possible primary disorder may include CBC, erythrocyte sedimentation rate (ESR), rapid plasma reagin, antinuclear antibody, human leukocyte antigen B27, fluorescent treponemal antibody absorption test, PPD, CXR, and Lyme titer.

Comments and Treatment Considerations
A hypopyon is an ophthalmologic emergency and requires emergent referral to an ophthalmologist for IV antibiotics and possibly intravitreous antibiotics. Anterior uveitis and iritis are ophthalmologic urgencies that once diagnosed need very close

follow-up with an ophthalmologist. The initial treatment, which should be started only after consultation, consists of topical cycloplegic agents and topical steroids (e.g., prednisolone [Pred-Forte] 1% q4-6h). This regimen relieves the photophobia and suppresses the inflammatory response. Many cases will resolve in 2 to 4 weeks. Long-term complications include permanent synechiae, glaucoma, and permanent visual loss.

 ## INFANTILE GLAUCOMA

Infantile glaucoma is characterized by an increased intraocular pressure, leading to corneal enlargement and edema, optic nerve damage, and visual impairment in early infancy and childhood. Glaucoma that occurs in the first 3 years of life is classified as *infantile glaucoma. Juvenile glaucoma* refers to isolated ocular disease occurring in the older child and is extremely rare. Secondary glaucoma is associated with traumatic ocular injuries, systemic disease, or various genetic syndromes. Recognition of the signs and symptoms of infantile glaucoma will allow physicians to refer infants and children to the ophthalmologists at a time when vision may be preserved. Checking the red reflex should be part of all newborn examinations and any haziness or abnormalities should prompt referral to an ophthalmologist.

Symptoms
- Epiphora (tearing)
- Photophobia (hallmark of disease)
- Blepharospasm (forced closing of the eyelid) secondary to photophobia

Signs
- Corneal haze
- Corneal/global enlargement
- Cupping of optic disc

Workup
- Any child with suspected glaucoma should be evaluated by an ophthalmologist.

Comments and Treatment Considerations

Primary infantile glaucoma is reported to be bilateral in 58% to 80% of cases. In one study, more than 90% of children with infantile glaucoma had initial presentation of corneal edema, corneal enlargement, or both. A significant number of children (21%) have infantile glaucoma without the classic symptoms of epiphora, photophobia, and blepharospasm. In most infants an examination under anesthesia is performed by an ophthalmologist, and if the diagnosis of infantile glaucoma is made, surgery is usually performed under the same anesthesia.

CHEMICAL BURNS

Chemical injury to the eye is a true ocular emergency. If a chemical burn is suspected, immediate irrigation should begin (after testing for ocular pH level if immediately available) even before completing the full examination (see below). Alkali injuries (pH > 7) tend to be much more severe, with rapid penetration to the cornea, causing damage to the entire anterior segment. Acid burns (pH < 7) tend to be limited to the ocular surface.

Most chemical injuries in children are caused by organic solvents found in household cleaning agents. The factors that determine the degree of ocular damage are the pH level of the offending substance, the quantity of the substance, and the length of time of contact between the eye and the substance.

Symptoms
- Pain
- Photophobia
- History of exposure to a chemical irritant

Signs
- Mild acid or alkali burns
  - Conjunctival injections
  - Conjunctival swelling (chemosis)
  - Mild corneal epithelial erosions

- Severe alkali burns
  - Corneal opacification
- Severe acid burns
  - Corneal and conjunctival opacification
  - Corneal epithelium may slough, leaving a relatively clear stroma

Workup

- Ocular surface pH level before and after ocular irrigation (normal pH = 6.5 to 7.5).
- Eyelids should be everted to examine for solid irritants.
- Fluorescein examination to check for corneal disruption.

Comments and Treatment Considerations

If the patient is outside the office or the hospital, irrigation of the affected eye should begin immediately with any available source of water and continue for at least half an hour. In the hospital or clinic setting an initial ocular pH level should be measured and then irrigation should begin with isotonic normal saline. The irrigation should continue for approximately 20 minutes or until the involved eye has received 2 L of fluid. A second ocular surface pH level should then obtained and irrigation continued until the pH level is within the normal reference range. Alkali burns may require many liters of irrigation. Ophthalmology consultation is indicated in significant chemical injury. Treatment initiated by an ophthalmologist often includes topical steroids, ascorbate, citrate, antibiotics, and/or cycloplegic agents.

 HYPHEMA

Hyphema is a sign of ocular trauma and is defined by bleeding into the anterior chamber. It is most commonly the result of blunt trauma secondary to a ball, BB pellet, fist, or stick. The entire anterior chamber may be filled with blood or there may be small clots or microscopic RBC; therefore, careful inspection with slit-lamp examination (microhyphema) is necessary. Patients with hyphema must also be evaluated for the potential of a ruptured globe.

Symptoms
- Eye pain
- Young children may be somnolent

Signs
- Blood in anterior chamber (Fig. 12-2)
- One third of patients with hyphema have other injuries that need evaluation as directed by examination

Workup
- Consult ophthalmology.
- If history of trauma is not elicited in a child with hyphema, consider a bleeding disorder, abuse, or sickle cell disease/trait.

Comments and Treatment Considerations

Management of traumatic hyphema is variable and controversial. Hospital admission is often recommended and an ophthalmologist should be consulted. Bed rest with the head elevated 45 degrees should be prescribed. This position facilitates more rapid settling of the blood in the anterior chamber. An eye shield (not patch) should be applied.

Medications should be prescribed in consultation with ophthalmology and may include a cycloplegic agent such as homatropine or cyclopentolate, topical steroids, and/or antifibrinolytic agents. Cyclopentolate should be used only under supervision of an ophthalmologist, as it has been implicated in behavioral disturbances and psychotic reactions in pediatric patients. Homatropine is given as one drop of 2% solution and finger pressure is applied to the lacrimal sac for 1 to 2 minutes to decrease the risk of systemic absorption. Onset of cycloplegia with homatropine occurs within 30 to 90 minutes and persists for up to 48 hours. Salicylates and NSAIDs are avoided because they prolong bleeding time and may exacerbate bleeding.

Most uncomplicated hyphemas will resolve within 4 to 6 days. Rebleeding, glaucoma, and staining of the cornea with blood are the most important complications. The size of the hyphema is directly proportional to the incidence of secondary glaucoma and is inversely proportional to visual prognosis. Spontaneous rebleeding may occur 3 to 5 days after the injury and is frequently of greater magnitude than the original hemorrhage. Secondary hemorrhage also significantly reduces the visual prognosis.

CORNEAL ABRASIONS

Corneal abrasions are one of the most common ocular complaints seen in an emergency setting. When the corneal epithelium is abraded, it exposes the underlying basement layer and superficial corneal nerves, causing significant discomfort and pain. A full ophthalmologic examination, including flipping of the eyelid to rule out foreign body, is indicated. At times, patients may believe they have a retained foreign body in spite of a negative examination as the abrasion may produce a similar sensation.

Symptoms
- Eye pain and resistance to opening the eyes +++++
- Tearing
- Photophobia
- The child may have foreign body sensation
- Extensive abrasion can cause a significant decrease in visual acuity

Signs
- Irregularity in the reflection of the light on the corneal surface

Workup
- Visual acuity.
- The eye should be inspected for any signs of injury, foreign body, and entrance wound through the skin, lid, conjunctiva, or cornea.
- The diagnosis can be made with fluorescein dye applied as impregnated paper or a solution with topical anesthetic. The fluorescein will stain the areas where the epithelium is damaged. A cobalt blue–filtered light from an

ophthalmoscope provides acceptable visualization. Magnification by a Wood's lamp allows more detailed evaluation.

• If possible, examination under a slit lamp should be performed to determine the depth of the abrasion.

Comments and Treatment Considerations

Ophthalmic topical anesthetic, such as proparacaine 0.5% or tetracaine 0.5%, can be administered to improve patient tolerance of examination. Only one drop of these medications is needed for rapid anesthetic effect. Proparacaine has a duration of 15 to 20 minutes, but the anesthetic effect of tetracaine may last up to 3 hours. Do not use tetracaine in patients with sulfite sensitivity.

The defects generally heal within 1 to 3 days without any long-term complications. Topical antibiotic therapy, in the form of either ointment or solution, is used to prevent infection until healed. Either erythromycin ophthalmologic ointment or Neosporin ophthalmologic ointment dosed one to three times per day is acceptable. Contact lens wearers may have a greater likelihood of *Pseudomonas aeruginosa* infection and require aminoglycoside and antipseudomonal ophthalmologic preparations. Subsequent examination in 24 to 48 hours is necessary to rule out early infection and to ensure healing.

Recent studies have shown that patching does not result in faster healing time or improvement of symptoms. Cycloplegic agents such as homatropine 2% and cyclopentolate 1% may be used with caution to reduce severe pain and photophobia (see previous section for treatment of hyphema). Although topical anesthetics provide rapid and temporary pain relief, they are toxic to the cornea and can cause extended loss of epithelium, increasing the risk of corneal infection. Therefore a topical anesthetic should not be prescribed to any patient for continued use. Contacts should not be worn until healed.

OCULAR FOREIGN BODY

Corneal and conjunctival foreign bodies are relatively common causes of acute ocular pain and foreign body sensation. The symptoms are similar to those of corneal abrasions.

Symptoms

- Symptoms develop abruptly, and the child can often pinpoint the exact time of onset
- Foreign body sensation
- Eye pain
- Photophobia

Signs

- A red, tearing eye

Workup

- The palpebral conjunctiva of the lower eyelid and the inferior cul-de-sac should be examined by pulling down the lower lid and having the patient look upward. Examination of the palpebral conjunctiva of the upper lid and the upper cul-de-sac is more difficult. The upper lid can be everted by gently grasping the eyelid at the lash line and pulling it down while placing minimal counterpressure at the upper boarder of the eyelid with a cotton applicator. The patient should be instructed to look down during the procedure.
- Fluorescein may be helpful. A large tarsal foreign body may cause a large staining defect, whereas a small foreign body beneath the upper lid may cause fine superficial vertical staining.

Comments and Treatment Considerations

Before removing a foreign body in the conjunctiva, the clinician should examine the underlying sclera to rule out a penetrating injury. When a foreign body is found, it can usually be easily removed. Topical anesthetics, such as proparacaine 0.5% and tetracaine 0.5%, can be used (see the note in the earlier section Corneal Abrasions). If the foreign body appears to adhere only to the cornea or conjunctiva, it can be removed with foreign body spud, fine forceps, or the edge of a medium-bore needle (22 gauge). This is best done at the slit lamp with the physician's hand resting on the patient's cheekbone. In a younger uncooperative child or when a slit lamp is not available, a safer approach is to use a cotton-tip applicator with a bland ophthalmic ointment (Lacri-Lube) applied to the tip. If the conjunctiva and the retained foreign body are not easily movable over the underlying sclera, or if the foreign body appears fixed to deeper structures of the globe, an accompanying injury to the sclera should be suspected. If foreign body sensation persists after removal of the foreign body and no corneal abrasion is present, a second foreign body should be sought.

Once a conjunctival foreign body is removed and there is no evidence of corneal abrasion, further treatment is usually not indicated. Corneal foreign bodies should be treated the same as corneal abrasions (see earlier section Corneal Abrasions) with topical antibiotic ointment, consideration of cycloplegic agents, and follow-up in 24 to 48 hours.

 ## ACUTE CONJUNCTIVITIS

Acute conjunctivitis is the most common disease of the eye in childhood and may be allergic, viral, or bacterial in etiology. Conjunctivitis must always be distinguished from keratitis, which occurs when corneal structures are involved. In conjunctivitis, there is normal vision and absence of photophobia. Patients with significant visual loss (not resulting from tearing), cloudy corneas, or corneal ulcerations should be referred to an ophthalmologist. This discussion focuses on signs and symptoms of uncomplicated acute conjunctivitis in healthy infants and children beyond the neonatal period based on etiology. Issues specific to the newborn are discussed separately in the next section.

BACTERIAL CONJUNCTIVITIS

In children, acute conjunctivitis is predominately caused by bacteria rather than viruses. The common pathogens are non-typable *Haemophilus influenzae, Staphylococcus aureus*, and *Streptococcus pneumoniae*. Other uncommon pathogens include *Neisseria gonorrhoeae, Neisseria meningitidis*, and *Moraxella catarrhalis*.

Symptoms

- Conjunctival erythema
- Purulent discharge, which may cause matting of the eyelashes and difficulty opening the eyes upon awakening

Signs

- Bulbar and palpebral conjunctival erythema and chemosis (Fig. 12-3)
- Purulent discharge, which may be minimal or diffuse
- Occasional lid swelling
- Some patients may have concomitant otitis media (conjunctivitis-otitis syndrome)

Workup

- In clinical practice the treating physician most often makes a presumptive diagnosis of bacterial conjunctivitis and treats empirically.
- Culture of purulent material can be obtained for culture but is not routinely necessary except in the newborn (see next section).
- Gram stain is usually not helpful.

Comments and Treatment Considerations

A topical ophthalmologic antibiotic is recommended for 5 to 7 days. Routinely used ophthalmologic antibiotics include

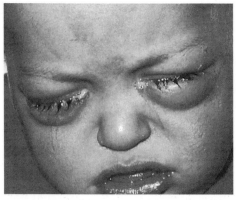

Fig. 12-3 Acute bacterial conjunctivitis. Copious amounts of mucopurulent discharge have made the upper and lower eyelids adherent to each other. Chemosis of the upper and lower lids may also make opening of the eyelids difficult. See Color Insert. (From Zitelli B, Davis H: *Atlas of pediatric physical diagnosis*, 4th ed, St. Louis, 2002, Mosby.)

polymyxin B sulfate–bacitracin zinc (Polysporin), trimetho-prim sulfate–polymyxin B sulfate (Polytrim), and those con-taining erythromycin (Ilotycin) or bacitracin. Usual dosing for ophthalmologic antibiotic ointments suggests applying between one quarter and one half of an inch to the affected lower conjunctival sac(s) three to four times per day.

In children with conjunctivitis-otitis syndrome, systemic oral antibiotic appropriate for treating otitis media is generally suf-ficient to cure conjunctivitis without additional topical therapy (see Chapter 22, Irritability). The use of an oral antibiotic should also be considered in the young child with conjunctivi-tis who is likely to develop conjunctivitis-otitis syndrome.

Parents should be counseled on the infectious nature of con-junctivitis and advised not to return children to school or day care until they have completed 24 hours of antibiotic therapy. All affected bedding and linens should be thoroughly washed with detergent and hot water. Children not improving in 5 to 7 days should be referred to an ophthalmologist.

VIRAL CONJUNCTIVITIS

Approximately 20% of acute conjunctivitis cases in children are caused by *Adenovirus*. Although viral conjunctivitis can present similarly to bacterial conjunctivitis, some features may help distinguish the two. Bacterial conjunctivitis tends to be more common in preschool children, more likely to be bilateral, and present with purulent discharge. Less common but impera-tive to diagnose is herpes simplex virus (HSV)–associated ker-atoconjunctivitis usually caused by HSV type 1.

HERPES SIMPLEX VIRUS

Although uncommon, conjunctivitis/keratitis caused by HSV is an ocular emergency and must be appropriately diagnosed to prevent permanent corneal damage.

Symptoms
- Conjunctival erythema
- Periorbital vesicular skin eruptions
- Symptoms usually unilateral

Signs
- Follicular conjunctivitis
- Vesicles on eyelids may be present
- Ipsilateral preauricular lymphadenopathy

Workup
- Corneal involvement can be nonspecific or can consist of classic dendritic keratitis. Fluorescein stain may show dendritic staining pattern on the cornea or conjunctiva (Fig. 12-4).

Comments and Treatment Considerations
In HSV ocular infections treatment should be initiated in consultation with an ophthalmologist. Usual treatment options include DNA inhibitors such as vidarabine ophthalmologic ointment 3% or trifluridine ophthalmologic solution 1%. Vidarabine ointment half an inch applied to the conjunctival sac five times per day (q3h while awake) is the preferred treatment in children. Trifluridine may be tried if vidarabine is not successful. Topical corticosteroids are contraindicated. Recurrence rates may be as high as 30% to 50%. For children with recurrent ocular lesions, oral suppressive therapy with acyclovir dosed at 80 mg/kg/day PO divided q6h (max 3200 mg/day, 800 mg/dose) may be of benefit.

ADENOVIRUS
Adenoviral ocular infections manifest as one of three classic forms: pharyngoconjunctival fever (PCF), epidemic keratoconjunctivitis (EKC), and nonspecific follicular conjunctivitis. PCF occurs more commonly in children than adults and is associated with upper respiratory tract infection, regional lymphadenopathy, and fever. Community outbreaks of *Adenovirus*-associated PCF have been attributed to exposure to water from contaminated swimming pools and fomites such as shared towels. EKC occurs most commonly in the 20- to 40-year-old age-group. Presentation includes foreign body sensation, preauricular lymphadenopathy, and diffuse superficial keratitis. EKC has been associated with nosocomial transmission in ophthalmologists' offices. Nonspecific follicular conjunctivitis is mild and self-limiting.

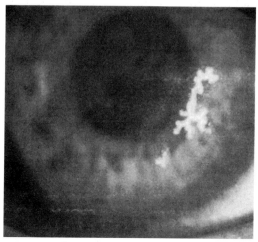

Fig. 12-4 Herpes keratitis. Dendritic pattern with fluorescein uptake. (From Palay D, Krachmer J: *Ophthalmology for the primary care physician*, St. Louis, 1997, Mosby.)

Symptoms

- Conjunctival erythema (Fig. 12-5)
- Purulent or mucous/serous discharge
- Dramatic lid swelling and sandy foreign body sensation are associated with EKC
- Upper respiratory tract infection, pharyngitis, and fever are associated with PCF

Signs

- Follicular conjunctivitis
- Preauricular lymphadenopathy

Workup

- Diagnosis is primarily based on clinical findings. Laboratory diagnosis is rarely necessary.

Comments and Treatment Considerations

Viral conjunctivitis is generally self-limited. If the patient clearly has viral conjunctivitis, antibiotic treatment is not indicated.

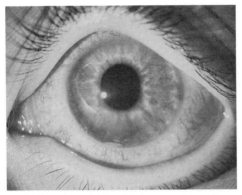

Fig. 12-5 Viral conjunctivitis with hyperemia and a watery discharge. See Color Insert. (From Zitelli B, Davis H: *Atlas of pediatric physical diagnosis*, 4th ed, St. Louis, 2002, Mosby.)

However, since differentiating between bacterial and viral conjunctivitis is difficult, antibiotic ointment is often prescribed (see earlier section). Cold saline drops may be beneficial. Symptoms may persist for 7 to 10 days, and given the contagious nature there is controversy over when it is appropriate to return to day care or school. Certainly children with red weeping eyes should be excluded until tearing stops. Children symptomatic after 10 days should be referred to an ophthalmologist.

ALLERGIC CONJUNCTIVITIS

Allergic conjunctivitis is due to an IgG-mediated reaction causing vascular dilatation and chemosis of the conjunctiva. It is usually seasonal, recurrent, and bilateral, presenting with watery eyes and significant pruritus. There may be a scant stringy mucoid discharge as well. The presence of pruritus is the usual hallmark and differentiates it from bacterial and viral conjunctivitis. Treatment is usually symptomatic and consists of topical H_1 antagonists such as emedastine (Emadine), mast-cell inhibitors, or a combination such as olopatadine (Patanol). Emedastine is dosed at one drop of 0.05% solution to affected eye(s) up to four times per day. Olopatadine is dosed at one to two drops of 0.1% solution to affected eye(s) twice a day. Both can be used in patients 3 years or older.

 ## NEWBORN CONJUNCTIVITIS

Ophthalmia neonatorum is conjunctivitis that occurs in neonates within the first 4 weeks of life, most often acquired during vaginal delivery. The major causes include *Chlamydia trachomatis*, *N. gonorrhoeae*, and chemically induced.

CHLAMYDIAL CONJUNCTIVITIS

Chlamydial conjunctivitis is the most commonly identified cause of ophthalmia neonatorum. Symptoms usually develop by 2 weeks of age.

Symptoms
- Mild to moderate conjunctival erythema
- Scant mucoid discharge to copious purulent discharge

Signs
- Injected conjunctiva with greater involvement on the palpebral rather than bulbar conjunctiva
- No follicular reaction or preauricular lymphadenopathy

Workup
- Definitive diagnosis can be made by isolating the organism in tissue culture. Conjunctival scrapings are preferred over the discharge because chlamydiae are obligate intracellular organisms.
- Nucleic acid amplification methods, such as polymerase chain reaction and lipase chain reaction, are more sensitive than cell culture and more specific and sensitive than DNA probe, direct fluorescent antibody tests, or enzyme immunoassays.
- Giemsa stain identifies the characteristic basophilic intracytoplasmic inclusion bodies within epithelial cells. This test is highly specific, but the sensitivity varies from 22% to 95%.

Comments and Treatment Considerations

Infants with chlamydial conjunctivitis may have other associated manifestations including pneumonia, otitis media, rhinitis, proctitis, and vulvitis. Chlamydial pneumonia is preceded by chlamydial conjunctivitis in approximately 50% of cases. Treatment of chlamydial conjunctivitis includes oral erythromycin ethylsuccinate dosed at 50 mg/kg/day PO divided q6h for 14 days and will cover the ophthalmic and systemic infection. When appropriate systemic therapy is used, topical ophthalmologic treatment appears to offer no further benefit. Alternatively, azithromycin 20 mg/kg/day PO q day × 3 days has been used successfully when concern for pyloric stenosis or drug-drug interactions is present. The mother and her sexual partner(s) should also be treated presumptively even if they are asymptomatic.

GONOCOCCAL CONJUNCTIVITIS

Routine neonatal ocular prophylaxis and the routine screening and treatment of pregnant women for gonorrhea have reduced the incidence of neonatal gonococcal conjunctivitis in United States. However, it remains one of the most important causes of ophthalmia neonatorum worldwide. The incubation period is usually 2 to 7 days.

Symptoms
- Erythematous conjunctiva
- Grossly purulent discharge
- Symptoms usually bilateral

Signs
- Severe, grossly purulent conjunctivitis

Workup
- Gram stain of conjunctival scrapings show gram-negative intracellular diplococci.
- Culture of eye discharge should be obtained.
- Tests for concomitant infection with *C. trachomatis*, congenital syphilis, and HIV should be considered.

Comments and Treatment Considerations

Gonococcal conjunctivitis can progress to ulceration of the cornea and globe within 24 hours of infection. Therefore, presumptive diagnosis must be made and treatment should be initiated on the basis of the results of a Gram stain. The infant should be hospitalized for immediate irrigation with saline to continue at frequent intervals until eye discharge is eliminated. Recommended antibiotic therapy is a single dose of ceftriaxone at 25 to 50 mg/kg (max 1 g/dose) IV or IM × 1 dose. Alternatively, a single dose of cefotaxime 100 mg/kg IV/IM may be used in hyperbilirubinemic infants. Topical antibiotic is unnecessary when recommended systemic antibiotic treatment is given. The mother and her sexual partner(s) also need appropriate management for *N. gonorrhoeae* and possible associated STDs.

CHEMICALLY INDUCED CONJUNCTIVITIS

Chemically-induced conjunctivitis is rarely seen since erythromycin ointment replaced silver nitrate as the standard ophthalmic antibiotic used in the routine prophylaxis of the newborn. Chemical conjunctivitis may occur secondary to either therapy but is less likely with erythromycin. The neonate presents with a mildly purulent conjunctivitis during the first 24 hours of life, usually resolving within 48 hours.

 ## CONGENITAL NASOLACRIMAL DUCT OBSTRUCTION

Congenital nasolacrimal duct obstruction occurs in up to 6% of newborns. The lacrimal drainage system is obstructed at the distal end, just proximal to the entrance into the nasal cavity (Fig. 12-6). Symptoms usually manifest in the first few weeks of life with persistent tearing (epiphora) and crusting on the eyelashes.

Symptoms

- Epiphora that can be variable in severity from a large tear meniscus on lower lid to overt epiphora

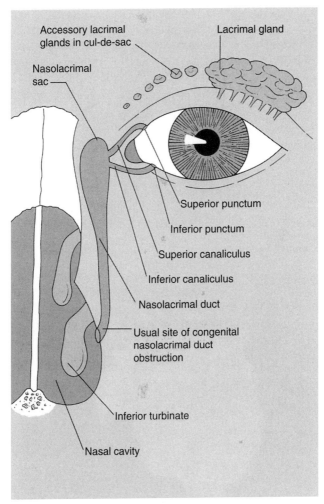

Fig. 12-6 Lacrimal secretory and collecting system. (From Zitelli B, Davis H: *Atlas of pediatric physical diagnosis,* 4th ed, St. Louis, 2002, Mosby.)

- Mucoid discharge in the medial canthal area may vary from clear or whitish to yellowish (Fig. 12-7)
- Secondary infection can occur with greenish purulent discharge
- Crusting of the eyelashes upon awakening

Signs
- Epiphora
- Mucoid discharge
- In severe cases injected conjunctiva, erythema, and edema of the eyelids may occur

Workup
- An easy test can be done by pressing gently over the lacrimal sac. If mucoid or purulent material is expressed

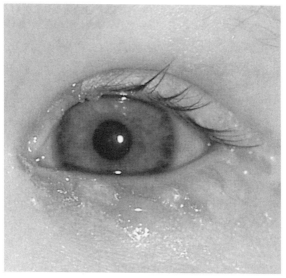

Fig. 12-7 Obstruction of the left nasolacrimal duct has led to the development of mucopurulent discharge and tearing. (See Color Insert.) (From Zitelli B, Davis H: *Atlas of pediatric physical diagnosis,* 4th ed, St. Louis, 2002, Mosby.)

from the puncta, the diagnosis is confirmed. If material cannot be expressed, the test does not rule out nasolacrimal duct obstruction.

- The fluorescein dye disappearance test works well in infants to diagnose obstruction. The test is performed by placing one drop of 0.5% proparacaine ophthalmologic solution, followed by one drop of 2% fluorescein or a moistened fluorescein paper strip into the conjunctival cul-de-sac of each eye. After 5 minutes, the eyes are examined with a cobalt blue light. In a normal lacrimal system all the dye should be cleared from the tear meniscus.

Comments and Treatment Considerations

Many studies have shown that symptoms of congenital naso-lacrimal duct obstruction resolve before the age of 12 months in more than 90% of patients. Most patients can be managed medically with massage and topical antibiotics. The massage should be performed in the medial canthal area. Initially the motion should milk any discharge from the sac by applying gentle pressure and stroking upward. After this, downward pressure should be applied to the nasolacrimal sac. The downward strokes should be performed three or four strokes at a time and the entire maneuver should be performed several times a day. Topical antibiotic should be reserved for evidence of bacterial superinfection or conjunctivitis. The decision to proceed with nasolacrimal probing by a pediatric ophthalmologist is based on severity of symptoms, age, and parental concerns.

REFERENCES

American Academy of Pediatrics: *2000 red book: report of the Committee on Infectious Diseases*, 25th ed, Elk Grove Village, Ill, 2000, American Academy of Pediatrics.

Bloom JN: Traumatic hyphema in children, *Pediatr Ann* 19:368-371, 1990.

Bodor FF: Conjunctivitis-otitis syndrome, *Pediatrics* 69:695-698, 1982.

Catalano RA: Eye injuries and prevention, *Pediatr Clin North Am* 40:827-839, 1993.

Centers for Disease Control and Prevention: Sexually transmitted diseases treatment guidelines 2002, *MMWR Morb Mortal Wkly Rep* 51(RR-6), 2002

Englanoff JS: Eye pain and redness. In: Davis MA et al, editors: *Signs and symptoms in emergency medicine: literature-based approach to emergent conditions*, Missouri, 1999, Mosby.

Forbes BJR: Management of corneal abrasions and ocular trauma in children, *Pediatr Ann* 30:465-472, 2001.

Frey T: Pediatric eye trauma, *Pediatr Ann* 12;487-497, 1983.

Gigliotti F: Acute conjunctivitis of childhood, *Pediatr Ann* 22(6):353-356, 1993.

Gigliotti F, Williams WT, Hayden FG, Hendley JO: Etiology of acute conjunctivitis in children, *J Pediatr* 98:531-536, 1981.

Hammerschlag MR: Neonatal conjunctivitis, *Pediatr Ann* 22:346-351, 1993.

Kaiser PK and the Corneal Abrasion Patching Study Group: A comparison of pressure patching versus no patching for corneal abrasions due to trauma or foreign body removal, *Ophthalmology* 102:1936-1942, 1995.

Lavrich JB, Nelson LB: Disorders of the lacrimal system apparatus, *Pediatr Clin North Am* 40:767-776, 1993.

Leibowitz HM: The red eye, *N Engl J Med* 343(5):345-351, 2000.

Levin AV: Eye emergencies: acute management in the pediatric ambulatory care setting. *Pediatr Emerg Care* 7:367-377, 1991.

Levin AV: Ophthalmic emergencies. In Fleisher GR, Ludwig S, editors: *Textbook of pediatric emergency medicine*, 4th ed, Philadelphia, 2000, Lippincott Williams & Wilkins.

Matoba A: Ocular viral infections, *Pediatr Infect Dis* 3(4):358-368, 1984.

Meisler DM, Beauchamp OR: Disorders of the conjunctiva. In Nelson LB, editor: *Harley's pediatric ophthalmology*, 4th ed, Philadelphia, 1998, WB Saunders.

Nelson LB, Calhoun JH, Menduke H: Medical management of congenital nasolacrimal duct obstruction, *Ophthalmology* 92:1187-1190, 1985.

Ogawa GS, Gonnering RS: Congenital nasolacrimal duct obstruction, *J Pediatr* 119:12-17, 1991.

O'Hara MA: Ophthalmia neonatorum, *Pediatr Clin North Am* 40:715-725, 1993.

Onofrey BE: Management of corneal burns, *Optom Clin* 4:31-40, 1995.

Rubin SE, Catalano RA: Ocular trauma and its prevention. In Nelson LB, editor: *Harley's pediatric ophthalmology*, 4th ed, Philadelphia, 1998, WB Saunders.

Seidman DJ, Nelson LB, Calhoun GL, et al: Signs and symptoms in the presentation of primary infantile glaucoma, *Pediatrics* 77:399-404, 1986.

Shingleton BJ: Eye injuries, *N Engl J Med* 325:408-413, 1991.

Siegel JD: Eye infections encountered by the pediatrician, *Pediatr Infect Dis J* 5(6):741-748, 1986.

Tingley DH: Consultation with the specialist: eye trauma: corneal abrasions, *Pediatr Rev* 20:320-322, 1999.

Wagner RS: Glaucoma in children, *Pediatr Clin North Am* 40:855-867, 1993.

CHAPTER 13

Failure to Thrive

ANDREW J. CAPRARO

F*ailure to thrive* (FTT) refers to physical growth in an infant
or child that is significantly less than that his or her peers as
defined by standard growth charts of the National Center of
Health Statistics. It is a relatively common problem, representing 3% to 5% of all pediatric hospital admissions, and can be
seen in as many as 10% of children in a primary care setting.
Most often the patient with FTT is an infant, but FTT may
occur at any age. Multiple studies have shown that there are
long-standing cognitive and developmental deficits in those
children with FTT who are not treated.

The underlying causes of FTT are numerous, so the evaluation and workup of these patients can be daunting and vexing to
the physician.

DEFINITION

Though a common problem, there has been no consensus definition for FTT. It is widely defined as a child who is growing below
the 3rd or 5th percentile on more than one occasion or a child
whose weight crosses two major percentiles downward on the
standard growth charts (Fig. 13-1). In general, patients with FTT
have relatively spared height and head circumference for age.
However, these parameters may be affected in long-standing
FTT. Infants who are small for gestational age are considered
an exception to this definition. Preterm infants should be plotted on growth charts at their corrected age, rather than chrono-
logic age to help avoid labeling them "FTT."

The diagnoses leading to FTT have traditionally been split
into organic and nonorganic categories. *Organic FTT* refers to
poor growth in a child as the result of an underlying physiologic
condition such as a chronic disease (including cystic fibrosis,

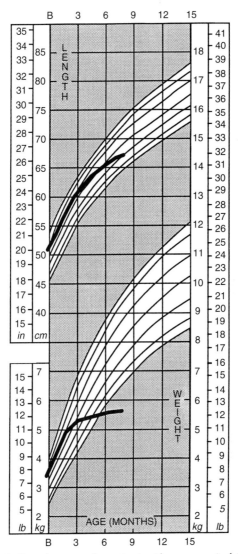

Fig. 13-1 Growth curve of a patient with nonorganic failure to thrive. The growth pattern is not specific and can be seen in hypocaloric diets resulting from a variety of causes, including malabsorption and overuse of energy. (From Gartner JC, Zitelli B: *Common and chronic symptoms in pediatrics*, St. Louis, 1997, Mosby.)

congenital heart disease, and renal disease). Organic etiologies may involve any organ system (Table 13-1). *Nonorganic FTT* refers to psychosocial or environmental conditions that lead to poor growth in a child. Examples of these circumstances include poor parent-infant bonding, financial burden, neglect, and abuse. Organic and nonorganic causes may occur together as well (Tables 13-1 and 13-2).

EVALUATION

The clinician must remember that FTT is a sign and not a diagnosis. The physician must evaluate the patient with FTT and seek the underlying cause. A thorough history and physical examination will guide the physician through an orderly workup of the patient.

Table 13-1   Organic Causes of Failure to Thrive

Gastrointestinal	Gastroesophageal reflux, pyloric stenosis, malrotation, Hirschsprung's disease, malabsorption, milk protein intolerance, cleft palate, hepatitis, pancreatitis
Cardiac	Congenital heart disease leading to congestive heart failure
Pulmonary	Cystic fibrosis, tracheoesophageal fistula, upper airway compromise (e.g., tonsillar hypertrophy)
Renal	Renal tubular acidosis, diabetes insipidus, chronic renal insufficiency
Neurologic	Cerebral hemorrhages, hydrocephalus, degenerative disorders
Endocrine	Hypothyroidism, diabetes mellitus, pituitary insufficiency, adrenal insufficiency or excess
Metabolic	Inborn errors of metabolism
Infectious	HIV disease, tuberculosis, parasitic infections
Miscellaneous	Lead poisoning, chromosomal abnormalities, malignancy

Table 13-2 Potential Etiologies of Failure to Thrive Based on Symptom	
Sign/Symptom	Differential
Poor feeding	Psychosocial difficulties, dysmorphic anomalies (cleft palate, tracheoesophageal fistula), hypertonia/hypotonia, myopathies
Dyspnea while feeding	Congenital heart disease
Vomiting	Gastroesophageal reflux, anatomic obstruction, intracranial mass
Diarrhea	Bacterial diarrhea, malabsorption (CF), protein intolerance, parasitic infection
Poor stooling/chronic constipation	Hirschsprung's disease
Chronic/recurrent infections	HIV disease, urinary tract infections, tuberculosis

HISTORY

A very detailed history should be obtained in a nonjudgmental manner with the caregivers of the patient. The history may point to the diagnosis (Tables 13-1 and 13-2). By definition, FTT is a chronic process. Acute processes may coexist with FTT, even exacerbating the condition. For example, intercurrent infections may worsen poor weight gain due to chronic inadequate caloric intake.

Natal History

The physician should begin with the gestation of the child. The health and weight gain of the mother during the pregnancy are important details that should also be obtained.

Dietary History

The dietary history is of primary importance. The physician should take a very detailed look at all aspects of feeding. If the patient is being breast-fed, the physician needs to ask questions about milk let down and nursing technique. The timing of the feeds needs to be measured. Is the mother taking any medications that may interfere with nursing? If the patient is formula-fed, the physician needs to ask questions about the volume of feeds and the timing. Is the formula being prepared correctly or is the formula more dilute than it should be? Has the child started solid foods yet? These questions help the physician discover if the caloric intake of the patient is appropriate. Observing the caregivers feeding the patient is also very useful for the clinician.

Feeding Behavior

The behavior of the patient during feeds should be elucidated. What position is the child in when being fed? Does there seem to be an anatomic impediment to feeding? Is there a significant pattern of vomiting or stooling around the feeds? Does the patient seem sated after feedings? Does the patient grow fatigued during feeds or become diaphoretic? These questions help the physician begin to formulate a differential diagnosis. Vomiting and irritability may represent gastroesophageal reflux disease (GERD). Nonbilious forceful vomiting may indicate pyloric stenosis. Poor stooling since birth may lead to a diagnosis of Hirschsprung's disease. Fatigue and diaphoresis are hallmarks of congenital heart disease.

Psychosocial History

The physician also should obtain a full psychosocial history of the family. It is here that the diagnosis of nonorganic FTT may come to the forefront of the differential. The physician needs to ask about the caregivers' psychological well-being and any financial stresses that may exist.

Developmental History

Developmental history of the child, particularly the acquisition of milestones, should be discussed. Family history of short stature, malabsorption, or constitutional delay should be sought.

REVIEW OF SYSTEMS

Because FTT can be due to organic causes affecting any organ system, a very detailed review of systems should be obtained.

Physical Examination

The physical examination of a patient with FTT must always begin with accurate measurements of the patient's height, weight, and head circumference that are then plotted on appropriate growth charts. Past measurements, if known, should also be plotted to see whether a pattern of growth arrest or weight loss exists. If all three parameters are under the 5th percentile, the clinician should consider an organic etiology. In the patient with nonorganic FTT, head circumference is relatively spared initially.

The physical manifestations of the patient's poor growth are numerous and include the loss of subcutaneous fat, decreased muscle mass, dermatitis, and alopecia. A complete physical examination should be performed. Findings involving the cardiopulmonary (e.g., murmurs), gastrointestinal (e.g., vomiting, diarrhea, masses), or nervous systems (e.g., incoordinated feeding, increased tone) should be investigated further.

Physical findings consistent with non-organic FTT include poor hygiene, a dull affect, excessive oral self-stimulation, and signs of developmental delay.

Further Evaluations

Laboratory tests should be performed judiciously and based on pertinent findings in the history and physical. In most cases laboratory testing is not helpful. Berwick et al. (1982) found that only 0.8% of all tests showed an abnormality. However, a CBC, set of electrolytes, and UA are often performed as an initial screen. The family should be instructed to track caloric intake with a detailed food diary and frequent weight checks (frequency based on degree of FTT).

Patients with significant FTT or questions concerning parental care/neglect may need to be admitted to the hospital for a trial of inpatient feeding. Hospital admission for FTT continues to be a controversial subject. Indications include severe malnutrition, the need for further evaluation for organic causes, and evaluation of the caregiver-child dyad. If neglect or abuse is considered, social services should be consulted.

In addition, testing based on clinical history and physical examination findings may include an ECG and CXR for the child with suspected heart disease, thyroid function tests for the child presumed to have an endocrinologic abnormality, and pH probe and endoscopy for the patient with suspected GERD or other gastrointestinal abnormality. PPD placement and HIV testing are useful in the patient with chronic infections. Sweat testing for cystic fibrosis should be performed on a child with malabsorptive gastrointestinal symptoms.

REFERENCES

Bauchner H: Failure to thrive. In *Nelson textbook of pediatrics*, 15th ed, Philadelphia, 1996, WB Saunders.

Berwick DM, et al: Failure to thrive: diagnostic yield of hospitalization, *Arch Dis Child* 57:347-351, 1982.

Fleisher GR: *Synopsis of pediatric emergency medicine*, 3rd ed, Philadelphia, 1996, Lippincott Williams & Wilkins.

Frank D et al: Failure to thrive, *Pediatr Clin North Am* 35:1187-1206, 1988.

Frank D et al: Failure to thrive: mystery, myth, and method, *Contemp Pediatr* 10:114, 1993.

Schwartz I: Failure to thrive: an old nemesis in the new millennium, *Pediatr Rev* 21:257-264, 2000.

Zenel J: Failure to thrive: a general pediatrician's perspective, *Pediatr Rev* 18:371-378, 1997.

CHAPTER 14

Fever

MARVIN B. HARPER

Fever as part of a presenting complaint is one of the most common reasons for an urgent pediatric visit and accounts for approximately one third of all pediatric ED visits. Although fever in the pediatric patient is usually associated with a benign viral syndrome, it may be the initial presentation of serious bacterial illness. As a result, the physician must remain vigilant to identify the rare case of life-threatening infection.

Although infection is by far the most common cause of fever in children, one must remember that fever may occur as the result of many noninfectious causes. These causes may include tissue injury, dehydration, malignancy, drugs, vaccines, as well as genetic, metabolic, endocrine, immunologic, rheumatologic, and inflammatory disorders. Children with fever and immunosuppression are at increased risk for serious infection (see Chapter 21, Immunocompromised Patients: Special Considerations).

When present, localizing signs or symptoms will determine the need for further diagnostic evaluation in many children (see chapters associated with the localizing symptoms such as Chapter 1, Abdominal Pain, for the child with abdominal pain); however, some children will have a fever with no source or clear explanation. When no signs or symptoms point to a specific infection (the patient with a fever and "no source"), then the age of the child, duration of fever, and the general appearance of the child will be the branch points to guide further evaluation. The degree of fever can also be helpful, although some infants (typically younger than 2 weeks) and some older children (e.g., those with underlying illness or malnutrition) may have difficulty in mounting a fever.

Signs and Symptoms

- Poor perfusion or hypotension is an ominous sign and should raise the concern for serious pathology (see Chapter 19, Hypotension).
- Neurologic abnormalities or altered mental status is concerning for serious infection, particularly involving the CNS (see Chapter 3, Altered Mental Status). With a rapid increase to high fever, chills and rigors are common and may be confused with seizure activity. Some children with high fevers may experience hallucinations and some children who are genetically predisposed may have true febrile seizures (see Chapter 32, Seizures).
- Tachycardia is commonly associated with fever. An increase of approximately 10 to 20 beats per minute per degree centigrade is common. Tachycardia with an increase beyond 10 to 20 beats per minute per degree centigrade should prompt a search for other causes (see Chapter 34, Tachycardia).
- Tachypnea is also commonly associated with fever. A respiratory rate increase of approximately four breaths per minute per degree centigrade can be attributed to fever, but increases beyond this should prompt further evaluation for a respiratory source (see Chapter 30, Respiratory Distress).
- Neck rigidity should raise the concern for meningitis (see Chapter 3, Altered Mental Status). Other causes of neck pain and fever are covered in Chapter 27, Neck Pain/Masses.
- Rash, especially petechiae or purpura, may represent life-threatening infectious disease, even though viral syndromes are the most common cause of the infectious rash (see Chapter 29, Rash). It is common for young children to have some acrocyanosis with relatively cool peripheral extremities, particularly when the fever is rising. Infants commonly have some mottling.
- Abdominal pain associated with fever is commonly caused by infections such as group A streptococcal pharyngitis, pneumonia, bacteremia, urinary tract infection (UTI), appendicitis, and infectious colitis (see Chapter 1, Abdominal Pain).

- Hyperthermia and anticholinergic symptoms or evidence of another toxidrome should provoke consideration of a possible ingestion (see Chapter 35, Toxic Ingestion, Approach To).
- Arthritis or joint complaints may present with fever. It is imperative to consider a septic joint etiology in these patients (see Chapter 24, Joint Pain and Swelling). In children with localized bone pain and fever, the possibility of osteomyelitis should be considered (see Chapter 25, Limp).

Comments and Treatment Considerations

Support the ABCs including intubation as indicated. Assess overall state of circulation and, if signs of sepsis are present, ensure adequate access, and provide fluid support (see Chapter 20, Hypotension/Shock). Consider external cooling for temperature >103.5° F with aggressive cooling for temperatures >105° F. Assess patient for any signs of serious infection or risk based on age and consider empiric antibiotic coverage (see recommendations by age, later in this chapter).

Certain patients are known to be at high risk of bacterial infections. These patients, such as those with malignancy, HIV, asplenia, sickle cell disease, neutropenia, drug-induced immunosuppression, and hypogammaglobulinemia, require special attention (see Chapter 21, Immunocompromised Patients: Special Considerations).

EVALUATION OF THE PATIENT WITH FEVER AND NO SOURCE, BY AGE-GROUP

THE WELL-APPEARING NEONATE AND VERY YOUNG INFANT: 0 TO 3 MONTHS OF AGE

A small increase in temperature is used for empiric diagnostic testing of very young infants because they are at increased risk of bacterial infection and may not yet have the ability to mount a high fever. The temperature measurement suggesting the need for empiric testing of the otherwise well-appearing infant younger than 2 to 3 months of age has generally been defined as $\geq 38.0°$ C. The routine evaluation of the infant with such a fever has been the subject of much study and debate. What is very clear is that such infants deserve a careful prompt physical examination, and that despite normal physical evaluation findings, approximately 7% will have a UTI, 2% will have bacteremia, and about 0.5% will have bacterial meningitis.

Workup

- CBC and blood culture.
- Sterile UA and urine culture via suprapubic tap or catheterization.
- CSF cell count, glucose and protein concentration, Gram stain, and culture.
- CXR in a patient with respiratory abnormalities or empirically if WBC >20,000.
- Consider stool studies.
- Consider HSV CNS infection. Polymerase chain reaction (PCR) of CSF for HSV.

Comments and Treatment Considerations

The risk of bacteremia and meningitis is highest in the first month of life. Infants in this age-group are generally admitted for IV therapy with ampicillin dosed at 200 to 300 mg/kg/day IV divided q6-12h (interval depends on age as follows: days of life [DOL] 1 to 14 q12h, DOL 15 to 28 q8h, and >1 month q6h) and gentamicin dosed at 4 mg/kg/day IV q24h pending the results of urine, blood, and CSF cultures. When a low WBC count is noted in the very young infant, the risk of bacteremia, sepsis, and/or meningitis increases substantially.

In the second or third month of life many clinicians use published guidelines that identify infants at low risk of meningitis, UTI, and bacteremia to determine management (Fig. 14-1). Infants meeting low-risk criteria are managed as outpatients with or without a single dose of ceftriaxone 50 mg/kg IV or IM pending the results of culture. It must be remembered that serious bacterial infections can and do occur among well-appearing infants meeting low-risk criteria, albeit infrequently.

Neonatal HSV infection presents with fever in the first several weeks of life. One should consider adding acyclovir 60

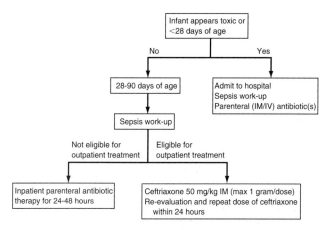

Sepsis work-up includes blood culture, urine culture, and CSF culture.

Eligibility criteria for outpatient treatment

>=28 days of age
Previously healthy
Non-toxic clinical appearance
Family can be easily contacted (e.g., accurate phone number)
No focal bacterial infection on examination (except otitis media)
Peripheral blood WBC count <20,000/mm³
Normal urinalysis (negative dipstick or <10 WBC/hpf)
When heme positive diarrhea present <5 WBC/hpf in stool
CSF WBC count <10/mm³

Fig. 14-1 An algorithm for the management of the previously healthy infant 0 to 90 days of age with fever ≥38° C without source evident on physical examination. (Adapted from Baskin MN, O'Rourke EJ, Fleisher GR: *J Pediatr* 120(1): 22-27, 1992.)

mg/kg/day IV divided q8h to the regimen of any ill-appearing patient. Those infants with a maternal history of herpes infection, lesions consistent with herpes infection, or abnormal neurologic examination results absolutely should receive acyclovir as dosed above and a CSF specimen should be sent for HSV PCR. Adequate hydration is essential during acyclovir therapy to prevent nephrotoxicity.

It is common for a tactile temperature to be reported by the parents and for the infant to be afebrile at the time of the patient visit. Bonadio and colleagues reported that infants younger than 2 months with only a tactile fever reported at home were half as likely to have fever measured in the ED or hospital as infants who had temperatures measured by rectal thermometry at home. Therefore some of these infants, but not all, have true fever. Some experts recommend observing the child over a few hours and repeat the temperature measurement in the ED. If no fever is detected, the guardian is instructed on the use of a rectal thermometer and sent home, to return if a measured temperature of ≥38° C is noted or the child appears ill.

The question regarding the effect of bundling on temperature in neonates is a common one. If the finding of fever is borderline, 38° C or 38.1° C, isolated, and unexpected (child coming in for unrelated reason and otherwise well), it is not unreasonable to unbundle the baby. If there is a rapid return to a temperature <38° C, it may be acceptable to disregard the single recording of fever.

THE WELL-APPEARING INFANT 3 TO 6 MONTHS OF AGE

The well-appearing febrile infant 3 to 6 months of age continues to be at risk for UTIs, although the rate of bacteremia declines substantially. Unfortunately, this is also the peak age-group for pneumococcal meningitis. For infants in this age-group who do not have passively acquired maternal antipneumococcal antibody, bacteremia progresses to meningitis much more frequently (see Chapter 3, Altered Mental Status). The full impact of the heptavalent conjugate pneumococcal (Prevnar) vaccine on the occurrence of pneumococcal meningitis is unclear, but the overall rate of invasive pneumococcal disease has decreased by 70% among children younger than 2 years. The threshold temperature for empiric testing at this age is generally regarded as 39° C.

Workup

- CBC and blood culture in any patient who has not completed the primary pneumococcal conjugate vaccine series (minimum of three vaccinations usually given at 2, 4, and 6 months).

- Sterile UA and urine culture via suprapubic tap or catheterization.
- Consider further studies based on clinical examination findings.

Comments and Treatment Considerations

If the WBC count exceeds 15,000 cells/mm^3, a single dose of ceftriaxone 50 mg/kg IV/IM may be given pending the results of cultures. If there is no clinical suspicion for meningitis, a lumbar puncture is not routinely necessary at this age.

THE WELL-APPEARING OLDER INFANT AND YOUNG CHILD 6 MONTHS TO 5 YEARS

In the well-appearing child 6 months to 5 years who has been fully vaccinated (including the conjugate pneumococcal vaccine) according to U.S. guidelines, there is no need for empiric blood testing. The most common infections not clinically evident on physical examination are pneumonia and UTIs.

Workup

- UA and urine culture should be obtained in all females younger than 2 years, all males younger than 1 year, children with a history of UTI, children with particularly high fever, fever lasting >2 days, and those children with a known leukocytosis.
- CXR should be obtained in those children with high or prolonged fever, a known leukocytosis, or respiratory symptoms.

Comments and Treatment Considerations

Infants and children at low risk of UTI may be suitably screened with a urinalysis. The urinalysis has at best an 80% chance of detecting a UTI and is therefore not suitable for use if there are any risk factors making a UTI more likely.

When a viral illness is suspected and causes for concern are eliminated, it is important to emphasize that antibiotics are not needed to treat fevers. It is also important to acknowledge that the patient is indeed sick and likely suffering from an infection, but to explain why antibiotic use is not helpful. Regardless of the outcome of the visit, a clear plan for the family to manage the child, signs and symptoms to report back to the clinician, and parameters for subsequent evaluation by a clinician should be discussed.

THE SCHOOL-AGE CHILD AND ADOLESCENT

Viral illnesses predominate in the school-age child and adolescent. Localizing signs or symptoms usually determine the need for further diagnostic evaluation (see chapters associated with the localizing symptoms such as Chapter 1, Abdominal Pain, for children with abdominal pain).

Workup

Empiric testing should seldom be required if the child is well appearing. Testing should be entirely directed by symptoms or if the fever becomes prolonged (>5 days). In these cases a screening CBC count can be useful to identify the patient with leukocytosis or possible malignancy (leukemia). Additionally, one should consider Kawasaki disease and other chronic causes of fever discussed later in this chapter.

Comments and Treatment Considerations

As a rule, antibiotics should not be prescribed empirically unless a specific bacterial infection is identified (see the previous section for children 6 months to 5 years of age).

 ## *CHRONIC FEVER*

Most children evaluated for fever are younger than 3 years and have had a fever for <2 days. Children with a high fever for 5 days are relatively uncommon and should automatically raise concern for the diagnosis of Kawasaki disease (KD). When the duration of fever exceeds 7 days, the diagnostic evaluation changes to search for more chronic infections or noninfectious sources. A complete discussion of the management of the patient with chronic fever is beyond the scope of this chapter. However, when appropriate, investigations for mononucleosis, cytomegalovirus, HIV, hepatitis, sinusitis, pneumonia, and abdominal abscess should be initiated. By the time the fever has persisted for 2 weeks, baseline testing should include a CBC, ESR, CXR, and UA. Specimens should be collected for culture of urine and blood. A history of patient or guardian travel, exposures to animals, exposure to other individuals with acute or chronic illness, and unusual or severe infections will serve to broaden the differential diagnosis. Collagen vascular diseases, drug-induced fevers, thyrotoxicosis, familial Mediterranean fever, and malignancy should all be considered.

 ## KAWASAKI DISEASE

Kawasaki disease (KD) is a vasculitis of unknown etiology that has been defined as having 5 consecutive days of fever without another explanation that is associated with at least four of the following symptoms (Fig. 14-2):

- Bilateral, nonexudative conjunctival injection
- At least one of the following: mucous membrane changes, injected or fissured lips, injected pharynx, or "strawberry tongue"
- At least one of the following: extremity changes: erythema of the palms or soles, edema of the hands or feet, or periungual desquamation
- Polymorphous exanthem
- Acute nonsuppurative cervical lymphadenopathy (at least one node ≥1.5 cm in diameter)

If left untreated, patients are at risk of coronary aneurysms. It should be noted that individually the signs of KD can be subtle and very nonspecific. Furthermore, there is no diagnostic test that absolutely confirms the diagnosis. As such, the practitioner needs to be vigilant in examining any pediatric patient with "prolonged" fever.

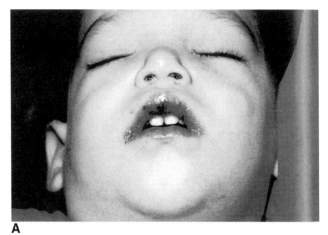

A

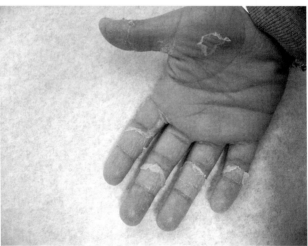

B

Fig. 14-2 Patient with Kawasaki disease. **A,** Dry, fissured lips. See Color Insert. **B,** Desquamation of palms. (Courtesy Anthony J. Mancini, MD, Chicago.)

Workup

- CBC showing leukocytosis and thrombocytosis.
- ESR or C-reactive protein elevation.
- UA showing sterile pyuria (the WBCs are monocytes, which may appear on Gram stain but will not be leukocyte esterase positive).
- Liver function tests and bilirubin level may show elevation (hydrops of the gallbladder has been associated with KD).
- Cardiac echocardiogram (evidence of ectasia or aneurysm virtually confirms the diagnosis).
- Ophthalmologic examination (which can reveal anterior uveitis).

Comments and Treatment Considerations

Recognizing KD is critical to prevent or ameliorate coronary artery aneurysms or ectasia, which if left untreated, occur in about 20% of patients. In Japan, where the disease was first described, KD is the leading cause of myocardial infarction in the pediatric age-group. Risk factors for developing coronary aneurysms with KD include male gender, age younger than 1 year, prolonged period of inflammation (including fever for >10 days), and recurrence of fever after treatment. In the first 6 months of life the classic features of disease may not be appreciated and the diagnosis of "atypical Kawasaki syndrome" should be considered, particularly because this age-group is at high risk of coronary artery involvement.

Many tertiary pediatric centers have cardiologists or rheumatologists with specific expertise in KD who should be consulted. An echocardiogram performed by an experienced pediatric practitioner should be ordered. Treatment generally consists of IV immune globulin (IVIG) and oral aspirin. IVIG is typically given as a single infusion of 2 g/kg IV over 8 to 12 hours. Premedication with an antihistamine, antipyretic, and/or hydrocortisone may be necessary. Epinephrine should be immediately available to treat anaphylactic reactions (see Chapter 29, Rash). Children who remain febrile after 24 to 48 hours after the initial IVIG dose may receive a second infusion. Aspirin is started at "high dose" 80 to 100 mg/kg/day PO divided q6h during the acute phase of the disease. It is changed to "low dose" (3 to 5 mg/kg/day PO every day) for its antiplatelet effect upon resolution of fever. Aspirin is usually discontinued after 6 to 8 weeks if the coronary arteries are normal. The patient with fever after two doses of IVIG or coronary artery abnormalities should be followed by a pediatric rheumatologist or cardiologist.

 ## NEUROLEPTIC MALIGNANT SYNDROME

Neuroleptic malignant syndrome can be induced by several medications including haloperidol, phenothiazines, lithium, and reserpine. The features can appear quite similar to malignant hyperthermia, although a different mechanism is believed responsible.

Signs
• Muscular rigidity
• Mental status changes

Workup
• Creatine kinase.
• UA for possible myoglobinuria.

Comments and Treatment Considerations
Treatment is generally supportive with cooling, monitoring, and in severe cases the administration of dantrolene (see the treatment considerations for malignant hyperthermia in the next section), bromocriptine, or even neuromuscular blockade. The offending medication should be discontinued.

 ## MALIGNANT HYPERTHERMIA

Malignant hyperthermia occurs in genetically susceptible patients as the result of administration of inhaled anesthetic agents or succinylcholine. The onset of fever can occur immediately or several hours after exposure. Differential diagnosis includes sepsis, thyroid storm, and pheochromocytoma.

Signs
- Muscle rigidity (may include masseter spasm)
- Tachycardia
- Tachypnea
- Acidosis
- Ventricular arrhythmia
- Hyperthermia

Comments and Treatment Considerations

Management consists of discontinuation of the offending agent, hyperventilation, and dantrolene at an initial dose of 2 to 2.5 mg/kg IV bolus with repeated doses as needed every 5 minutes up to a total dose of 10 mg/kg. Because dantrolene is necessary for the successful treatment of these patients, it may be necessary to have a single clinician focus on the mixing and administration of this drug while others attend the acute issues of care. The 20-mg vial of dantrolene must be reconstituted with 60 ml of sterile water for injection *only* and may not be further diluted with normal saline or dextrose in water. Use extreme caution in patients maintained on calcium channel blockers, because dantrolene may precipitate cardiovascular collapse. After dantrolene use, observation for at least 24 hours in an intensive care unit is recommended. Dantrolene therapy is continued post-crisis until CPK levels begin to drop (4 to 8 mg/kg/day divided qid for 1 to 3 days).

 ## HEATSTROKE

The diagnosis of heatstroke should be considered in any patient coming to the ED with a temperature (usually >40.5° C) and a recent history of heat exposure or notable exertion. The onset can be very rapid (generally minutes to a couple of hours) and it is often difficult to initially appreciate this diagnosis.

Symptoms

Symtoms are generally vague and nonspecific.
- Weakness
- Dizziness

- Nausea
- Vomiting
- Anorexia
- Frontal headache
- CNS symptoms (drowsiness, disorientation, anxiety, or irritability/psychosis)

Workup

- PT, PTT, and disseminated intravascular coagulation (DIC) panel.
- Liver function tests.
- Creatine kinase.
- Electrolytes, including BUN and SCr.
- pH level.
- Lactate.

Comments and Treatment Considerations

General supportive critical care management must be instituted in parallel with cooling measures. The degree of neurologic injury is likely a product of the height and duration of temperature elevation. Cases of complete recovery despite very high rectal temperatures (46° C) have been reported.

Cooling should be begun emergently because delay is associated with increased mortality and morbidity. Ice water immersion appears to be the most successful modality for rapid cooling and may secondarily have the benefit of causing peripheral vasoconstriction that may assist in the management of associated hypotension. In the ED setting, evaporative cooling using circulating fans and cold water is commonly employed in addition to the application of ice packs. In some cases gastric and rectal lavage can be helpful but should not be the primary modality of cooling.

Concerning complications include DIC, elevation in transaminases, rhabdomyolysis, acute renal failure, hypocalcemia, lactic acidosis, and cardiovascular collapse. Shivering or shaking chills should not be seen and would suggest another cause for the temperature elevation.

DRUG FEVER

The term *drug fever* is generally used in relation to the administration of a medication in usual therapeutic doses with the development of fever occurring as a side effect. Most often this type of fever will begin approximately 7 to 10 days after initiation of the medication but can occur at any time. Penicillins, sulfonamides, phenytoin, furosemide, salicylates, antihistamines, barbiturates, procainamide, quinidine, methyldopa, isoniazid, allopurinol, and cimetidine are among the medications commonly cited as causing drug fevers. Most often the fever will resolve within 2 days of withdrawal of the medication, but this is not universally the case.

It should be noted that some drugs cause hyperthermia as a direct result of either excessive heat production associated with agitation, muscular hyperactivity, or seizures or increased muscle tone. Examples of drugs that can do this include amphetamines, cocaine, LSD, PCP, tricyclic antidepressants, antihistamines, monoamine oxidase inhibitors, and strychnine.

Other medications such as adrenergic receptor agonists and those with anticholinergic effects may impair the ability to dissipate heat and in times of heat exposure or exertion may result in some degree of hyperthermia (see Chapter 35, Toxic Ingestion, Approach To).

REFERENCES

Bachur R, Perry H, Harper M: Empiric chest radiographs in febrile children with leukocytosis, *Ann Emerg Med* 33(4):480, 1999.

Bachur RG, Harper MB: Predictive model for serious bacterial infections among infants younger than 3 months of age, *Pediatrics* 108(2):311-316, 2001.

Baker MD: Evaluation and management of infants with fever, *Pediatr Clin North Am* 46(6):1061-1072, 1999.

Baskin MN, O'Rourke EJ, Fleisher GR: Outpatient treatment of febrile infants 28 to 89 days of age with intramuscular administration of ceftriaxone, *J Pediatr* 120(1):22-27, 1992.

Bonadio WA, Hegenbarth M, Zachariason M: Correlating reported fever in young infants with subsequent temperature patterns and rate of serious bacterial infections. *Pediatr Infect Dis J* 9(3): 158–160, 1990.

Hall SC: General pediatric emergencies: malignant hyperthermia syndrome, *Anesth Clin North Am* 19(2):367-382, 2001.

Jaskiewicz JA, McCarthy CA, Richardson AC, et al: Febrile infants at low risk for serious bacterial infection—an appraisal of the Rochester criteria and implications for management. Febrile Infant Collaborative Study Group, *Pediatrics* 94(3):390-396, 1994.

Kuppermann N: Occult bacteremia in young febrile children, *Pediatr Clin North Am* 46(6):1073-1109, 1999.

Lee GM, Fleisher GR, Harper MB: Management of febrile children in the age of the conjugate pneumococcal vaccine: a cost-effectiveness analysis, *Pediatrics* 108(4):835-844, 2001.

Shaw KN, Gorelick M, McGowan KL, et al: Prevalence of urinary tract infection in febrile young children in the emergency department, *Pediatrics* 102(2):e16, 1998.

CHAPTER 15

Fractures Not to Miss

ANDREA STRACCIOLINI

Trauma is a common reason for children to seek medical attention. Fortunately, most childhood injuries are not severe due to a variety of factors, including lower forces involved in the mechanism of injury and the greater elasticity of bone, cartilage, and soft tissues as compared to adults. However, because the skeleton is immature and needs to maintain potential for growth, a missed diagnosis can cause significant morbidity. Metaphyseal fractures of the extremities in children younger than 2 years are strongly suggestive of nonaccidental trauma (see Chapter 2, Abuse/Rape).

This chapter provides an overview of bony injuries seen in children, including descriptions of fractures in general, as well as specific bone and joint injuries. Cervical injuries are covered in Chapter 36, Trauma.

GENERAL FRACTURE TYPES

SALTER-HARRIS FRACTURES

The most significant difference between pediatric and adult fractures is due to the presence of the growth plate (physis) in the long bones of children. Identification of fractures involving the growth plates is essential because of the potential implications for impaired growth. Furthermore, because of the presence of these growth plates, the pattern of long bone injuries in children is quite different from that in adults. First, growth plates act as shock absorbers, and as a result comminuted fractures are rare. Second, growth plates are weaker than ligaments, so sprains are uncommon in children. Finally,

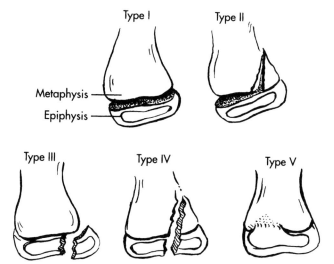

Fig. 15-1 Salter-Harris classification of growth-plate fractures in children. (From Davis M, Votey, S, Greenough PG: *Signs and symptoms in emergency medicine,* St. Louis, 1999, Mosby.)

growth plates allow for greater modification after injury or, in other words, children's bones can straighten themselves out.

Growth-plate injuries are classified according to the Salter-Harris system (Fig. 15-1).

- Salter-Harris type I: Epiphyseal separation through the physis: may or may not be displaced; if undisplaced, the radiographs may show no abnormalities.
- Salter-Harris type II: A triangular fragment of the metaphysis remains attached to the epiphysis (Thurston-Holland sign), with the separation also through the physis.
- Salter-Harris type III: Physeal separation that passes through the epiphysis and into the joint; this leads to an intraarticular fracture; possible joint incongruity may occur if not anatomically reduced.
- Salter-Harris type IV: Fracture passes through the metaphysis, growth plate, and epiphysis into the joint; as

with type III injuries, an anatomic reduction is necessary for continued growth and joint congruity.
- Salter-Harris type V can be diagnosed only in retrospect and is due to a compression injury of the physis that leads to permanent injury.

Symptoms
- Pain with motion of the extremity
- Neurologic symptoms including tingling and numbness with significant displacement

Signs
- Swelling
- Deformity
- Tenderness over physis
- Joint incongruity
- Growth disturbance because of growth-plate arrest (late sign if untreated)

Workup
- Two views on x-ray of the injured area.

Comments and Treatment Considerations
Orthopedic consultation should be obtained for any patient with a growth-plate injury with the possible exception of a Salter I fracture. Growth-plate injuries that have neurovascular impairment are a true orthopedic emergency. Patients who are neurovascularly intact can often be splinted in an anatomically neutral position and can follow up with orthopedics on an urgent basis.

Familiarity of the location and appearance of growth plates is essential in identifying Salter-Harris fractures. A "normal" growth plate can have a contour that appears irregular and may be misdiagnosed as a fracture. One can always obtain comparison views of the contralateral extremity to help differentiate between fractures and growth plates.

Finally, all growth-plate injuries have the potential to impair longitudinal growth, especially types III, IV, and V. Orthopedic follow-up in these patients is essential.

GREENSTICK AND BOWING FRACTURES

Because bone is more plastic in children and the periosteum is quite thick, greenstick (fracture through only one side of the cortex) and bowing (persistent plastic deformation) fractures are seen in children. These fractures typically will not remodel without orthopedic reduction to achieve acceptable anatomic and cosmetic result.

TORUS (BUCKLE) FRACTURES

Because of the more plastic nature of children's bones, torus (or buckle) fractures are also common in children. These fractures occur at the metaphysis from a compressive load, which causes the cortex to buckle (Fig. 15-2). These fractures are typically quite stable, and because they do not involve the physis directly, they do not have implications for longitudinal growth. These fractures are usually treated by casting, although the injury may be splinted in an anatomically neutral position with orthopedic follow-up.

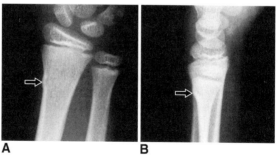

A **B**

Fig. 15-2 Torus fracture of the distal radius resulting from a fall on an outstretched arm. **A,** An anteroposterior radiograph of the wrist shows a minor torus or buckle fracture of the radius. **B,** The lateral radiograph shows the dorsal location of the deformity. This injury can be expected to completely remodel. (From Zitelli B, Davis H: *Atlas of pediatric physical diagnosis*, 4th ed, St. Louis, 2002, Mosby.)

SUPRACONDYLAR FRACTURES

Supracondylar fractures are the most common fractures of the elbow in children younger than 8 years. The mechanism of injury involves a fall onto an outstretched hand and the olecranon forcefully abuts the olecranon fossa, causing disruption of the anterior cortex with posterior displacement of the distal fragment. Because of the proximity of the neurovascular structures, orthopedic consultation is required for all supracondylar fractures.

Supracondylar fractures are further classified as follows:
- Type I undisplaced
- Type II displaced in extension with intact posterior cortex
- Type III displaced with no cortical contact
  - Posteromedial rotation of the distal fragment
  - Posterolateral rotation of the distal fragment

Symptoms
- Pain with motion of the joint
- Neurologic symptoms, including paresthesias; present in 10% to 18% of displaced supracondylar fractures

Signs
- Pallor of the extremity with vascular compromise—late finding in compartment syndrome
- Weak or absent pulse is not uncommon and is most often the result of arterial spasm; it may be a late finding in compartment syndrome or arterial injury
- Soft-tissue tenting and dimpling are also signs of soft-tissue injury, which suggest reduction should be performed promptly
- Loss of two-point discrimination >6 mm with nerve injury (should always be compared to the contralateral side)
- Loss of vibratory perception with nerve injury may be a more sensitive test when there is only mild to moderate nerve compression, in which case two-point discrimination may be normal
- Loss of sympathetic innervation from nerve dysfunction may cause the skin to become dry in the area of distribution

Workup

- Anteroposterior (AP) and true lateral radiographs are required (Fig. 15-3).

Comments and Treatment Considerations

Type II and III supracondylar fractures are quite obvious on x-ray. The determination of the anterior humeral line (a line drawn down the anterior humeral cortex through the capitellum)

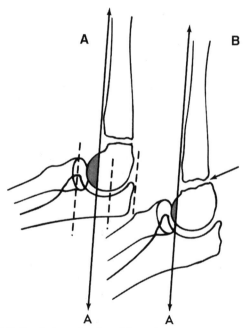

Fig. 15-3 Depiction of a "true" lateral view to assess possible supracondylar fracture. **A,** Normal: One third of capitellum lies anterior to anterior humeral line. **B,** Less than one third of capitellum lying anterior to humeral line indicates a probable supracondylar fracture *(arrow). A,* Anterior humeral line. (From Davis M, Votey, S, Greenough PG: *Signs and symptoms in emergency medicine,* St. Louis, 1999, Mosby. Courtesy Michael F. Rodi, MD.)

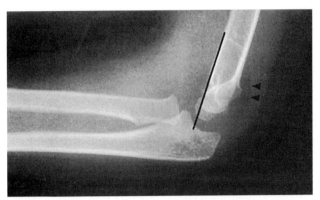

Fig. 15-4 Lateral view of elbow shows supracondylar fracture in a child. The posterior fat pad is displaced (*arrowheads*), indicating hemarthrosis. The anterior humeral line is abnormal, indicating posterior displacement of the distal humerus (*line*). (From Davis M, Votey, S, Greenough PG: *Signs and symptoms in emergency medicine,* St. Louis, 1999, Mosby. Courtesy Michael Zucker, MD, Los Angeles, CA.)

and Baumann's angle (formed by the growth plate of the capitellum and the long axis of the humeral shaft) is useful in detecting subtle type I fractures. Furthermore, the presence of a posterior fat pad on radiograph suggests hemarthrosis secondary to intraarticular injury and a type I fracture (Fig. 15-4).

All supracondylar fractures require orthopedic consultation, especially in the case of an open fracture or if there is evidence of neurovascular impairment. Type I fractures may simply require immobilization, whereas type II and III fractures generally require operative reduction and alignment.

✚ *MONTEGGIA FRACTURE DISLOCATION OF THE ELBOW*

The Monteggia fracture dislocation is a fracture of the proximal third of the ulna associated with a dislocation of the radial head (Fig. 15-5). The Monteggia fracture accounts for 2% of elbow

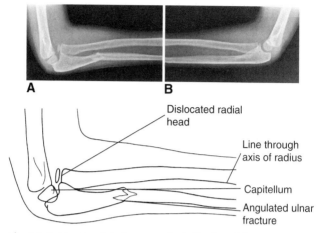

A   **B**

Dislocated radial head

Line through axis of radius

Capitellum

Angulated ulnar fracture

Fig. 15-5 Monteggia's fracture. **A,** A displaced fracture of the proximal right ulna is accompanied by dislocation of the radial head. A line drawn through the long axis of the radius would intersect the distal humerus above the level of the capitellum. **B,** The comparison view of the left arm shows the normal position of the radial head. (From Zitelli B, Davis H: *Atlas of pediatric physical diagnosis,* 4th ed, St. Louis, 2002, Mosby. **A** and **B** Courtesy Department of Radiology, Children's Hospital of Pittsburgh, Pittsburgh, PA.)

fractures in children. Fractures of the radius or ulna often are accompanied by dislocation of the radial head or the distal radioulnar joint (DRUJ). Mechanisms of injury that result in an anterior or lateral dislocation of the radial head include: hyperextension of the elbow with a fall on the outstretched hand, hyperpronation of the elbow with a fall on the outstretched hand, and a direct blow to the posterior aspect of the forearm. Hyperextension of the elbow is believed to be the most common mechanism of injury in children. Because of the proximity of the elbow to the brachial artery and the ulnar, median, and radial nerves, a detailed neurovascular examination is essential to rule out injuries to these structures.

Symptoms
- Pain

Signs
- Deformity
- Swelling of the joint and area overlying fracture
- Absence of finger extension at the metacarpophalangeal joints and inability to extend the thumb at the interphalangeal joint if injury has occurred to the interosseous nerve
- Decreased sensation on the distal dorsal aspect of the thumb with injury to the sensory branch of the radial nerve
- Tenderness with palpation of the proximal ulna and in the region of the displaced radial head, which may be visible or palpable just beneath the skin

Workup
- AP and lateral radiographs of the entire radius and ulna that include the wrist and elbow joints are essential.

Comments and Treatment Considerations
A line drawn through the long axis of the radial neck must bisect the capitellum in all views to rule out a radial head or DRUJ dislocation (Fig. 15-6). Comparison radiographs of the opposite elbow are often helpful in children. One needs to maintain a high index of suspicion of a possible dislocation, especially with a plastic deformation (bowing fracture) of the ulna. Orthopedic consultation is essential.

 ## GALEAZZI FRACTURE-DISLOCATION

The Galeazzi injury is a fracture of the shaft of the radius with an associated dislocation of the distal radioulnar articulation. Most patients with this type of injury are older than 10 years of age. The injury often is a greenstick type of fracture with angular displacement. Generally the dislocation of the DRUJ is evident clinically and radiographically. The main stabilizer of the DRUJ is the triangular fibrocartilage complex (TFCC). There can be no dislocation of the DRUJ without disruption of the TFCC. The

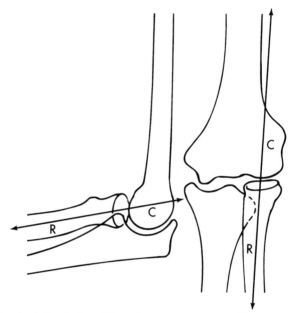

Fig. 15-6 Depiction of "true" anteroposterior and lateral views of the elbow to assess possible dislocation of the radial head. *R*, Radius; *C*, capitellum. *Arrows* represent the radiocapitellar line drawn through the shaft of the radius; if the line does not pass through the capitellum, the radial head is likely dislocated. (From Davis M, Votey, S, Greenough PG: *Signs and symptoms in emergency medicine*, St. Louis, 1999, Mosby. Courtesy Michael F. Rodi, MD.)

function of the TFCC is to limit the rotational movements of the radius and ulna relative to each another. In the neutral position, the distal radius and ulna are compressed against each other. The most likely mechanism of injury is a fall on the outstretched hand combined with extreme pronation of the forearm.

Symptoms
• Pain that localizes to the ulnar side of the wrist

Signs

- Tenderness around the TFCC with compression of the DRUJ
- "Clicking" at the extremes of pronation and supination
- Distal radius and ulna instability on range of motion. Physical exam may demonstrate crepitus, grinding, or laxity of the DRUJ
- Ulnar dorsal dislocation
  - Increased dorsal prominence over the distal ulna compared with the unaffected side
  - Forearm fixed in pronation
  - Pain with supination of the wrist
- Ulnar volar dislocation
  - Furrow on the dorsal-ulnar side of the wrist
  - Prominence on the volar aspect
  - Fixed in supination
  - Pain over the DRUJ

Workup

- AP and lateral views of the wrist, forearm, and elbow; a true lateral radiograph of the wrist is the critical film to be obtained, which can reveal an ulnar styloid base fracture. Radiographs should be evaluated for widening of the DRUJ space on the AP view, dislocation on the lateral view, or >5-mm radial shortening (relative to the ulna).
- CT scan of the wrist if high clinical suspicion; should be performed on both the injured and the uninjured side with the same degree of forearm rotation for comparison.

Comments and Treatment Considerations

Most Galeazzi dislocation fractures yield poor results with closed reduction and cast immobilization. Orthopedics consultation is imperative because open reduction/internal fixation with stabilization of the radius fracture using a dynamic compression plate is suggested.

 SCAPHOID FRACTURES

The scaphoid fracture is the most common carpal bone injury in children. Most of these fractures occur in adolescence during the last stages of endochondral ossification. The mechanism of injury is falling on the outstretched hand. Diagnosis of the nondisplaced scaphoid fracture can be difficult.

Symptoms
- Pain with range of motion of the wrist

Signs
- Anatomic snuffbox/scaphoid tenderness
- Swelling of the radial aspect of the wrist

Workup
- Optimal plain radiographs should include at least two orthogonal views of the wrist but may be negative even in the presence of a significant fracture.
- Scaphoid view, with the wrist in ulnar deviation is useful.
- Comparison view of the contralateral uninjured wrist may be helpful.
- MRI or bone scan can confirm the diagnosis in patients in whom there is a high clinical suspicion of injury but with negative findings on plain film.

Comments and Treatment Considerations
If clinical suspicion is high and radiographs show no abnormalities, prescribe immobilization of the wrist for 1 or 2 weeks and reimage to make the diagnosis. All real or suspected scaphoid fractures should be immobilized in a short-arm thumb spica cast. Because pediatric scaphoid fractures are rarely displaced, scaphoid fractures in children usually heal with nonoperative treatment with a short-arm thumb spica cast. Osteonecrosis is uncommon in children.

 ANKLE FRACTURES

Acute trauma to the ankle can result in soft-tissue or bony injury. Physeal fractures are the most common ankle injuries seen in children because the physes are weaker than the adjacent bones and ligaments. The most common injuries are inversion injuries.

One must be aware that inversion injuries in children frequently involve the foot. Fractures of the foot that are often missed are covered in the following sections.

LISFRANC'S JOINT FRACTURES

Lisfranc's joint fractures occur in the proximal portion of the second metatarsal and involve the volar and medial aspects of Lisfranc's joint. The more proximally recessed middle cuneiform forms the base of this articulation, with adjacent cuneiforms locking the proximal head of the second metatarsal into a rigid socket. As a result, this joint is prone to injury. The patient comes to the emergency department with pain on ambulation over the mid-dorsum of the foot and swelling and tenderness over the proximal second metatarsal. The diagnosis can be difficult and is often delayed, requiring radiographs, CT, and bone scan.

MAISONNEUVE FRACTURE

The deltoid ligament is disrupted and forces travel up the syndesmosis to the proximal leg. Forces exit laterally, resulting in high fibular fracture, and this can be missed if one obtains ankle films only and does not examine the proximal leg. This results in a seriously unstable ankle joint. Orthopedic consultation is required if one suspects this injury.

METATARSAL FRACTURES

Fractures of the fifth metatarsal often occur with inversion injuries. The Jones fracture is less common in children and involves a transverse fracture of the proximal diametaphyseal junction involving the fourth to fifth metatarsal articulation caused by forefoot adduction. The Jones fracture is minimally displaced.

More commonly in children the peroneus brevis tendon is pulled taut and avulses (fractures) the base of the fifth metatarsal. The presence of the apophysis of the base of the fifth metatarsal on radiographs may confuse evaluation but can be clarified by examination of comparison radiographs of the opposite uninvolved foot. The proximal fifth metatarsal has a poor blood supply and is at significant risk of nonunion. The use of crutches and partial weight bearing until pain subsides are usually sufficient treatment for these types of injuries.

TODDLER'S FRACTURE

A toddler's fracture classically refers to an oblique nondisplaced fracture of the tibia. There is often (but not always) a history of relatively minor trauma, followed by a complaint of limp.

Symptoms
- Pain
- Limp or refusal to walk or bear weight
- Fussiness

Signs
- Swelling, most often minimal
- Tenderness with gentle twisting

Workup
- X-ray of the lower extremity: In addition to AP and lateral views, an oblique view is often required to make the diagnosis.
- Bone scan is often done when symptoms (i.e., limp) persist in the absence of other radiographic findings.

Comments and Treatment Considerations

Immobilization (i.e., casting) provides symptomatic relief, although no treatment may be necessary if the injury is thought to have occurred weeks ago.

 ## *CLAVICULAR FRACTURE*

Clavicular fractures are one of the most commonly encountered musculoskeletal injuries in children younger than 10 years. Clavicular fractures are classified according to the location of the injury: outer end (lateral), midportion (shaft), and inner end (medial). Most of these fractures occur in the midportion near the juncture of the double curves that form the clavicle. The most common mechanism of injury is the result of a blow to the shoulder girdle followed by a fall on an outstretched arm. These fractures can also occur during the birth process, especially in newborns weighing >3800 g. The fractures are usually nondisplaced or minimally displaced. These fractures heal rapidly, usually within 7 to 10 days.

Symptoms
• Pain, especially with motion of shoulder ++++

Signs
Newborns
• Difficulty identifying the margins of the affected clavicle
• Crepitus on palpation of the clavicle
• Overlying hematoma
• Infants head tilted toward side of fracture
• Refusal to feed from one breast versus the other
• Pain with range of motion of the upper extremity
• Asymmetric Moro's reflex with pseudoparalysis of the limb
• Midshaft bump (approximately day 10 of life)

Children
• Hematoma and swelling over the fracture site
• Tenting of overlying skin
• Shoulder may droop in the forward position to splint the fracture
• Palpable and visible globular mass of new bone at fracture site during healing phase

Workup
• X-ray of clavicle.

Comments and Treatment Considerations
Treatment for toddlers and juveniles usually involves immobilization of the extremity for comfort using a sling or figure-of-eight clavicle strap. As healing occurs a globular mass of new bone forms about the fracture ends that is palpable and visually prominent. Complete fractures with side-to-side

bayonet apposition exhibit the greatest healing response. The remodeling potential of the child results in near-anatomic restoration of shape within 12 months. Older juveniles and teens have less remodeling potential and a greater possibility of a residual bump at the fracture site. The differential diagnosis for clavicular fractures in newborns includes fracture of the proximal humerus, spinal nerve root avulsions, and brachial plexus injury. In the neonate or older infant acute osteomyelitis of the proximal humerus and septic shoulder joint must be considered.

RADIAL HEAD SUBLUXATION (NURSE MAID'S ELBOW)

Radial head subluxation (nursemaid's elbow) is not a true fracture, but a subluxation of the radial head from the annular ligament. The patient has pain because of the course of the ulnar nerve behind the radial head. The mechanism of injury is a quick jerk (traction) of the forearm, wrist, or hand. The injury can also be seen as a result of a fall. The injury usually occurs in children between the ages of 6 months and 5 years.

Symptoms
- Pain with movement of the arm
- Not moving the arm (pseudoparalysis)
- No or minimal complaints if the arm is not moved

Signs
- Child holds arm out with forearm in pronation and elbow in extension
- No point tenderness, swelling, or neurovascular compromise

Workup
- The diagnosis is made clinically.
- X-ray to rule out underlying bony injury if a clear mechanism cannot be obtained from the history.

Comments and Treatment Consideration

The subluxed radial head can be reduced in a variety of methods. The most common is a quick supination and flexion of the elbow joint while providing gentle traction on the forearm. A subtle "click" can be felt over the radial head as it is reduced. The patient should be using the arm within several minutes of the reduction, although some children may continue to refuse due to the "memory" of the pain prior to reduction. One should have a low index of suspicion to image the elbow if the patient does not start moving the arm after two or three attempts at reduction and a short period of observation. As children age, a bony lip forms at the radial head, making this injury exceedingly uncommon in children older than 5 years. X-rays should definitely be obtained in this older age-group.

REFERENCES

England SP, Sundberg S: Management of common pediatric fractures, *Pediatr Clin of North Am* 43(5):991-1011, 1996.

Le TB, Hentz VR: Hand and wrist injuries in young athletes, *Hand Clin* 16(4):597-606, 2000.

Light T: Carpal injuries in children, *Hand Clin* 16(4):513-521, 2000.

Lins RE, Simovitch RW, Waters PM: Pediatric elbow trauma, *Orthop Clin North Am* 30(1):119-131, 1999.

Marsh JS, Daigneault JP: Ankle injuries in the pediatric population, *Curr Opin Pediatr* 12:52-60, 2000.

Micheli LJ, Sohn RS, Solomon R: Stress fracture of the second metatarsal involving Lisfranc's joint in ballet dancers, *J Bone Joint Surg* 67-A(9):1372-1375, 1985.

Nicolaidis SC, Hildreth DH, Lichtman DM: Acute injuries of the distal radioulnar joint, *Hand Clin* 16(3):449-458, 2000.

Pizzitullo PD: *Pediatrics orthopedics in primary care*, New York, 1997, McGraw-Hill.

Rockwood CA, Kaye EW, Beaty JH: *Fractures in children*, 4th ed, vol 3, Philadelphia, 1996, Lippincott–Raven Press.

Skaggs D, Pershad J: Pediatric elbow trauma, *Pediatr Emerg Care* 13(6):425-434, 1997.

CHAPTER 16

Gastrointestinal Bleeding

RON KAPLAN

Gastrointestinal bleeding (GIB) is a relatively common complaint in the pediatric population. In contrast to adults, most children with GIB do not have significant hemorrhage or evidence of hemodynamic instability. However, potentially life-threatening causes of GIB do occur.

The initial approach to the child with GIB requires assessment of the severity of bleeding and beginning emergency therapy for significant blood loss. Obtaining history, physical examination results, and laboratory study results aid in diagnosis and management. Signs of significant blood loss include tachycardia, pallor, prolonged capillary refill time, and as a late ominous sign, hypotension. If evidence of significant blood loss is found, immediate management should begin even before further evaluation of etiology (see the section Emergent Management of Gastrointestinal Bleeding, later in this chapter).

Children with bleeding diatheses or known thrombocytopenia are a special consideration (see Chapter 6, Bleeding and Bruising), although initial management is unchanged. It is imperative to test vomitus or stool in cases of suspected GIB by Gastroccult or Hemoccult, respectively, because many dyes, drugs, and foods can mimic the color of blood or melena. Common offenders include Jell-O gelatin, Kool-Aid, other fruit juices, beets, iron, dark chocolate, bismuth, drugs, and licorice.

As appropriate resuscitative measures are instituted, the severity of the bleeding and the level of bleeding within the gastrointestinal (GI) tract are determined. GIB is classified as upper GIB (UGIB) when the site of bleeding is proximal to the ligament of Treitz or lower GIB (LGIB) when the bleeding occurs distal to the ligament. Chronic or recurrent bleeding is not discussed in detail and often requires consultation with a gastroenterologist and endoscopy or colonoscopy for diagnosis.

Specific diagnoses are suggested by age, history, physical examination, and laboratory test results. Specific treatment is tailored to the underlying diagnosis.

 ## EMERGENT MANAGEMENT OF GASTROINTESTINAL BLEEDING

The first priority is attention to the ABCs and assessment of hemodynamic stability. Two large-bore intravenous catheters should be placed and blood emergently sent for type and cross-match in addition to baseline laboratory testing (see the later sections). Crystalloid is the initial fluid indicated for volume replacement. Either 0.9% normal saline or lactated Ringer's solution at 20 ml/kg is appropriate and may be repeated to a total of 60 to 80 ml/kg until the patient is stable or packed red blood cells (PRBCs) can be started. Patients with large or ongoing hemorrhage or persistent hemodynamic instability despite 40 to 60 ml/kg of crystalloid will require blood transfusion. O-negative blood may be needed unless time allows for matched blood (see Chapter 6, Bleeding and Bruising, and Chapter 20, Hypotension/Shock, for treatment recommendations). Octreotide may be considered for patients with ongoing UGI bleed dosed as: 1 mcg/kg (max 50 to 100 mcg) initial bolus followed by 1 mcg/kg/hr (max 50 mcg/hr to start) continuous infusion; titrate infusion rate to response; taper dose by 50% every 12 hrs when no active bleeding occurs for 24 hrs. Infusion may be discontinued when dose is 25% of initial dose.

Attention should be given to correcting coagulopathies with specific clotting factors or fresh frozen plasma (see Chapter 6, Bleeding and Bruising). A surgeon or gastroenterologist should be emergently consulted to aid in identification of ongoing blood loss.

UPPER GASTROINTESTINAL BLEEDING

UGIB may originate from the mouth, nasopharynx, esophagus, stomach, biliary tree, or duodenum. An upper GI source may be obvious in the patient with hematemesis or coffee-ground emesis but should also be considered in the patient with melena because blood from an upper GI source will eventually be seen in the stool.

Etiologies to Consider
- Mucosal gastroesophageal lesions account for 95% of cases of UGIB and include esophagitis, gastritis, Mallory-Weiss tear, peptic ulcer disease, and duodenitis.
- In newborns, consider swallowed maternal blood, hemorrhagic disease of the newborn if prophylactic vitamin K was not administered at birth, or history of umbilical catheterization complicated by thrombosis.
- Oropharyngeal, tracheal, or pulmonary bleeding may be confused with UGIB and may include epistaxis, hemoptysis, oral or posterior pharyngeal bleeding, and, rarely, swallowed foreign bodies.
- Esophageal or gastric varices, especially in patients with underlying disease such as portal hypertension or liver disease.
- Toxic effect of ingestion or drugs such as aspirin, NSAIDs, alcohol, or steroids.

Symptoms
- Hematemesis indicates active UGIB
- Coffee-ground emesis suggests UGIB that may or may not be ongoing
- Melena suggests bleeding from the upper GI tract or proximal small bowel
- Hematochezia may be seen with massive UGIB because blood is a cathartic

Signs
- Occult or gross blood in stool
- Signs of hypovolemia such as tachycardia, increased capillary refill, and eventually hypotension (ominous)
- Pallor (sign of anemia)

- Signs of bleeding diatheses such as easy bruising, or mucosal bleeding
- Signs of liver disease such as hepatomegaly, jaundice, or ascites

Workup

- Blood for type and crossmatch.
- CBC, remembering that hematocrit is an unreliable index of acute blood loss, but a baseline value is useful to assess for severe anemia and for later comparison. A low mean corpuscular volume and hypochromic microcytic anemia suggest chronic mucosal bleeding.
- Other laboratory studies to consider are coagulation studies, liver function tests, *Helicobacter pylori* antigen, and Apt test in newborns. The Apt test in newborns will differentiate swallowed maternal blood from fetal blood and requires very small amounts, which may be dried and scooped off a cloth or diaper.
- Nasogastric lavage if significant UGIB is suspected, to assess amount of blood in stomach and ongoing losses.
- Abdominal films are not generally helpful unless perforation is suspected.

Comments and Treatment Considerations

After hemodynamic stability has been obtained (see the earlier section on emergency management of GIB), the cause of bleeding must be sought. Most cases of UGIB in children (95%) come from mucosal lesions and are self-limited. Admission with IV therapy with an H_2 antagonist such as ranitidine 3 to 4 mg/kg/day IV divided q6-8h (max 50 mg/dose) may be warranted. Endoscopy may be necessary to determine the site of bleeding and for therapeutic measures in patients with large UGIB, those with ongoing UGIB, or those who required transfusion. If endoscopy cannot determine the site of bleeding, arteriography or labeled RBC studies may be necessary. Consultation as needed with a gastroenterologist or surgeon is recommended.

Patients with acute, minor self-limited UGIB with no evidence of hemodynamic instability or ongoing hemorrhage may safely be discharged from the emergency department with instructions for appropriate follow-up. Patients with suspected gastritis or ulcer disease should be given an H_2 antagonist such as ranitidine 4 to 6 mg/kg/day PO divided bid (max 150 mg/dose) or a proton pump inhibitor such as omeprazole 0.7 to 3.5 mg/kg/day PO divided qd-bid (max 20 mg/dose). If *H. pylori* positive, an effective antibiotic regimen along with a proton pump inhibitor should be prescribed for 10 to 14 days. One example includes amoxicillin 25 to 50 mg/kg/day PO divided bid (max 1000 mg/dose) plus clarithromycin 15 mg/kg/day PO divided bid (max 500 mg/dose) plus omeprazole as dosed above. Consultation with a pediatric gastroenterologist is recommended.

LOWER GASTROINTESTINAL BLEEDING

LGIB can present with melena, hematochezia, and "currant jelly" or maroon stool. Melena typically represents old blood that has been oxidized, hematochezia represents fresh blood, and currant jelly or maroon blood is indicative of bowel ischemia.

Etiologies to Consider

- Infectious gastroenteritis is the most common cause of LGIB among all ages, commonly seen with bacterial enterocolitis or hemolytic uremic syndrome (HUS) (see Chapter 10, Diarrhea, and Chapter 38, Vomiting).
- In newborns, consider the life-threatening diagnosis of midgut volvulus, especially if bleeding is associated with bilious emesis, abdominal pain, and distention (see Chapter 1, Abdominal Pain). Other etiologies include swallowed maternal blood (see the previous section), allergic colitis from milk protein sensitivity, Hirschsprung's disease (especially in infants who do not pass meconium in the first 24 to 48 hours), and necrotizing enterocolitis (NEC) with 10% of cases occurring in full-term infants.
- Pseudomembranous colitis associated with *Clostridium difficile* toxin may be seen in patients with recent antibiotic use.

- Intussusception may occur at any age but most commonly occurs in children older than 3 months and less than 2 years (see Chapter 1, Abdominal Pain).
- Juvenile colonic polyps may be seen at any age; 30% to 40% are palpable on rectal examination. Many are benign and multiple, causing painless rectal bleeding.
- Inflammatory bowel disease (Crohn's and ulcerative colitis) should be considered in children older than 10 years, particularly with abdominal pain and recurrent bleeding.
- Meckel's diverticulum, which manifests as painless bright red or maroon blood per rectum.
- Henoch-Schönlein purpura (HSP), primarily in children 3 to 7 years of age, may present with melena or bloody stools, which in 20% of cases precede the characteristic rash (see Chapter 6, Bleeding and Bruising).
- Intestinal abnormalities such as bowel duplications and GI vascular malformations (see Chapter 1, Abdominal Pain).
- Anal fissures are a benign cause usually recognizable on examination.

Symptoms
- Fever and vomiting (infectious etiologies)
- Lethargy and/or abdominal pain are suggestive of intussusception
- Anorexia, weight loss, abdominal pain, and recurrent bloody stools are suggestive of inflammatory bowel disease
- Dietary history may suggest milk protein intolerance
- History of constipation is suggestive of risk for anal fissures

Signs
- Occult or gross blood in stool
- Signs of hypovolemia such as tachycardia, increased capillary refill time, and eventually hypotension (ominous)
- Pallor (sign of anemia)
- Signs of bleeding diatheses such as easy bruising, mucosal bleeding

- Skin manifestations such as the characteristic rash of HSP (see Chapter 6, Bleeding and Bruising), eczema with milk allergy, or freckles with familial polyposis

Workup

- Identical to evaluation for UGIB, see earlier section.
- Arteriography may be considered with ongoing bleeding that has not been localized.
- Stool cultures and assays for *C. difficile* toxin, as indicated by history.

Comments and Treatment Considerations

After stabilization of hemodynamic status (see earlier section on emergency management of acute GIB), the cause of bleeding should be sought. The most common cause of LGIB in children of all ages is infectious gastroenteritis. Minimal workup and supportive treatment is usually sufficient (see Chapter 10, Diarrhea). Routine antibiotic treatment is not recommended in patients with presumed bacterial colitis until HUS has been ruled out because antibiotics may worsen the course of HUS (see Chapter 10, Diarrhea). Removal of cow's milk and/or soy protein from the diet is often all that is needed in infants with suspected milk protein sensitivity. Newborns represent a unique group and consultation with neonatology or gastroenterology should be obtained for any newborn with significant blood loss, concern for NEC, or recurrent unexplainable bleeding.

Nasogastric lavage is indicated in certain patients with apparent LGIB to rule out massive UGIB as a cause of hematochezia. Specific tests may be indicated to diagnose certain conditions such as a radionucleotide scan to diagnose Meckel's diverticulum and air contrast or barium enema to diagnose intussusception. Air contrast or barium enema is usually therapeutic and diagnostic for intussusception (see Chapter 1, Abdominal Pain). Endoscopy may be necessary to establish the site of bleeding and to obtain intestinal biopsy specimens in patients with ongoing LGIB in order to establish diagnoses such as inflammatory bowel disease. Arteriography or labeled RBC studies may be necessary with ongoing bleeding that has not been localized. Consultation as needed with a gastroenterologist or surgeon is recommended.

REFERENCES

Durbin DR, Liacouras CA: Gastrointestinal emergencies. In Fleisher GR, Ludwig S, editors: *Textbook of pediatric emergency medicine*, 4th ed, Philadelphia, 2000, Lippincott Williams & Wilkins.

Gryboski JD: Peptic ulcer disease in children, *Pediatr Rev* 12:15-21, 1990.

Kharasch SJ: Gastrointestinal bleeding. In Fleisher GR, Ludwig S, editors: *Textbook of pediatric emergency medicine*, 4th ed, Philadelphia, 2000, Lippincott Williams & Wilkins.

Latt TT, Nicholl R, Domizio P, et al: Rectal bleeding and polyps, *Arch Dis Child* 69:144-147, 1993.

Luks FI, Yzabeck S, Perreault G, et al: Changes in presentation of intussusception, *Am J Emerg Med* 10:574-576, 1992.

Teach SJ, Fleisher GR: Rectal bleeding in the emergency department, *Ann Emerg Med* 23(6):1252-1258, 1994.

Vinton NE: Gastrointestinal bleeding in infancy and childhood, *Gastroenterol Clin North Am* 23:93-122, 1994

CHAPTER 17

Headache

ANA MARIA PAEZ

Headache is a common complaint in children. Epidemiologic studies have indicated that by the age of 15, up to 75% of children will have had a complaint of a significant headache. Isolated headache is a relatively unusual presentation in pediatrics; it is more commonly seen with other symptoms such as fever, vomiting, and sore throat. Although most headaches are benign, there is a small subset of patients in whom headache may be attributed to life-threatening illness. The challenge of the physician is to distinguish between the clinical features of benign headache and those of more serious illness.

In childhood and adolescence, migraine and tension headache are the two most common types of chronic or recurrent headache. In a retrospective study of children presenting to a pediatric ED with headache, 39% were diagnosed with viral illness, sinusitis (16%), migraine (16%), posttraumatic headache (6%), pharyngitis (5%), and tension headache (5%). Other more serious causes of headache include infection (meningitis), increased intracranial pressure (ICP), hypertension, and tumor (see Chapter 3, Altered Mental Status; Chapter 14, Fever; and Chapter 19, Hypertension). Fortunately, these causes are less common and usually can be ruled in or out by careful history and examination. Diagnostic imaging and laboratory testing are seldom required.

Clinical features that should prompt further investigation include increased severity and frequency of headache, morning or nocturnal occurrence, lack of relieving or triggering factors, headache associated with vomiting of increased severity and frequency, lack of familial migraine history, irritability, lethargy, papilledema, and neurologic abnormalities.

Headaches in a child with a ventricular shunt require careful evaluation for possible shunt malfunction (see Chapter 3, Altered Mental Status).

INFECTION

Whenever headache presents with associated fever, infection must be considered. Several causes including meningitis, encephalitis, pharyngitis, sinusitis, and viral illness must be included in the differential diagnosis (see Chapter 3, Altered Mental Status; Chapter 14, Fever; and Chapter 27, Neck Pain/ Masses).

INCREASED INTRACRANIAL PRESSURE

Headache may be the result of increased ICP, which can be a potentially life-threatening process. The differential is broad and includes trauma, tumor, drugs, and abuse. Appropriate emergency therapeutic interventions to reduce ICP should be instituted immediately. Idiopathic intracranial hypertension (pseudotumor cerebri) is discussed later in this chapter (see Chapter 2, Abuse/Rape; Chapter 3, Altered Mental Status; and Chapter 36, Trauma).

HYPERTENSION

Hypertension, of any etiology, may present with headache and may reflect a potential hypertensive crisis (see Chapter 19, Hypertension).

TUMOR

Undiagnosed brain tumor is a major concern for clinicians and families of pediatric patients with headache, and delayed diagnosis is common. Morning headaches with vomiting are concerning symptoms associated with brain tumors. (See Chapter 3, Altered Mental Status).

✚ *MIGRAINE*

Migraine headaches are recurrent headaches separated by long, symptom-free intervals. The prevalence of migraine varies between 2.7% and 10% among children depending on the age and diagnostic criteria used. The sex ratio is approximately 1:1, with a mild preponderance in boys younger than 12 years.

Migraine headache is extensively underestimated in the pediatric population. The diagnosis is clinical and the lack of specific biological markers or imaging often reduces this entity to behavioral or psychological illness. Its presentation is slightly different from that in adults. It is usually of shorter duration, often lasting less than 1 hour, and is less frequently preceded by an identifiable aura (<50% of children with migraine report an aura). It is also more commonly frontal and bilateral in children, versus unilateral in adults. Triggers are less easily identified than in adults but can include emotional stress, lighting changes, minor head trauma, nitrates (lunch meats), and tyramine (cheeses). Migraines in children appear to be associated with a medical history of motion sickness, dizziness, vertigo, and paroxysmal events. A family history of migraine can also be very helpful in making the diagnosis. The risk of migraine is approximately 70% if both parents have migraines and 45% if only one parent is affected. This risk increases if there is a family history of severe migraines. Migraines can usually be managed effectively with abortive therapy in the ED; furthermore, once identified, prophylaxis may be warranted.

Symptoms

- Moderate to severe incapacitating headache typically described as "pounding" or "throbbing" +++++
- Nausea and/or vomiting ++++
- Abdominal pain +++
- Aura (visual most common) +++

- Photophobia ++
- Phonophobia ++
- Symptoms usually relieved by sleep ++++

Signs
- No focal neurologic deficits ++++
- Transient hemiplegia +
- Transient ophthalmoplegia +

Workup
- Diagnosis of migraine is made based on history and is supported by the absence of abnormalities on examination.
- Head CT or MRI scanning if focal neurologic deficits are found on examination, not previously associated with a migraine attack.
- EEG is generally not helpful. Nonspecific EEG abnormalities are found in 20% to 90% of children with migraines.

Comments and Treatment Considerations
Once the diagnosis of acute migraine attack is made, symptomatic therapy should not be delayed. A variety of medications are available to abort or symptomatically treat the headache; however, most treatment interventions have been developed from research data extrapolated from adult studies. Recent preliminary studies in children have shown similar beneficial effects; however, larger, randomized, double-blinded, controlled studies are necessary to further investigate their effectiveness and safety in children.

The currently accepted initial treatment approach centers on the use of analgesics, antiinflammatory, and antiemetic medications (Table 17-1).

Commonly used medications include ibuprofen, acetaminophen, ketorolac, antiemetics, and narcotics. For many children, acetaminophen or ibuprofen combined with best rest may be sufficient. When oral intake is limited secondary to nausea or vomiting, parenteral ketorolac (Toradol) may be given. Ketorolac is an antiinflammatory agent that does not

Table 17-1   Agents for Acute Treatment of Migraine Headache

Drug	Dose
Analgesics	
Acetaminophen	10-15 mg/kg/dose (max 1000 mg/dose, 4000 mg/day) PO/PR q4-6h
Ibuprofen	10 mg/kg/dose (max 800 mg/dose) PO q8h
Ketorolac	0.5-1 mg/kg (max 30 mg IV or 60 mg IM) single dose; multiple dose 0.5 mg/kg/dose (max 30 mg/dose) IV q6h or 10 mg PO q4-6h if > 50 kg
Antiemetics	
Metoclopramide	0.1 mg/kg/dose (max 10 mg/dose) IV q4-6h; high-dose metoclopramide 1 mg/kg/dose (max 50 mg/dose) IV/PO q4-6h may be pretreated with diphenhydramine 1 mg/kg/dose (50 mg/dose) IV/PO
Prochlorperazine	0.15 mg/kg/dose (max 10 mg/dose) IV × 1 dose, then change to PO or IM q6h (IV administration is changed to IM or PO dosing as soon as possible at the lowest effective dose due to concerns of increased extrapyramidal side effects)
Promethazine	0.25-1 mg/kg/dose (max 25 mg/dose) PO/PR/IV/IM q4-6h
Ondansetron	0.15 mg/kg/dose (max 4 mg/dose) PO/IV q8h
Specific antimigraine agents	
Dihydroergotamine	Adolescents: 1 mg IV/IM/SC; may repeat × 1 dose after 1 hr, max 2 mg/day, max 6 mg/wk
Sumatriptan	50 mg PO for BSA of 0.75-1.5 m^2; 100 mg PO for BSA >1.5 m^2; adolescents 6 mg SC or 20-mg nasal spray
Rizatriptan	Adolescents: 5-10 mg PO (orally disintegrating wafer)

cause the respiratory depression or sedation seen with opioids. A dose of 30 mg of ketorolac has been demonstrated to be as effective as 4 mg of morphine in adult pain studies. When nausea and vomiting are severe, antiemetic medications such as prochlorperazine (Compazine), metoclopramide (Reglan), and promethazine (Phenergan) are useful. In addition to their antiemetic effect, these agents often provide some relief of headache and allow the patient both to rest comfortably and to tolerate other oral agents. Prochlorperazine was initially used solely for its antiemetic effect, but the possibility of a dopaminergic mechanism in migraines highlighted its potential use as a direct treatment of migraine. It has been observed to be effective for intractable headache in adults, and a preliminary study has shown similar effectiveness in the treatment of intractable migraine in the pediatric population. In select patients with unrelieved pain, narcotic therapy may be needed.

Ergot preparations are specifically indicated for aborting migraine attacks at their onset. They must be used early in the headache, preferably at the onset of the prodrome to be effective. Strict usage guidelines must be employed to avoid side effects and they are contraindicated with concurrent use of protease inhibitors, monoamine oxidase inhibitors, selective serotonin reuptake inhibitors, and serotonin 5-HT_1 receptor agonists (the "triptans").

The 5-HT_1 agonists are a new class of pharmacologic agents that have proven useful in the treatment of migraine in adults. Different routes of administration and formulations are available. There are several ongoing studies to determine the safety profile and efficacy in the pediatric population. Consultation with a neurologist is recommended before beginning prophylactic therapy.

Prophylactic treatment should be considered in children in whom migraine is frequent and severe. Among the medications used for chronic suppressive therapy are β-blockers, antidepressants, antihistamines, and anticonvulsants. Many of these drugs are under investigation for use in children and as a rule should be started after consultation with a neurologist and require close follow-up. Nonpharmacologic measures, such as dietary modification and stress management, may also aid in the prevention of migraines.

 ## CLUSTER HEADACHE

Cluster headaches are a type of vascular headache that tend to occur in "clusters" with long pain-free periods. Onset is typically during the second and third decade of life, making them a rare cause of headache in children. Symptoms are usually unilateral, consisting of nonthrobbing pain behind the eye, lacrimation, conjunctival injection, rhinorrhea, sweating, and flushing. Prodromes and vomiting are rare. There is no genetic predilection. Treatment usually needs to be prophylactic because symptoms, though severe, usually last only 60 to 90 minutes and analgesics often do not have time to take effect.

 ## IDIOPATHIC INTRACRANIAL HYPERTENSION (PSEUDOTUMOR CEREBRI)

Idiopathic intracranial hypertension or pseudotumor cerebri is a poorly understood cause of increased ICP. It is a diagnosis of exclusion and should be considered in any patient with headache and papilledema and may occur without any other neurologic complaints. It can present at any age during childhood, but most commonly occurs in adolescent girls, especially those who are obese. Most cases are idiopathic, but it has been associated with infections (otitis media and mastoiditis), endocrine disorders (hyperthyroidism, Addison's disease), medications (hypervitaminosis A, tetracyclines, steroid withdrawal), and minor head trauma.

Symptoms
- Headache ++++
- Nausea
- Vomiting
- Dizziness
- Double or blurred vision

- Decreased visual acuity
- Irritability (in infants)

Signs
- Papilledema ++++
- Sixth nerve palsy (rare)

Workup
- Head CT or MRI scanning to rule out mass lesion or hydrocephalus. Ventricles will appear normal or small.
- LP reveals elevated opening pressure (>200 mm H_2O) but normal cell count and chemistries.

Comments and Treatment Considerations

Once other causes of increased ICP have been ruled out, treatment is directed at removal of or lowering production of CSF. Discontinue offending medications, if needed. Therapeutic LPs may be performed to remove CSF. Treatment with acetazolamide (Diamox), dosed at 5 to 15 mg/kg/day PO divided q12h (common initial dose 250 mg PO bid) is then started to reduce CSF production. Long-term monitoring of visual function is particularly important in patients with long-standing disease. Consultation with a neurologist is recommended.

 TENSION HEADACHE

Tension headache is probably the most common recurrent headache experienced by children. It is thought to be caused by recurrent episodes of neck muscle tension or spasms leading to muscle soreness. It is usually associated with prolonged periods of mental or emotional stress. It is unlikely in younger children but is often seen in adolescents, especially in older girls. It is important to differentiate tension headaches from migraine headaches. Tension headaches are less intense and seem to interrupt the patient's daily activity less than migraines. Although the pain may be present upon awakening, the pain usually does not awaken patients from sleep. Tension headaches usually occur at the end of the day and are not associated with nausea and vomiting. As with all illness presenting with headache, more serious causes of headache must be considered before making the diagnosis of tension headache.

Symptoms
- Diffuse headache, with symmetric "band-like" distribution, usually at the end of the day and associated with stress ++++
- Not associated with nausea or vomiting +++++
- Fatigue ++

Signs
- No focal neurologic deficits +++++
- Neck muscular tenderness to palpation ++

Workup
- Diagnosis of tension headache is made based on history and is supported by the absence of abnormalities on examination.

Comments and Treatment Considerations

Once the diagnosis of tension headache is made, identification of the predisposing, precipitating, and perpetuating factors should be sought. Most tension headaches respond to simple analgesia (acetaminophen or ibuprofen), rest, and removal of the stress. Nonpharmacologic modalities, such as relaxation techniques, may also be beneficial in the prophylaxis and treatment of recurrent tension headache.

Analgesic abuse and polypharmacy are common problems seen more frequently in teenagers and adults with chronic headaches. The development of a drug-rebound headache syndrome can confound the clinical diagnosis of tension and migraine headaches. The patient's history will show that he or she is taking excessive amounts of analgesics. These drugs may initially alleviate the pain but after several days may become responsible for the ongoing headache. These patients must be managed carefully with a program of slow drug withdrawal, which may require an inpatient setting.

SINUS INFECTIONS

Acute sinusitis is a common infection that can present with headache. It has been estimated that as many as 1 billion episodes (viral, bacterial, and other) occur each year in the U.S. population. Presentation of sinusitis in children differs slightly from that in adolescents and adults. Children have a continuously changing anatomy and a higher incidence of viral upper respiratory tract infections than adults. It is believed that acute bacterial sinusitis complicates approximately 0.5% to 5.0% of viral respiratory tract infections. Overlap and similarities in these two entities make diagnosis difficult, leading to significant overdiagnosis and treatment. Treatment is directed at the most likely pathogens: nontypeable *Haemophilus influenzae, Streptococcus pneumoniae,* and *Moraxella catarrhalis.*

Symptoms
- Nasal discharge or congestion for >10 days +++++
- Cough ++++
- Headache ++ (more common in adolescents)
- Facial pain ++ (more common in adolescents)

Signs
- Fever +++
- Purulent rhinorrhea ++++
- Tenderness over sinuses ++
- Discrepancy of two sides on transillumination of sinuses ++

Workup
- Clinical diagnosis of acute bacterial sinusitis requires nonspecific upper respiratory tract signs and symptoms for >10 to 14 days or more severe upper respiratory tract signs and symptoms (fever > 39° C, facial swelling, facial pain). Radiographic studies are seldom indicated. CT is more sensitive and specific than plain radiography but requires greater radiation exposure.
  - Sinus x-ray is recommended only occasionally, because it has low sensitivity and specificity. It may appear abnormal (air-fluid levels, opacification, and/or mucosal

thickening >4 mm) with the common cold. Consider if recurrent episodes, suspected complications, or unclear diagnosis. Must be interpreted with caution.
- Sinus CT scan should be obtained if complicated sinusitis is suspected.
- MRI if concern of cavernous sinus thrombosis.
- CBC is not helpful. Approximately 60% to 80% of children with sinusitis have normal white blood cell count.

Comments and Treatment considerations

In an attempt to minimize emerging antibiotic resistance, the Centers for Disease Control and Prevention and the American Academy of Pediatrics recently published principles for judicious use of antibiotics in common respiratory tract infections, including acute sinusitis. A 10- to 14-day course of amoxicillin, dosed at 60 to 100 mg/kg/day PO divided q8h (max 3 g/day), is a good initial choice. However, because many of these organisms are now resistant to amoxicillin, a β-lactamase–stable antibiotic such as amoxicillin-clavulanate or the cephalosporin cefuroxime axetil could be considered if patients do not clinically improve within 48 to 72 hours. Though frequently used, current evidence offers no clear indication for the use of decongestants and antihistamines in the treatment of acute sinusitis. Furthermore, the use of topical decongestants for >3 days should be avoided because they can cause rebound congestion. Antiinflammatory drugs, such as ibuprofen or acetaminophen, can be given for relief of pain.

Most sinus infections are benign with or without treatment; however, ethmoid, sphenoid, and frontal sinusitis can lead to serious sequelae. Possible complications include meningitis, periorbital or orbital cellulitis, epidural or subdural empyema, facial cellulitis, and cavernous sinus thrombosis. Broad-spectrum intravenous antibiotics, such as a third-generation cephalosporin, should be started if complicated sinusitis is suspected. Patients with complicated sinusitis and/or resistant infections should be evaluated by otolaryngologist as soon as possible. Antral puncture or aspiration for identification of the bacterial organism may be indicated in these cases.

REFERENCES

Annequin D, Tourniaire B, Massiou H: Migraine and headache in childhood and adolescence, *Pediatr Clin North Am* 47(3):617, 2000.

Burton LJ, Quinn B, Pratt-Cheney JL, Pourani M: Headache etiology in a pediatric emergency department, *Pediatr Emerg Care* 13:1, 1997.

Hershey AD, Powers SW, Lecates S, Bentti AL: Effectiveness of nasal sumatriptan in 5 to 12 year old children, *Headache* 41:693, 2001.

Ioannidis JP, Lau J: Technical report: evidence for the diagnosis and treatment of acute uncomplicated sinusitis in children: a systematic review, *Pediatrics* 108:E57, 2001.

Jacobs RF: Judicious use of antibiotics for common pediatric respiratory infections, *Pediatr Infect Dis J* 19:938, 2000.

Kabbouche MA, Bentti Vockell AL, LeCates SL, et al: Tolerability and effectiveness of prochlorperazine for intractable migraine in children, *Pediatrics* 107:E62, 2001.

Molofsky WJ: Headaches in children, *Pediatr Ann* 27:615, 1998.

Pakalnis A: New avenues in treatment of paediatric migraine: a review of the literature, *Fam Pract* 18:101, 2001.

Winner P, Rothner D, Saper J, et al: A randomized, double-blind, placebo-controlled study of sumatriptan nasal spray in the treatment of acute migraine in adolescents, *Pediatrics* 106:989, 2000.

CHAPTER 18

Hematuria

KEVIN J. WALSH

Red blood cells can enter the urinary tract at any point along its path from kidney to bladder to urethra. Classically the presence of >5 RBCs/hpf is considered abnormal and warrants evaluation. Up to 1% of healthy school-age children may have hematuria on a single specimen and have no significant urinary pathology. However, any positive test result must be considered in context to determine whether any further testing is needed. Brown or tea-colored urine is more common when bleeding occurs in the renal parenchyma and bright red urine tends to point to post-glomerular bleeding. A diagnosis for a presenting symptom of hematuria may not be made initially; however, it is important to recognize and treat conditions that may be serious and progressive.

An initial workup should include a urine dipstick and microscopy because some foods and medications can discolor the urine; phenazopyridine (Pyridium) is notorious (Table 18-1). Additionally, myoglobinuria must be ruled out.

 TRAUMA

Gross hematuria following blunt abdominal or pelvic trauma requires careful evaluation, most commonly with abdominal CT scanning and surgical consultation. Retrograde urethrogram is required if urethral injury is suspected before placement of a Foley catheter in a trauma patient. If the CT scan shows no abnormalities, the hematuria clears, or is only microscopic, close observation and follow-up for subsequent testing is acceptable (see Chapter 36, Trauma).

Table 18-1   Medicine and Foods that Can Cause Red-Appearing Urine

Medicines	Foods
Anthraquinone dyes	Beets
Aspirin	Blackberries
Cascara	Paprika
Daunorubicin	Rhubarb
Deferoxamine	
Dihydroergotamine mesylate	
Fluorescein sodium	
Furazolidone	
Methyldopa	
Phenazopyridine	
Phenolphthalein	
Phenothiazines	
Phensuximide	
Phenytoin	
Rifabutin	
Rifampin	
Senna	
Salicylazosulfapyridine	
Sulfasalazine	

 ## COAGULATION DISORDER

Renal bleeding may be seen in any disorder of coagulation (see Chapter 6, Bleeding and Bruising).

 ## HEMOLYTIC UREMIC SYNDROME

Hemolytic uremic syndrome (HUS) is the most common cause of acute renal failure in children. It is a multisystem disease commonly caused by infection with *Escherichia coli O157* and may present as thrombocytopenia, microangiopathic hemolytic anemia, and renal dysfunction. Patients may exhibit gross or microscopic hematuria (see Chapter 10, Diarrhea).

GLOMERULONEPHRITIS

The nephritides cover a wide spectrum of diseases ranging from relatively benign postinfectious to rapidly progressive crescentic glomerulonephritis. Their presentations overlap and diagnosis often requires a stepwise evaluation, nephrologic consultation, and surgical biopsy. The initial physician presented with a patient with hematuria and proteinuria must obtain baseline studies, particularly to identify postinfectious glomerulonephritis and then to identify those patients at risk of rapid progression.

Children with glomerulonephritis range from being asymptomatic with a routine urinalysis showing hematuria and proteinuria to critically ill with oliguria and renal failure. In addition, a number of systemic diseases and genetic syndromes are commonly associated with renal involvement.

Acute postinfectious glomerulonephritis is discussed separately because of its common occurrence and frequent evaluation before referral to a nephrologist.

ACUTE GLOMERULONEPHRITIS

Most children with acute postinfectious glomerulonephritis have few presenting symptoms; however, a child may rarely be hypertensive. Commonly, there is an acute onset of hematuria with or without proteinuria. RBC casts can be seen on a fresh urine specimen but often are missed on routine urinalyses, which are run in batches in most hospital laboratories. Acute glomerulonephritis is most commonly a complication of infection caused by group A β-hemolytic streptococci.

Symptoms
- Gross hematuria ++/+++
- Tea- or cola-colored urine
- Edema ++++
- History of preceding pharyngitis (1 to 2 weeks prior) or skin infection (3 to 6 weeks prior)

- Abdominal pain
- Headache or confusion associated with hypertension

Signs
- Hematuria (gross or microscopic) +++++
- Decreased urine output
- Hypertension +++

Workup
- UA showing hematuria, proteinuria, and possibly RBC casts.
- Urine culture to rule out infection.
- CBC, electrolytes, BUN, and SCr to assess renal function.
- Total protein and albumin concentrations.
- C3 level <50% of normal ++++.
- Streptolysin-O enzyme positive (more commonly positive after pharyngitis) +++/++++.
- Streptozyme assay (testing for multiple streptococcal antigens) positive +++++.
- C4 antinuclear antibody (ANA) to suggest other types of nephritis.

Comments and Treatment Considerations

It is essential to identify patients with elevated blood pressure and initiate appropriate treatment (see Chapter 19, Hypertension). Meticulous follow-up must be arranged for all patients but particularly for any patient with hypertension or even mildly abnormal renal function. Children typically have very low BUN and creatinine measurements; what is considered a normal value for an older patient may demonstrate a two- to three-fold increase in a younger patient. Antibiotics with adequate streptococcal coverage should be prescribed for any patient whose initial infection was not treated. Please see Chapter 26, Mouth Pain, for antibiotic recommendations for streptococcal infection. Steroids and cytotoxic agents have not been shown to be beneficial and may be harmful.

Spontaneous improvement for children diagnosed with postinfectious disease usually begins within 1 to 2 weeks, with resolution of edema in 5 to 10 days and hypertension in 2 to 3 weeks, although urinalysis findings may remain abnormal for 2 to 3 years. Rarely complications such as progressive renal failure, congestive heart failure, or hypertensive encephalopathy may occur.

Any child not clearly improving or who develops hypertension or evidence of renal dysfunction should be referred to a pediatric nephrologist for further evaluation and management. These patients will often require renal biopsy for diagnosis.

 ## WILMS' TUMOR

Microscopic or gross hematuria may be present in 10% to 25% of children with Wilms' tumor (see Chapter 1, Abdominal Pain).

 ## UROLITHIASIS

Though more common in adults, kidney stones account for significant pediatric illness. Hematuria will be present in up to 90% of children with kidney stones. The prevalence of disease is increased in some geographic areas (e.g., the southeast United States and southern California). Stones may be made up of calcium (60%), struvite, cystine, or uric acids. Calcium stones may be seen in patients with hypercalciuria, but serum calcium concentration is usually normal. Struvite stones are commonly associated with specific urinary pathogens such as *Proteus*, *Pseudomonas*, *Klebsiella*, *Serratia*, *Mycoplasma*, and *Staphylococcus*. In addition, some medications, other chronic disease states, and rare metabolic disorders are associated with stone formation.

The classic history of intermittent, crampy flank and/or abdominal pain radiating anteriorly suggests this diagnosis but may not be present in the younger patient.

Symptoms
- Abdominal and/or flank pain (may radiate to groin) +++
- Urinary frequency

- Dysuria
- White race ++++
- Urinary retention
- Family history of nephrolithiasis +++
- Medication use that predisposes to stone formation such as diuretics, anticonvulsants, or protease inhibitors
- History of urinary tract infections (UTIs) with pathogens known to be associated with stone formation

Signs

- Hematuria ++++
- Fever++
- Pain +++
- Tachycardia
- Increased blood pressure
- Costovertebral angle and flank tenderness

Workup

- Urinalysis demonstrating microscopic hematuria.
- Urine culture because some patients may have a predisposing, concurrent, or secondary infection.
- BUN and creatinine to access renal function.
- Blood pressure.
- The current radiologic study of choice is abdominal CT (Fig 18-1).
- Abdominal plain film will commonly demonstrate the stone (95% of stones are radiopaque) but has been replaced by CT scans and ultrasound (Fig 18-2).
- Consider urinary calcium/creatinine ratio (≥0.21 indicates hypercalciuria).

Comments and Treatment Considerations

Hydration and pain control are the focus of management. Younger children will often not have the severe pain classically seen in the older patient. Admission for intravenous hydration and analgesia is necessary when the child is unable to tolerate oral fluids and medications. Ketorolac dosed at 0.5 mg/kg/dose IV q6h (max 30 mg/dose) is often an effective analgesic, although it should not be used if there is evidence of renal insufficiency. Narcotics analgesics such as morphine 0.05 to

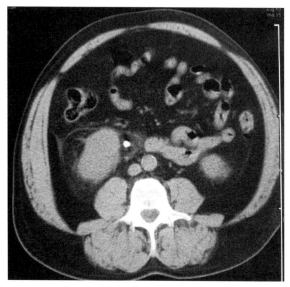

Fig. 18-1 Axial CT image without contrast (dedicated stone protocol) demonstrating a large right ureteropelvic junction calculus with associated perinephric inflammatory reaction (fat stranding). (From Haudrigan MT: *Emerg Clin North Am* 19(3): 2001.)

0.1 mg/kg/dose IV q3h prn or hydromorphone 0.015 mg/kg/dose IV q4-6h prn may also be used. Empiric antibiotics should be added with urology consultation if a coexisting infection is suspected. Small stones (<5 mm) usually pass spontaneously if there are no anatomic abnormalities of the genitourinary system. Urology consultation for possible surgical intervention and follow-up is important in patients with evidence of obstruction or larger stones.

✳ *URINARY TRACT INFECTIONS*

Uninary tract infection (UTI) is defined as a bacterial infection at any level of the urinary tract most commonly involving either

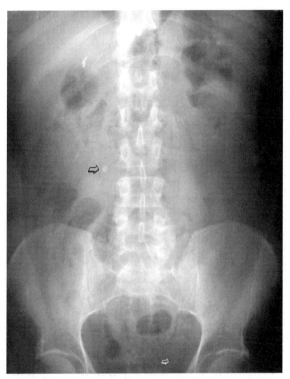

Fig. 18-2 Large right ureteral stone just distal to the uretero-pelvic junction (UPJ) *(arrow outlined in black)*, small left ureter-vesicular junction (UVJ) stone *(arrow outlined in white)*, and bilateral nephrolithiasis. (From Haudrigan MT: *Emerg Clin North Am* 19(3): 2001.)

the bladder (cystitis) or the renal parenchyma (pyelonephritis). Most infections occur as a result of ascending infection with the exception of hematogenous spread in the bacteremic newborn. The most common pathogen is *E. coli* but other pathogens include *Enterococcus*, group B streptococci (mostly infants), *Klebsiella*, *Enterobacter*, *Proteus*, and *Pseudomonas*. For practical purposes, differentiating between upper and lower tract disease is often difficult in the younger patient; therefore it is standard practice to consider all febrile UTIs in children as potentially involving the renal parenchyma. An attempt is made to simplify the presentation of this complex topic, but it should be noted that there are many diagnosis, treatment, and follow-up controversies.

Symptoms

- Newborns may have only fever, jaundice, irritability, and poor feeding
- Older children
  - Irritability
  - Fever +++
  - Dysuria, frequency, and/or urgency
  - Nausea and/or vomiting
  - Malodorous urine
  - Shaking chills
  - Predisposing condition such as genitourinary reflux, meningomyelocele, or an anatomic abnormality of urinary tract

Signs

- Fever
- Abdominal pain (the bladder is an abdominal organ in infants and toddlers; therefore generalized abdominal pain, as well a suprapubic pain can be associated with UTIs)
- Flank/costovertebral angle tenderness

Workup

- UA with microscopy looking for signs supportive of infection such as the following:
  - Leukocyte esterase (LE) positive ++++
  - Nitrate positive +++
  - WBCs (>5/hpf on an unspun sample or >10/mm^3 on a spun sample) ++++
  - RBCs
  - The combination of LE, nitrate, or WBC positive +++++
  - A high pH level is often seen with *Proteus* infection and nitrates are indicative of *E. coli* infections.

- Sterile urine culture collected via suprapubic tap, catheterization, or in the older patient a clean voided specimen (CVS). Girls can be asked to sit backwards on the toilet during collection to minimize contamination.
- Consider CBC and blood culture (recommended in all febrile children younger than 3 months with suspicion of UTI).
- Blood pressure measurement.

Comments and Treatment Considerations

Positive culture results remain the gold standard. Single colony growth >100,000 colony-forming units (cfu)/hpf on CVS, >10,000 cfu/hpf on catheterization (some authors propose >50,000), and any bacterial growth on suprapubic tap constitute a positive result. Specimens obtained from a urine bag should not be sent for culture (with rare exception) because these samples are often contaminated and may confuse patient management. A renal nuclear scan can confirm the diagnosis of pyelonephritis but is seldom necessary because management for febrile UTI and pyelonephritis is identical.

Infants and young children who ultimately are diagnosed with a UTI can present with fever without a source. Additionally, the urine dip can be negative in some patients who then have positive urine cultures; whether this represents true UTI, early UTI, contamination, or colonization is controversial. Given these issues, current conservative recommendations for fever evaluation without a source include sending a sterile urine culture in all febrile infants younger than 3 months, in all boys younger than 12 months, and in girls younger than 2 years (some authors recommend 3 years). Some experts advocate using a urinalysis as an initial screening tool then sending a sterile specimen for culture only if urinalysis is suggestive of infection; however, this method will miss those UTIs in patients with normal urinalysis findings.

Vomiting, toxic appearance, or the inability to tolerate oral medications are all indications for admission and intravenous antibiotics. Children younger than 3 months with evidence of a UTI are usually admitted for parenteral therapy pending urine culture and blood culture results.

Outpatient Antibiotic Choices

Trimethoprim-sulfamethoxazole 6 to 12 mg of trimethoprim/kg/day PO divided bid (max 160 mg of trimethoprim/dose)

OR

First-generation Cephalosporin such as:
Cephalexin 25 to 50 mg/kg/day PO divided q6-8h (max 500 mg/dose)

OR

Fluoroquinolone (for patients >18 years of age) such as:
Ciprofloxacin 20 to 30 mg/kg/day PO divided bid (max 750 mg/dose)

Parenteral Therapy Choices

Ampicillin 100 to 200 mg/kg/day IV divided q6-12h (dose-dependent on age, see Chapter 14, Fever)

AND

Gentamicin 4 to 7.5 mg/kg/day IV divided q8-24h (dose-dependent on age)

OR

Ceftriaxone 50 to 100 mg/kg/day IV divided q12-24h (max 2 g/dose)

Because of increasing ampicillin and cephalosporin resistance, some experts recommend using ampicillin, gentamicin, and a third-generation cephalosporin for ill-appearing hospitalized patients with pyelonephritis. Therapy should be tailored to the narrowest spectrum drug after culture identity and sensitivities are known.

UTI can be the first indication of a congenital abnormality in urinary tract anatomy or function. In some studies the rate of vesicoureteral reflux among children younger than 1 year exceeds 50%. Failure to diagnose the underlying condition can lead to chronic scarring and renal failure. Any child younger than 5 years, all male patients, and any prepubertal female patient older than 5 years with recurrent UTI should have an ultrasound and follow-up voiding cystourethrogram (VCUG). There are data supporting that an ultrasound need not be obtained after a urine infection if the child had a prenatal ultrasound after 32 weeks of gestation and questioning the value of VCUG because prophylactic antibiotics may not reduce renal scarring in patients with reflux; however, additional studies are needed before we can change current practice.

A ultrasound may be obtained initially and the VCUG delayed until after resolution of infection; however, some authors have proposed obtaining a VCUG during infection while the child is on therapeutic antibiotics. If the VCUG is delayed, then a child should be placed on prophylactic antibiotics at one half to one third of the normal therapeutic dose until study results can be obtained. Children with abnormal ultrasound and/or VCUG findings should remain on prophylactic antibiotics until evaluated by a urologist who can then dictate further management and follow-up. Some children will eventually require surgical correction for vesicoureteral reflux.

 ## SICKLE CELL

Sickle cell hemoglobinopathies are associated with recurrent gross hematuria.

 ## EXERCISE

Vigorous exercise may cause transient microscopic hematuria. Subsequent urinalysis after exercise restriction for 3 to 5 days will usually normalize the urinalysis findings and confirm the diagnosis.

REFERENCES

Byington CL, Rittichier KK, Bassett KE, et al: Serious bacterial infections in febrile infants younger than 90 days of age: the importance of ampicillin-resistant pathogens, *Pediatrics* 111(5):964-968, 2003.

Chong CY, Tan AS, Ng W, et al: Treatment of urinary tract infection with gentamicin once or three times daily, *Acta Paediatr* 92(3):291-296, 2003.

Committee on Quality Improvement and Subcommittee on Urinary Tract Infection: Practice parameter: the diagnosis, treatment, and evaluation of the initial urinary tract infection in febrile infants and young children, *Pediatrics* 103(4):843-852, 1999.

Elder JS, Peters CA, Arrant BS, et al: Pediatric vesicoureteral reflux guideline panel summary report on the management of primary vesicoureteral reflux in children, *J Urol* 157:1846-1851, 1997.

Gorelick MH, Shaw KN: Screening tests for urinary tract infections in children: a metal-analysis, *Pediatrics* 104(5):1-7, 1999.

Hoberman A, Charron M, Hickey RW, et al: Imaging studies after a first febrile urinary tract infection in young children, *N Engl J Med* 348(3):195-202, 2003.

Hoberman A, Wald ER: Urinary tract infections in young febrile children, *Pediatr Infect Dis J* 16(1):11-17, 1997.

Hoberman A, Wald ER, Hickey RW, et al: Oral versus initial intravenous therapy for urinary tract infections in young febrile children, *Pediatrics* 104(1):79-86, 1999.

Hrick D, Chung-Park M, Sedor JR: Glomerulonephritis, *N Engl J Med* 339:888-899, 1998.

Ingelfinger JR et al: Frequency and etiology of gross hematuria in a general pediatric setting, *Pediatrics* 59(4):557-561, 1977.

Keren R, Chan E: A meta-analysis of randomized, controlled trial comparing short- and long-course antibiotic therapy for urinary tract infections in children, *Pediatrics* 109(5):1-6, 2002.

Merguerian PA, Chang B: Pediatric genitourinary tumors, *Curr Opin Oncol* 14:273-279, 2002.

Newman TB: Urine testing and urinary tract infections in febrile infants in office settings, *Arch Pediatr Adolesc Med* 156:44-54, 2002.

Shaw KN, Gorelick M, McGowan KL, et al: Prevalence of urinary tract infections in febrile young children in the emergency department, *Pediatrics* 102(2), 1998.

CHAPTER 19

Hypertension

YIANNIS L. KATSOGRIDAKIS

Though very rare, a pediatric patient may come to the ED with symptoms and signs of hypertensive emergency, which is defined as elevated blood pressure with evidence of end-organ dysfunction that needs to be emergently managed. Most commonly, blood pressure (BP) elevation in the ED is secondary to a primary process such as a painful injury.

Most pediatric patients with hypertension are asymptomatic and identified on routine screen or presentation for other issues. These asymptomatic patients fall into a spectrum of urgency based on the degree of hypertension. The decision to pharmacologically treat the elevated BP is based on the height of repeated BP readings and suspected etiology.

Hypertension is defined as an average systolic and/or diastolic BP in or above the 95th percentile for age, sex, and height, with measurements obtained on at least three occasions using an appropriately sized cuff (Table 19-1). The cuff must be wide enough to cover two thirds of the length of the upper arm (a cuff that is too narrow will result in falsely elevated measurements) and wide enough to completely encircle the arm's circumference. Approximately 1% of children and adolescents will have hypertension with repeated measurements.

Once diagnosed, a focused hypertension history should be taken. This should include symptoms attributable to hypertension, including neonatal history such as the use of umbilical lines, growth pattern, history of renal or urologic disorders, use of medications with vasopressor effects, and use of oral contraceptives. Symptoms suggestive of an endocrine etiology are weight loss, diaphoresis, flushing, fevers, palpitations, and a family history of primary hypertension. Finally, a family history

Table 19-1 Classification of Hypertension in Boys and Girls, According to Height

BP	Age (yr)	Height Percentile for Boys				Height Percentile for Girls			
		5th	25th	75th	95th	5th	25th	75th	95th
Systolic	1	98	101	104	106	101	103	105	107
(mm Hg)	3	104	107	111	113	104	105	108	110
	6	109	112	115	117	108	110	112	114
	10	114	117	121	123	116	117	120	122
	13	123	124	128	130	121	123	126	128
	17	132	135	138	140	126	127	130	132
Diastolic	1	55	56	58	59	57	57	59	60
(mm Hg)	3	63	64	66	67	65	65	67	68
	6	72	73	75	76	71	72	73	75
	10	77	79	80	82	77	77	79	80
	13	79	81	83	84	80	81	82	84
	17	85	86	88	89	83	83	85	86

Data adapted from the National High Blood Pressure Education Program Workshop: Update on the 1987 task force report on high blood pressure in children and adolescents, *Pediatrics* 98(4 Pt 1):649-658, 1996.

should focus on genetic disorders known to be associated with secondary hypertension.

The most common form of hypertension in children and adolescents is primary hypertension. Because this is a diagnosis of exclusion, the clinician should first attempt to identify common secondary causes of hypertension (Table 19-2). Hypertension secondary to renal disease may be amenable to therapy and result in normalization of BP.

�֍ *HYPERTENSIVE EMERGENCY*

Hypertension is considered an emergency when end-organ damage occurs as a result of increased BP. As a general guide, the BPs listed in Table 19-3 denote blood pressures that could

Table 19-2 Common Causes by Age-Group of Chronic Sustained Hypertension Seen in Clinic Populations

Age-Group	Cause
Newborn	Renal artery thrombosis, renal artery stenosis Congenital renal malformations Coarctation of the aorta Bronchopulmonary dysplasia
Infancy to 6 yr	Renal parenchymal diseases (includes renal structural and inflammatory lesions, as well as tumors) Coarctation of the aorta Renal artery stenosis
6-10 yr	Renal artery stenosis Renal parenchymal disease Primary (essential) hypertension
Adolescence	Primary (essential) hypertension Renal parenchymal disease

National High Blood Pressure Education Program Workshop: Report of the second task force on blood pressure control in children—1987, *Pediatrics* 79(1):1-25, 1987.

Table 19-3 Blood Pressures Indicating Hypertensive Emergencies

Age	Systolic Blood Pressure	Diastolic Blood Pressure
≤10 yr	≥160 mm Hg	≥105 mm Hg
≥10 yr	≥170 mm Hg	≥110 mm Hg

lead to end-organ damage and should be considered a possible hypertensive emergency when taken in a calm child on two to three repeated attempts.

Signs and symptoms vary based on the degree of hypertension and whether the presentation is acute, chronic, or acute on chronic but include the following:

Symptoms
- Headache
- Abdominal pain
- Nausea/vomiting
- Altered mental status
- Visual disturbance
- Seizure
- Stroke

Signs
- Spasm and tortuosity of retinal arteries
- Papilledema and/or fundal hemorrhage
- Heart murmur
- CHF
- Hematuria
- Lower motor neuron facial palsy

Workup
- BP and cardiac monitoring.
- In the patient with altered mental status, head CT without contrast to rule out hemorrhagic CNS lesions or mass.
- UA to look for protein or red blood cell casts indicating renal involvement.
- Urine culture to rule out infection.
- Electrolytes to rule out endocrine abnormality.
- BUN and SCr to assess renal function.
- ECG to detect evidence of cardiac ischemia.
- CXR to rule out CHF.

Comment and Treatment Considerations
In most cases, no treatment is needed as blood pressure elevation is due to pain, fever, or a stressful environment. In the very rare circumstance where emergent treatment is needed due to end-organ damage, pharmacologic therapy should be directed at lowering the mean arterial pressure by 20% to 25%. Intravenous drugs should be initiated if there is any evidence of end-organ involvement. Sodium nitroprusside is the usual drug of choice in malignant hypertension given the ease of

titration (see Table 19-4 for recommended drug therapy options). Close BP monitoring is mandatory to prevent overcorrection of the hypertension, which can have castrophic consequences. Provide supportive care as needed. This may potentially include oxygen, intravenous access, continuous cardiac monitoring, a Foley catheter, arterial line, and admission to an intensive care unit. A pediatric nephrologist should be consulted.

For hypertensive urgencies (hypertension that is not associated with life- or organ-threatening manifestations), the oral route may be used (Table 19-5) with close follow-up.

Table 19-4   Hypertensive Emergency Therapy Options

Drug	Dose
Sodium nitroprusside	Initial continuous infusion 0.5-1 mcg/kg/min, may be increased stepwise to 10 mcg/kg/min maximum
Labetalol*	Initial 0.2-0.5 mg/kg/dose (max 20 mg/dose) IV bolus, followed by additional intermittent doses increased incrementally every 10 min until response achieved, up to 1 mg/kg/dose (max 300 mg total) or continuous infusion 0.4-1.5 mg/kg/hr (max 3 mg/kg/hr)
Hydralazine	Initial 0.1-0.2 mg/kg/dose (max 20 mg/dose) IV q4-6h prn, dose may be repeated after 20 min if no response (max 40 mg total/dose)
Esmolol*	500 mcg/kg IV load (must dilute to ≤ 10 mg/ml) given over 1-2 min; then initiate continuous infusion at 200 mcg/kg/min. May increase by 50-100 mcg/kg every 5-10 min as needed to a max of 1000 mcg/kg/min

National High Blood Pressure Education Program Workshop: Update on the 1987 task force report on high blood pressure in children and adolescents, *Pediatrics* 98(4 Pt 1):649-658, 1996.
*Beta blockers, such as labetalol and esmolol, should not be used as first-line agents for hypertension secondary to sympathomimetic toxic exposures.

Table 19-5   Oral Therapies for Hypertensive Urgencies

Drug	Dose
Nifedipine	0.25-0.5 mg/kg/dose (max 10 mg/dose) PO q4-6h prn
Minoxidil	0.1-0.2 mg/kg/dose PO × 1, usually given with a β-blocker to minimize minoxidil-induced tachycardia

 ## RENOVASCULAR LESIONS

Renovascular lesions, such as renal artery stenosis and coarctation of the aorta, result in hypertension through stimulation of the renin-angiotensin-aldosterone system.

RENAL ARTERY THROMBOSIS/STENOSIS

Renal artery thrombosis is an especially important consideration in neonates and young infants. Important history includes prior umbilical artery catheters. Renal artery stenosis is usually associated with moderate to malignant hypertension. It may also be associated with Williams' syndrome and neurofibromatosis.

Symptoms
- Asymptomatic
- Failure to thrive
- Headaches
- Dizziness
- Epistaxis
- Visual problems
- Vomiting

Signs
- Wide changes in BP
- Tachycardia
- Abdominal bruit

- Hypertensive funduscopic changes (arteriolar narrowing, tortuosity, arteriovenous nicking)
- Bell's palsy
- Neurologic deficits
- Cardiomegaly
- Heart failure

Workup
- Renal US and renal angiography for definitive diagnosis.
- CBC.
- Electrolytes, BUN, SCr, UA, and urine culture to assess renal function and rule out possible infection.
- ECG, CXR, and echocardiogram to assess cardiac end-organ dysfunction.

Comments and Treatment Considerations
Patients with renal artery thrombosis/stenosis and hypertension require ongoing BP control and possible percutaneous or surgical treatment. Hypertensive emergencies and urgencies should be treated as needed (see Tables 19-4 and 19-5 for therapy options). A nephrologist and pediatric surgeon should be consulted.

COARCTATION OF THE AORTA
Coarctation of the aorta is the second most common cause of secondary hypertension after renal disease. Constrictions of the aorta of varying degrees may occur at any point but are most commonly seen just below the origin of the left subclavian artery at the origin of the ductus arteriosus. Depending on the degree of constriction, an acutely ill presentation may occur in the newborn period while minimal symptomatology and high BP on routine examination may be found later in life. More than 70% of patients will have a bicuspid aortic valve.

Symptoms
- Asymptomatic
- Decreased activity
- Decreased feeding

- Vomiting
- Failure to thrive
- Cyanosis

Signs

- Upper extremity hypertension
- Systolic BP gradient between the arms and legs of >10 mm Hg
- Cardiac murmur consistent with a bicuspid aortic valve
- Decreased or absent femoral pulses
- Cardiomegaly
- CHF
- Hypertensive funduscopic changes (arteriolar narrowing, tortuosity, arteriovenous nicking)
- Bell's palsy
- Neurologic deficit

Workup

- Echocardiogram is usually diagnostic.
- Four-extremity BP looking for a decrease in pulse pressure in the lower extremities as compared to the upper extremities.
- ECG usually normal in a young patient but may show left ventricular hypertrophy in an older patient.
- CXR may show cardiac enlargement and pulmonary congestion in severe disease.
- Electrolytes, BUN, SCr, UA, and urine culture to assess renal function and rule out possible UTI.

Comments and Treatment Considerations

Neonates with symptoms and signs suggestive of coarctation of the aorta and associated shock require immediate supportive care. Initiation of alprostadil (also called prostaglandin E_1 [PGE_1]) should be done to keep the ductus arteriosus open (see Chapter 9, Cyanosis). If possible, a pediatric cardiologist should be consulted before starting prostaglandins but should not delay therapy. Patients presenting later in life are usually asymptomatic and do not require urgent BP therapy.

Early detection and repair of coarctation of the aorta is important because late repair is associated with premature cardiovascular disease. Cardiac catheterization and angiography may be needed if lesion and collateral blood flow is not well visualized on echocardiography.

CONGENITAL RENAL ANOMALIES

Possible etiologies include asymmetric renal disease (unilateral small kidney), malformations (including bilateral polycystic kidneys, hypoplasia, and obstruction of ureteropelvic junction), and hydronephrosis.

Symptoms
- Asymptomatic
- Failure to thrive
- Frequent urinary tract infections or fevers of unknown etiology

Signs
- Tachycardia
- Wide changes in BP
- Edema
- Abdominal mass/palpable kidneys
- Hypertensive funduscopic changes (arteriolar narrowing, tortuosity, arteriovenous nicking)
- Bell's palsy
- Neurologic deficits
- Cardiomegaly
- Heart failure

Workup
- Renal US and/or renal nuclear scan for definitive diagnosis.
- CBC looking for hemolysis and anemia.
- Electrolytes, BUN, SCr, UA, and urine culture to assess renal function and rule out possible infection.

- ECG and echocardiogram to assess cardiac end-organ dysfunction.

Comments and Treatment Considerations

Hypertension should be treated as needed (see the previous table under malignant hypertension for therapy options). Therapy will be based on the anomaly detected. A pediatric nephrologist and surgeon should be consulted.

 ## CATECHOLAMINE EXCESS

Catecholamine excess as a cause of hypertension in children is rare. Potential causes include pheochromocytoma, sympathomimetic overdose (cocaine, amphetamines, decongestant, or diet pills), withdrawal from sedative hypnotics (clonidine), or drug-food interactions with monoamine oxidase inhibitors.

Benzodiazepine therapy such as lorazepam or midazolam dosed at 0.05 to 0.1 mg/kg/dose IV (max 4 mg/dose lorazepam, max 10 mg/dose midazolam) may be adequate for reduction of BP in sympathomimetic overdose. Avoid β-blockers in patients with catecholamine excess (e.g., cocaine), because the unopposed alpha effect can cause significant vasoconstriction and end-organ damage.

 ## PRIMARY (ESSENTIAL) HYPERTENSION

Primary or essential hypertension is frequently associated with obesity and a family history of essential hypertension. A significant correlation exists between primary childhood hypertension and hypertension in adulthood; however, hypertension rarely causes heart failure, renal disease, or ocular abnormalities in children.

Symptoms
- Asymptomatic
- Headaches

- Dizziness
- Epistaxis
- Visual problems
- Vomiting
- Poor appetite and weight loss

Signs
- Obesity
- Hypertensive funduscopic changes (arteriolar narrowing, tortuosity, arteriovenous nicking)
- Bell's palsy
- Neurologic deficits
- Cardiomegaly
- Heart failure

Workup
- Consider renal imaging if diagnosis is in question to rule out renal disease and/or anomalies.
- CBC looking for hemolysis and anemia.
- Electrolytes, BUN, SCr, UA, and urine culture to assess renal function and rule out possible infection.
- Uric acid, which when high correlates with decreased renal blood flow and higher renal vascular resistance.
- ECG and echocardiogram to assess cardiac end-organ dysfunction.
- Fasting cholesterol, triglycerides, high-density lipoprotein, low-density lipoprotein levels to assess other risks factors for cardiac disease.

Comments and Treatment Considerations
Nonpharmacologic therapy should be the primary focus of therapy and consists of weight reduction, exercise, and dietary intervention. Pharmacologic therapy is indicated in symptomatic patients and those with persistent elevation of BP above the 99th percentile. Diuretics and β-blockers tend to be the mainstay of pharmacologic treatment for chronic hypertension in children, although angiotensin-converting enzyme inhibitors have shown encouraging results in certain

populations. Pediatric patients with essential hypertension are usually followed by pediatric nephrologists.

 ## WHITE COAT HYPERTENSION

White coat hypertension is an elevated BP measured during a stressful time for the patient. The stressor may simply be the presence of a medical professional.

Symptoms
- Asymptomatic
- *No* headaches

Signs
- Elevated BP measurements in the presence of a medical professional

Workup
- Focused hypertension history and physical examination to rule out other possible etiologies.
- Average repeated BP measurements using correct cuff size and technique under optimal setting.

Comments and Treatment Considerations

Workup indicated in those with persistently elevated BP and concerning history. Physical examination should be performed to rule out possible causes of secondary hypertension. Though seldom necessary, white coat hypertension may be distinguished from persistent hypertension by 24-hour ambulatory BP monitoring. This technique allows for multiple BP measurements in the patient's normal environment.

REFERENCES

Bartosh SM, Aronson AJ: Childhood hypertension. An update on etiology, diagnosis, and treatment, *Pediatr Clin North Am* 46(2):235-252, 1999.

Daniels SR: Consultation with the specialist. The diagnosis of hypertension in children: an update, *Pediatr Rev* 18(4):131-135, 1997.

Ing FF, Starc TJ, Griffiths SP, Gersony WM: Early diagnosis of coarctation of the aorta in children: a continuing dilemma, *Pediatrics* 98(3 Pt 1):378-382, 1996.

Kay JD, Sinaiko AR, Daniels SR: Pediatric hypertension, *Am Heart J* 142(3):422-432, 2001.

Lieberman E: Pediatric hypertension: clinical perspective, *Mayo Clin Proc* 69(11):1098-1107, 1994.

Louden M, Uner A: Hypertension. In Davis MA, editor: *Signs & symptoms in emergency medicine*, St Louis, 1999, Mosby.

National High Blood Pressure Education Program Workshop: Update on the 1987 task force report on high blood pressure in children and adolescents: a working group report from the National High Blood Pressure Education Program. National High Blood Pressure Education Program Working Group on Hypertension Control in Children and Adolescents, *Pediatrics* 98(4 Pt 1):649-658, 1996.

National High Blood Pressure Education Program Workshop: Report of the Second Task Force on Blood Pressure Control in Children—1987. Task Force on Blood Pressure Control in Children. National Heart, Lung, and Blood Institute, Bethesda, Maryland, *Pediatrics* 79(1):1-25, 1987.

Potter DE, Hoffman J: The circulatory system. In Rudolph CD, Rudolph AM, editors: *Rudolph's pediatrics*, 21st ed, New York, 2003, McGraw-Hill.

Sinaiko AR: Hypertension in children, *N Engl J Med* 335(26):1968-1973, 1996.

Sorof JM, Portman RJ: White coat hypertension in children with elevated casual blood pressure, *J Pediatr* 137(4):493-497, 2000.

CHAPTER 20

Hypotension/Shock

KATHERINE F. McGOWAN

Shock is defined as inadequate perfusion to meet the body's metabolic needs. Shock begins when there is an absolute or functional hypovolemia and the body attempts to compensate for the functional decrease in circulating volume. Pediatric patients initially maintain their cardiac output through an increase in heart rate. Therefore, in the pediatric population, unexplained tachycardia is one of the earliest signs of shock. Hypotension, or low blood pressure, is a late and ominous sign in the pediatric patient; hence, increased capillary refill time is a better initial physical sign of shock than a low blood pressure reading, which may occur only seconds before cardiopulmonary arrest.

The appropriate management of a child in shock requires the following:

- Prompt recognition of shock
- Early institution of general supportive care
- Rapid presumptive treatment (particularly where infection is a potential etiology) while determining the underlying etiology
- Correction of the underlying cause
- Management of complications and secondary injury

Multiple classifications of shock exist. One of the most common classification systems includes hypovolemic, distributive, cardiogenic, and other (including obstructive, adrenal insufficiency, and dissociative). It should be remembered that these classifications oversimplify the fact that many acutely ill patients have more than one classification contributing to their overall symptoms of shock (e.g., the septic patient with myocardial dysfunction). First the symptoms, signs, workup, and treatment recommendations common to all classifications are discussed and then the specific classes themselves.

SYMPTOMS

- History of poor oral intake or increased fluid losses (vomiting, diarrhea)
- History of blood loss or blunt trauma
- Fever
- History of cardiac disease or other chronic underlying disease

Signs

- Tachycardia +++++
- Altered mental status (initially irritability or lethargy, which may proceed to agitation, confusion, stupor, and coma) ++++
- Fever or hypothermia ++++
- Oliguria ++++
- Cool mottled extremities/prolonged capillary refill >2 seconds ++++
- Weak pulses +++
- Hypotonia ++
- Late ominous signs
  - Tachypnea or irregular respirations ++
  - Hypotension ++
  - Bradycardia ++

GENERAL WORKUP FOR SHOCK

Initial workup will be based on history and severity of symptoms. Consider the following:
- Blood type and crossmatch.
- CBC, remembering that initial hematocrit may not reflect acute blood loss; low or high WBC count can be concerning for infection or possible malignancy.
- Electrolytes, including BUN and SCr.
- ABG analysis for signs of metabolic acidosis.
- PT, PTT.
- Stool guaiac.
- UA, CXR, and cultures of urine, blood, and/or CSF, looking for signs of infection.

EMERGENT THERAPY FOR SHOCK

The priority is attention to the ABCs and assessment of hemodynamic stability. Two large-bore IV catheters should be placed, with blood emergently sent for type and crossmatch in addition to baseline laboratory testing (see later sections in this chapter). Crystalloid solutions are used initially for volume replacement. Typically, normal saline or lactated Ringer's solution at 20 ml/kg is rapidly infused and may be repeated up to a total of 60 to 80 ml/kg until the patient demonstrates hemodynamic stability or colloid can be started. Patients with large or ongoing hemorrhage or persistent hemodynamic instability despite 40 to 60 ml/kg of crystalloid will require colloid to assist in volume replacement. There is no absolute hematocrit or hemoglobin value for which transfusion is required; however, the patient with an acute blood loss and a hemoglobin value <7 g/dl will generally require a transfusion. O-negative blood may be needed unless time allows for matched blood. Attention should be given to correcting coagulopathies with specific clotting factors or fresh frozen plasma (see Chapter 6, Bleeding and Bruising).

Vasoactive agents should be considered only after adequate volume resuscitation. Dopamine is most often the first vasopressor added to support blood pressure in pediatric shock. Dose-related effects of dopamine include "renal" dose D_1-receptor activation at 1 to 5 mcg/kg/min, β_1-receptor agonism and subsequent increase in cardiac output at 5 to 10 mcg/kg/min, and α_1-receptor agonism resulting in increased systemic vascular resistance (SVR) at 10 to 20 mcg/kg/min. Any patient requiring dopamine for shock should be started at a dose of 10 to 15 mcg/kg/min after adequate fluid resuscitation, then titrated to effect. An epinephrine infusion may also be used to support the blood pressure when unresponsive to fluid and dopamine. The usual range for epinephrine infusion is 0.1 to 1 mcg/kg/min. Dobutamine is a potent β-agonist, most often used in cardiogenic shock states secondary to the significant increases in inotropy and minimal effect on peripheral resistance. Dobutamine infusions commonly range from 5 to 20 mcg/kg/min. Norepinephrine is primarily an α-agonist, resulting in increased SVR with less significant increases in cardiac inotropy. Neurogenic and some patients with septic shock may respond better to norepinephrine when refractory to fluid resuscitation. Norepinephrine infusions are commonly run at 0.05 to 2 mcg/kg/min. Extravasation of vasopressors can cause signifi-

cant tissue damage and necrosis. Central access and administration is recommended as soon as possible after beginning
vasopressor therapy.

Broad-spectrum antibiotic therapy should be initiated early if
there is a concern for sepsis and should not be delayed to obtain
diagnostic tests. Third-generation cephalosporins, such as ceftriaxone or cefotaxime, are usually excellent empiric antibiotics. If the
patient is immunocompromised, *Pseudomonas* coverage with an
antipseudomonal penicillin, ceftazidime, or a fluoroquinolone is
warranted. Infants younger than 3 months should receive ampicillin in addition to a cephalosporin or aminoglycoside to ensure
Listeria coverage. Any patient with a life-threatening infection
from presumed methicillin-resistant *Staphylococcus aureus* or
penicillin-resistant *Streptococcus pneumoniae* should receive vancomycin empirically until culture results are available (see Chapter
14, Fever, and Chapter 21, Immunocompromised Patients: Special
Considerations).

Once the etiology of shock is identified, consider the need
for the appropriate emergent consultation (e.g., general surgery,
gastroenterology, gynecology, infectious disease, etc.). Patients
treated for shock should be cared for in an ICU setting.

 ## *HYPOVOLEMIC SHOCK*

In hypovolemic shock the initial derangement is loss of circulating volume caused by either hemorrhagic or nonhemorrhagic
etiologies. Workup and treatment are considered simultaneously and initial therapy is begun often before a full evaluation
has been performed.

HEMORRHAGIC SHOCK

The etiology of hemorrhagic shock is usually clear when
there is obvious external blood loss. Blood loss can occur
from the skin and soft tissues (e.g., lacerations or surgical
incisions); through pleural, mediastinal, or abdominal
tubes/drains after surgery; upper and/or lower gastrointestinal tract bleeding; or vaginal bleeding. Blood loss can be
occult or internal after trauma or surgery. Some areas of the
body where trauma in children can lead to significant blood

loss not easily appreciated or not seen in older patients include scalp hematomas in infants, femur fractures with significant blood loss into the thigh, and retroperitoneal hemorrhage with pelvic fracture (see Chapter 36, Trauma).

Symptoms
- Weakness
- History of blood loss or trauma
- Back or abdominal pain (in the case of a ruptured aneurysm)

Signs
- Obvious blood loss
- Depressed level of consciousness
- Tachycardia
- Hypotension (late)
- Pallor
- Abdominal tenderness or distention in the case of intraperitoneal bleeding
- Expansile pulsatile abdominal mass in the case of an aneurysm
- Tachypnea/irregular respirations from acidosis

Workup and Treatment Considerations
See the previous section, Emergent Therapy for Shock, for emergent therapy and suggested workup, noting that vasopressors should not be used with ongoing hemorrhagic losses. Aggressive volume replacement including blood transfusion is the mainstay of therapy until definite care can be provided.

NONHEMORRHAGIC HYPOVOLEMIC SHOCK
Vomiting and diarrhea from infectious enteritis leading to dehydration and subsequent nonhemorrhagic hypovolemic shock is the most common cause of shock in children. The World Health Organization estimates that worldwide there are 5 to 10 million diarrheal-associated infant deaths annually. Other mechanisms of volume loss include burns, peritonitis, glycosuric diuresis, and sunstroke.

Symptoms
- History of poor fluid intake and/or increased fluid losses (vomiting, diarrhea)
- Decreased urine output
- Lethargy

Signs
- Poor skin turgor
- Dry mucous membranes
- Oliguria/anuria
- Increased capillary refill time
- Cool extremities
- Decreased alertness/lethargy
- Tachycardia
- Hypotension
- Tachypnea/irregular respirations

Workup and Treatment Considerations
See previous section, Emergent Therapy for Shock, for emergent therapy and suggested workup. Prevention of dehydration in the setting of infectious enteritis is the most important intervention in preventing subsequent shock states (see Chapter 10, Diarrhea).

 ## *DISTRIBUTIVE SHOCK*

Distributive shock occurs when vasodilation and pooling of blood in the peripheral vasculature ensue. The most common cause in children is sepsis but other etiologies are anaphylaxis, spinal cord injuries, and ingestions.

ANAPHYLACTIC SHOCK
Anaphylaxis is an immediate immunoglobulin E–mediated hypersensitivity reaction that is potentially life threatening. See the previous section, Emergent Therapy for Shock, and Chapter 29, Rash (section on Urticaria), for treatment recommendations.

SEPTIC SHOCK

Septic shock results from exposure of microbial components or toxins that trigger the inflammatory cascade. The most common bacterial organisms responsible for septic shock in infants and children are *S. pneumoniae*, *Neisseria meningitidis*, group B *Streptococcus*, *Listeria monocytogenes*, *Haemophilus influenzae* type b, gram-negative bacilli, *S. aureus*, *Pseudomonas aeruginosa*, and *Salmonella enteritidis* (see Chapter 11, Edema, Chapter 14, Fever, and Chapter 29, Rash).

Symptoms
- Fever
- Decreased urine output
- Lethargy

Signs
- Fever
- Ill or toxic appearance
- Oliguria/anuria
- Increased capillary refill time
- Cool extremities
- Decreased alertness/lethargy
- Tachycardia
- Hypotension
- Petechiae/purpura (common in menningococcemia)
- Tachypnea/irregular respirations from acidosis

Additional Workup Recommendations for Suspected Septic Shock
- Urinalysis and cultures.
- Gram stain of secretions, blood, urine, and CSF as indicated.
- Blood cultures.
- WBC (leukocytosis or leukopenia is common).
- CXR.
- CSF studies and cultures (if patient is stable and not coagulopathic or thrombocytopenic).
- Electrolytes including BUN/SCr and liver function tests.

- Coagulation studies (fibrinogen < 250 in meningococcemia is a poor prognostic indicator).
- Consider latex agglutination studies of CSF and/or urine, if antibodies given prior to obtaining cultures.

Workup and Treatment Considerations

See previous section, Emergent Therapy for Shock, for emergent therapy and suggested workup. Antibiotics are indicated as a mainstay of correcting the underlying cause of septic shock (see earlier section) and should not be unduly delayed in order to obtain cultures. Corticosteroids such as fludrocortisone and hydrocortisone have received more attention in the treatment of adult shock; however, the benefits in children in shock are not well elucidated. Steroids should be given to patients with a history of steroid dependence. Activated protein C infusions (Xigris) are generally used under strict protocol and do not routinely need to be started in the emergency department.

NEUROGENIC SHOCK

Primarily seen with associated trauma, neurogenic shock (a.k.a., spinal shock) is a centrally mediated process from loss of sympathetic function and often refractory to fluid resuscitation. The classic clinical presentation is a hypotensive but bradycardic patient with evidence of peripheral vasodilation as a result of lack of sympathetic tone.

Typically there is a significant mechanism of injury that is a result of either a violent impact to the head, neck, torso, or pelvis or a sudden acceleration or deceleration injury (e.g., high-speed motor vehicle collisions and falls from significant height). In patients with a concerning mechanism of injury, in addition to first addressing the ABCs, careful and meticulous attention must be paid to C-spine immobilization and appropriate splinting.

Symptoms

- Pain, numbness, and/or tingling
- Weakness
- Pain with movement
- Difficulty breathing (cervical or high thoracic injuries may cause paralysis of the respiratory musculature and breathing may be from the diaphragm alone)

Signs
- Relative bradycardia
- Hypotension
- Peripheral vasodilation/flush
- Gross deformity
- Tenderness
- Paralysis
- Hypothermia (resulting from peripheral vasodilation)
- Loss of or decreased sensation
- Incontinence
- Priapism

Workup
See Chapter 36, Trauma.

Comments and Treatment Considerations
Treatment of patients with suspected cervical spine injury includes stabilization via the ABCs, immobilization, pharmacologic therapy, and emergent neurosurgical consultation (see Chapter 36, Trauma).

Consider high-dose steroids in patients with suspected spinal cord injury at a dose of 30 mg/kg IV bolus of methylprednisolone over 15 minutes, followed 45 minutes later by a continuous infusion of 5.4 mg/kg/hr. However, recent studies have called into question this standard practice. Norepinephrine is the vasopressor of choice because of the significant peripheral vasoconstriction that occurs during infusion. Pediatric patients with neurogenic shock should be cared for in an ICU setting with pediatric neurosurgical consultation.

 ## CARDIOGENIC SHOCK

Cardiogenic shock is due to myocardial dysfunction or "pump" failure. Cardiogenic shock is most commonly seen in adult patients with acute myocardial infarction and is rare in the pediatric population. In children, the common etiologies of cardiogenic shock include viral myocarditis, arrhythmia, ingestions, postoperative complications of cardiac surgery, metabolic derangements (hypoglycemia), and congenital heart disease (see Chapter 8, Chest Pain, and Chapter 34, Tachycardia).

Symptoms
- History of congenital heart disease or heart surgery
- Difficulty or tiring with feeding
- Failure to thrive

Signs
- Rales on pulmonary examination
- Gallop
- Hepatomegaly
- Jugular venous distention
- Tachycardia/bradycardia
- Irregular heart rate
- Weak or absent pulses

Additional Workup Recommendations for Suspected Cardiogenic Shock
- CXR.
- ECG.
- Echocardiography.

Comments and Treatment Considerations
See earlier section, Emergent Therapy for Shock, for emergent therapy and suggested workup. The treatment of cardiogenic shock will vary a great deal based on underlying etiology. If cardiogenic shock is suspected, emergent consultation with a pediatric cardiologist is required. Consider the early use of vasopressors and inotropes.

 OTHER

Other etiologies of shock include obstructive (e.g., tamponade, tension pneumothorax, and pulmonary embolism), adrenal insufficiency, and dissociative (e.g., carbon monoxide poisoning or methemoglobinemia) processes. Obstructive etiologies and their treatment are discussed in Chapter 8, Chest Pain, and Chapter 30, Respiratory Distress. Carbon monoxide poisoning is discussed in Chapter 35, Toxic Ingestion, Approach To. Methemoglobinemia is discussed in Chapter 9, Cyanosis.

A rare patient with acute adrenal insufficiency can be hypotensive, hypovolemic, and in shock. Clues to diagnosis include a history of adrenal insufficiency, ambiguous genitalia, laboratory evidence such as hyponatremia, hyperkalemia, hypoglycemia, hypercalcemia, and/or metabolic acidosis, and exogenous use of long-term steroids. The diagnosis is particularly difficult in a male infant but needs to be considered if electrolytes show hyponatremia with hyperkalemia. Commonly, these patients will have undergone an additional stress such as acute infection or trauma. An endocrinologist should be consulted immediately and emergent management with fluid support and stress steroids should be initiated. Fluid support should consist of normal saline without potassium added until blood pressure and serum potassium level have normalized. Hydrocortisone 50 to 100 mg IV immediately and then as 50 mg/m^2/24 hr IV given continuously or divided q6h or methylprednisolone 7.5 mg/m^2/24 hr IV divided q8h. Admission to a pediatric ICU with pediatric endocrinology consultation is necessary for further management, diagnosis, and treatment planning.

REFERENCES

American College of Emergency Physicians and American Academy of Pediatrics: *APLS: The pediatric emergency medicine course*, 3rd ed, Washington, DC, 1998, ACEP/AAP.

American Heart Association and American Academy of Pediatrics: *Pediatric advanced life support, 1997–1999*, Washington DC, 1999, AHA/AAP.

Bell LM: Shock. In Fleisher GR, Ludwig S: *Textbook of pediatric emergency medicine*, 4th ed, Philadelphia, 2000, Lippincott Williams & Wilkins.

Bracken MB, Shepard ML, Collins WF, et al: A randomized controlled trial of methylprednisolone or naloxone in the treatment of acute spinal-cord injury study, *N Engl J Med* 332:1405-1411, 1990.

Fink MP: In Rippe JM, Irwin RS, Fink MP, Cerra FB, editors: *Intensive care medicine*, 3rd ed, Boston, Little, Brown, 1996.

Malley R, Huskins WC, Kuppermann N: Multivariable predictive models for adverse outcome of invasive meningococcal disease in children, *J Pediatr* 129(5):702-710, 1996.

Parillo JE: Approach to the patient with shock. In Goldman L, editor: *Cecil textbook of medicine*, 21st ed, Philadelphia, 2000, WB Saunders.

CHAPTER 21

Immunocompromised Patients: Special Considerations

BEN M. WILLWERTH

Children who are immunocompromised are at increased risk of life-threatening illness from infectious agents that often would be noninvasive in an immunocompetent child. Children can be immunocompromised because of a variety of chronic illnesses including sickle cell disease, human immunodeficiency virus (HIV), hypogammaglobulinemia, or severe combined immune deficiency. Other factors such as pharmacologic immunosuppression in solid organ transplant recipients, current or recent chemotherapy, recent bone marrow transplant, and asplenia can also cause an immunocompromised state. These children may require empiric antibiotics in the setting of a low-grade fever even without other signs of possible infection. Patients with absolute neutrophil counts (ANCs) <500 are at increased risk of infection and should be empirically treated with broad-spectrum antibiotics pending culture results. Immunocompromised patients may have less clinically apparent manifestations of acute infection because of treatments, including steroids. Additionally, these patients may deteriorate more quickly than one would expect in an immunocompetent host.

SEPSIS

Given their increased susceptibility to systemic infections, immunocompromised patients are at increased risk of developing sepsis. Early recognition and treatment of sepsis is critical to improve patient outcome (see Chapter 14, Fever, and Chapter 20, Hypotension/Shock).

Symptoms

- Fever +++
- Lethargy or irritability in infants
- Confusion/altered mental status
- May have shortness of breath, vomiting

Signs

- Tachycardia +++
- Tachypnea
- Late signs include hypotension and/or evidence of poor perfusion: delayed capillary refill, weak peripheral pulses, cool extremities, and/or oliguria
- Petechiae or purpura may be present +

Workup

- Blood cultures while obtaining intravenous access followed immediately by intravenous antibiotics.
- CBC to evaluate for neutropenia (ANC <500).
- Cultures of other potential sites of infection (urine, cerebrospinal fluid, stool, or wound drainage) as soon as possible but do not delay antibiotics to obtain these cultures. Positioning for lumbar puncture may cause respiratory compromise, so this procedure should be deferred in the patient with an unstable respiratory status.
- Electrolytes, which may show evidence of a metabolic acidosis.
- Renal function and coagulation studies.

Comments and Treatment Considerations

Septic shock should be aggressively treated in the standard fashion by initially evaluating and stabilizing the airway, breathing, and circulation. Antibiotics, intravenous fluid, and if necessary inotropic and vasoactive agents should be rapidly administered (see Chapter 20, Hypotension/Shock). Although the likely causative agent of septic shock varies according to patient population and origin of immunosuppression, initial antibiotic therapy in all cases should be broad spectrum. Some patients will have previously positive cultures that may help to direct antibiotic choice. Of the many antibiotic combinations available, two choices include the following: ceftazidime 150 mg/kg/day IV divided q8h (max 6 g/day) or piperacillin-tazobactam dosed at 300 mg of piperacillin component/kg/day IV divided q6-8h (max 18 g of piperacillin per day) plus gentamicin 6 to 7.5 mg/kg/day IV divided q8-24h.

If there is a possibility of central venous catheter (CVC) infection (see the following section for further details), either of the preceding options plus vancomycin 40 to 60 mg/kg/day IV divided q6-8h (max 2 g/day) should be prescribed.

Consultation with the infectious disease service and the appropriate specialist providing care for the underlying diagnosis should occur as early as possible when making management decisions but should not delay initial doses of antibiotics.

CENTRAL VENOUS CATHETERS: INFECTION

CVCs are often placed in certain groups of immunosuppressed children to provide intravenous access for transfusions, medications, or fluids. Although these catheters can be a nidus for infection in any patient, immunocompromised patients are particularly susceptible. Recognition and treatment of CVC infection may help prevent a more systemic infection, sepsis, and death.

Symptoms
- Fever
- May have erythema or discharge at catheter entry site

Signs
- Temperature >38-38.5° C on two measurements ++
- Discharge from line entry site
- Erythema around entry site or along CVC route
- Tenderness along CVC route

Workup

- Blood culture from CVC.
- Consider peripheral blood culture.
- Culture discharge from line entry site if present.
- CBC count with differential looking for leukocytosis or neutropenia defined as ANC <500.
- Surgical consult if CVC tunnel infection suspected.

Comments and Treatment Considerations

Patients with CVCs are at increased risk of infection from gram-positive organisms, particularly *Staphylococcus aureus* and *Staphylococcus non-aureus*. Some patients will have previously positive cultures that may help to direct antibiotic choice. In general, patients with suspected CVC infections should receive broad-spectrum intravenous antibiotics including vancomycin (see above) and should be admitted to the hospital.

Although many CVC infections can be successfully treated with antibiotics without removal of the catheter, at times the catheter will need to be removed to clear the infection. Consultation with the infectious disease service, the appropriate specialist providing care for the underlying diagnosis, and the surgeon who placed the line should occur as early as possible when making management decisions but should not delay initial doses of antibiotics.

FEVER: POSSIBLE OCCULT INFECTION

Fever in the immunocompromised patient may be the first sign of a life-threatening infection and must be addressed promptly and thoroughly. Fever in this population can be an indicator of viral, bacterial, or fungal infections or may be related to noninfectious etiologies such as transfusion of blood products. Laboratory testing and empiric treatment of possible occult infections should be tailored to the severity of immunosuppression. Patients with human immunodeficiency virus (HIV) and/or low CD4 cell counts, neutropenia from chemotherapy, recent bone marrow transplant, and multidrug pharmacologic immunosuppression should be tested and treated more aggressively.

Symptoms
- Fever
- No other symptoms need be present, but if present, they may help direct workup and management

Signs
- Temperature >38-38.5° C on two measurements
- Stable vital signs
- Nontoxic appearance

Workup
- Blood culture.
- CBC with differential evaluating for neutropenia (ANC <500).
- UA and urine culture (catheterization should be avoided in neutropenic patients if possible).
- CXR in patients with cough, respiratory distress, and/or hypoxia. Consider CXR in patients with sickle cell disease who are younger than 3 years.
- Throat culture in patients with sore throat or posterior pharyngeal findings consistent with strep throat.
- Stool cultures for *Salmonella*, *Shigella*, *Campylobacter*, *Yersinia*, and *Escherichia coli* if diarrhea present.
- Central venous line entry site culture if any exudate.

Comments and Treatment Considerations

Significantly immunocompromised patients should receive empiric broad-spectrum antibiotics in the emergency department with minimal delay. Antibiotic choice should also be tailored to local bacterial resistance patterns. Patients who meet low-risk criteria such as well-appearing patients with sickle cell disease who are older than 6 months, who have acceptable hematologic parameters, and who will reliably follow up, as well as well-appearing nonneutropenic oncology patients with reliable follow-up can typically be treated with ceftriaxone dosed at 50 mg/kg (max 2 g/dose) IV × 1 and discharged. Higher risk patients, including those with sickle cell disease and a focal bacterial infection such as pneumonia; oncology patients who are neutropenic; and HIV-positive patients with depressed CD4 cell counts, should be admitted for empiric broad-spectrum IV antibiotics with *Pseudomonas* coverage (see previous section). Consultation with the infectious disease service and the specialist providing care for the patient's underlying diagnosis should occur as early as possible when making management decisions.

VARICELLA AND VARICELLA EXPOSURES

Primary infection with varicella-zoster virus (VZV) causes chickenpox. Though generally a benign, self-limited disease, chickenpox can lead to disseminated life-threatening illness in the immunocompromised patient (see Chapter 29, Rash).

Symptoms
- Prodromal symptoms such as fever, malaise, anorexia, and headache may precede rash by 1 to 2 days
- Intensely pruritic vesicular rash develops 10 to 21 days after known exposure
- Disseminated disease may be suggested by cough (pneumonia), abdominal pain (hepatitis), and abnormal behavior (encephalitis)

Signs
- Fever
- Generalized, pruritic, vesicular rash, which may not be as typical as when seen in an immunocompetent host
- May be accompanied by signs of disseminated disease such as respiratory distress (pneumonia), abdominal tenderness (hepatitis), or altered mental status (encephalitis)

Workup
- Immunofluorescent antibody test performed on vesicular scrapings can confirm presence of VZV infection in cases in which the diagnosis is unclear.
- Testing for disseminated disease should be based on symptomology.

Comments and Treatment Considerations

Immunocompromised individuals should receive varicella-zoster immune globulin (VZIG) if they have had significant exposure to an infectious individual. The dose is 125 units for every 10 kg of body weight (min 125 units/dose, max 625 units/dose) IM × 1. No more than 2.5 ml of VZIG should be administered per site. Once disease is established, VZIG is no longer effective and should not be given. The recommended time frame for VZIG administration is within 48 hours but not >96 hours after exposure. Acyclovir dosed at 30 mg/kg/day IV divided q8h (use 60 mg/kg/day IV divided q8h for encephalitis) is recommended in immunocompromised patients with active disease begun at the first sign of rash. Appropriate hydration and dose modification in patients with renal insufficiency is necessary when treating with acyclovir. Consultation with the infectious disease service and the specialist providing care for the patient's underlying diagnosis should occur as early as possible.

 ZOSTER

As with primary varicella infection, recurrent varicella infection (zoster) can lead to disseminated life-threatening illness in the immunocompromised host.

Symptoms
- Sudden onset of skin lesions in localized region
- Often, but not always, pain in region of lesions

Signs
- Grouped vesicles on a erythematous base in a dermatomal distribution
- Thoracic dermatomes most commonly involved

Workup
- None needed if classic appearance present.
- May perform immunofluorescent antibody test for VZV if diagnosis is unclear.

Comments and Treatment Considerations

Immunocompromised patients with zoster infection should be admitted to the hospital for intravenous acyclovir (see dosing recommendations above). They are at risk of dissemination of VZV, leading to pneumonia, hepatitis, or encephalitis. Testing for these complications should be done if symptoms are present. Consultation with the specialist providing care for the patient's underlying diagnosis should occur as early as possible.

REFERENCES

Committee on Infectious Diseases: Varicella-zoster infections. In Peter G, editor: *2001 Red Book*, Elk Grove Village, Ill, 2001, AAP.

Dayan P, Pan S, Chamberlain J: Fever in the immunocompromised host, *Clin Pediatr Emerg Med* 1:138-149, 2000.

Egerer G, Goldschmidt H, Muller I: Ceftriaxone for the treatment of febrile episodes in nonneutropenic patients with hematooncologic disease of HIV infection: comparison of outpatient and inpatient care, *Chemotherapy* 47:219-225, 2001.

Furth S, Sullivan E, Neu A: Varicella in the first year after renal transplantation: a report of the North American Pediatric Renal Transplant Cooperative Study (NAPRTCS), *Pediatr Transplant* 1:37-42, 1997.

Nachman J, Honig G: Fever and neutropenia in children with neoplastic disease, *Cancer* 45:407-412, 1980.

Pizzo P: Fever in immunocompromised patients, *N Engl J Med* 341:893-900, 1999.

Schexnayder S: Pediatric septic shock, *Pediatr Rev* 20:303-307, 1999.

Riikonen P, Saarinen U, Lahteenoja K, et al: Management of indwelling central venous catheters in pediatric cancer patients with fever and neutropenia, *Scand J Infect Dis* 25:357-364, 1993.

Rizzari C, Palamone G, Corbetta A, et al: Central venous catheter-related infections in pediatric hematology-oncology patients: role of home and hospital management, *Pediatr Hematol Oncol* 9:115-123, 1992.

Rowland P, Wald E, Mirro J: Progressive varicella presenting with pain and minimal skin involvement in children with acute lymphoblastic leukemia, *J Clin Oncol* 13:1697-1703, 1995.

Takayama N, Yamada H, Kaku H: Herpes zoster in immunocompetent and immunocompromised Japanese children, *Pediatr Int* 42:275-279, 2000.

Wilimas J, Flynn P, Harris S, et al: A randomized study of outpatient treatment with ceftriaxone for selected febrile children with sickle cell disease, *N Engl J Med* 329:472-502, 1993.

CHAPTER 22

Irritability

DEWESH AGRAWAL

The irritable infant presents with excessive inconsolable crying or fussiness, the source of which is not obvious to the parents. The differential diagnosis of infant crying ranges from normal hunger reaction to severe life-threatening illness. Few, if any, symptoms in medicine are less specific than crying in an infant. Numerous studies have reported that normal healthy infants cry up to 3 hours daily.

The clinician evaluating an irritable infant thus is faced with the daunting task of deciphering the cause of the infant's distress. Unfortunately, a careful and orderly diagnostic approach including a thorough history and detailed physical examination will definitively identify the cause only about half of the time. Fortunately, this same approach should exclude all severe life-threatening causes of irritability. This chapter focuses on reviewing the evaluation and treatment of the more serious illnesses that present with an irritable infant.

 INCREASED INTRACRANIAL PRESSURE

See Chapter 3, Altered Mental Status.

 TORSION OF THE TESTES

See Chapter 31, Scrotal Pain or Swelling.

INFECTION/SEPSIS/MENINGITIS

See Chapter 14, Fever.

SUPRAVENTRICULAR TACHYCARDIA

See Chapter 3, Altered Mental Status, and Chapter 34, Tachycardia.

 ## INCARCERATED HERNIA

See Chapter 31, Scrotal Pain or Swelling.

 ## SKULL FRACTURE

See Chapter 2, Abuse/Rape, and Chapter 36, Trauma.

 ## OTHER FRACTURES

See Chapter 15, Fractures Not to Miss.

 ## ABUSE

See Chapter 2, Abuse/Rape.

 ## GASTROESOPHAGEAL REFLUX

See Chapter 38, Vomiting.

NEONATAL DRUG WITHDRAWAL

Infants born to mothers who abuse drugs may show symptoms of withdrawal. Commonly, these infants are identified in the newborn nursery; however, an infant may present for evaluation after discharge home, particularly if the mother has been trying to conceal her drug abuse problem. Before attributing signs of irritability to possible withdrawal, it is imperative to rule out other particularly life-threatening etiologies of irritability. No matter what the drug of abuse, social concerns need to be addressed and the child's safety ensured. The two most common withdrawal patterns are from opioids or cocaine.

NEONATAL NARCOTIC ABSTINENCE SYNDROME

The diagnosis of neonatal narcotic abstinence syndrome (NAS) should be suspected based on history and may be substantiated by neonatal meconium or urine drug testing; however, testing may prove negative if last maternal use was not recent.

Infants with NAS frequently exhibit symptoms of central nervous system irritability and gastrointestinal dysfunction. Seizures occur in 2% to 11% of infants. The degree of symptomatology is related to the amount and timing of maternal use, with approximately 50% to 60% of exposed infants requiring therapy. A scoring system of signs and symptoms (Fig. 22-1) has been developed to aid in the diagnosis and monitoring of the infant's clinical response to therapy. The abstinence scoring sheet weighs 31 items most commonly observed in an opioid-exposed infant. Higher scores are assigned to infants with more severe withdrawal symptoms. Infants with scores higher than 8 generally require medical therapy with a morphine equivalent or phenobarbital to lessen symptoms of withdrawal. The same scoring system is then used to wean the infant from this therapy. Comfort measures include swaddling, pacifier use, aspirating nasal secretions, providing soft sheets/sheepskin, and controlling noise/light exposure. Consultation with a neonatologist for admission and further management is recommended.

PERINATAL COCAINE EXPOSURE

Although cocaine use has begun to decline, it still represents a major public health problem, especially in urban centers. Cocaine is a highly psychoactive substance that readily crosses the placenta, generating numerous and variable effects on the developing fetus. Prenatal cocaine exposure produces selective alterations in the nigrostriatal dopaminergic system, which are felt to underlie the neurobehavioral alterations seen in exposed infants.

NEONATAL ABSTINENCE SCORING SYSTEM

SYSTEM	SIGNS AND SYMPTOMS	SCORE	AM						PM					COMMENTS
CENTRAL NERVOUS SYSTEM DISTURBANCES	Excessive high pitched (or other) cry	2												Daily weight:
	Continuous high pitched (or other) cry	3												
	Sleeps ,1 hour after feeding	3												
	Sleeps ,2 hours after feeding	2												
	Sleeps ,3 hours after feeding	1												
	Hyperactive Moro reflex	2												
	Markedly hyperactive Moro reflex	3												
	Mild tremors disturbed	1												
	Moderate-severe tremors disturbed	2												
	Mild tremors undisturbed	3												
	Moderate-severe tremors undisturbed	4												
	Increased muscle tone	2												
	Excoriation (specific area)	1												
	Myoclonic jerks	3												
	Generalized convulsions	5												
METABOLIC/VASOMOTOR/RESPIRATORY DISTURBANCES	Sweating	1												
	Fever ,101 (99-100.8 F/37.2-38.2 C)	1												
	Fever .101 (38.4 C and higher)	2												
	Frequent yawning (.3-4 times/interval)	1												
	Mottling	1												
	Nasal stuffiness	1												
	Sneezing (.3-4 times/interval)	1												
	Nasal flaring	2												
	Respiratory rate .60/min	1												
	Respiratory rate .60/min with retractions	2												
GASTROINTESTINAL DISTURBANCES	Excessive sucking	1												
	Poor feeding	2												
	Regurgitation	2												
	Projectile vomiting	3												
	Loose stools	2												
	Watery stools	3												
	TOTAL SCORE													
	INITIALS OF SCORER													

Fig. 22-1 Neonatal abstinence score sheet. (From Finnegan LP: Neonatal abstinence syndrome. In Nelson N (ed): *Current therapy in neonatal/perinatal medicine*, ed 2, Ontario, 1990, BC Decker.)

Symptoms

- Irritability ++++
- Excessive crying ++++
- Tremulousness ++++
- Excitability +++
- Sleep disturbance +++
- Poor feeding +++

Signs
- Hypertonia ++++
- Hyperreflexia +++
- Premature birth ++
- Low birth weight ++
- Microcephaly +
- Cerebral infarction and seizures +

Workup
- Urine toxicology screen.

Comments and Treatment Considerations
Because cocaine is a sympathomimetic stimulant, cocaine-addicted infants do not demonstrate the classic signs of opioid withdrawal. Cocaine withdrawal alone rarely requires pharmacologic treatment. However, if additional substances were being abused by the mother, then the neonate may show more serious withdrawal symptoms and require medical therapy (see earlier section).

Most cocaine associations are transient and resolve in infancy or early childhood. Whether such transient abnormalities place infants at increased risk of later neurodevelopmental impairments is not fully known. Controlled studies have found no cognitive differences related to prenatal cocaine exposure among young children, except as mediated through effects on head growth. However, cocaine-exposed children do appear to suffer from neurobehavioral abnormalities such as decreased attentiveness and emotional expressivity.

 ## ACUTE OTITIS MEDIA

Otitis media is the most common diagnosis in pediatric sick office visits, accounting for one third of all pediatric sick visits in the United States. The greatest prevalence is seen in infants 6 to 18 months of age. Sixty-two percent of children by 1 year of age have had an episode of acute otitis media (AOM), and seventeen percent have had three or more. By 3 years of age, >80% of children have had at least one episode, and 46% have had at least three episodes. Children have eustachian tubes, which are shorter, more horizontal, and with less cartilaginous support when compared to adults. This predisposes to reflux of nasopharyngeal secretions into the middle ear cavity and impedes drainage of the middle ear contents, setting the stage for otitis media.

AOM is best defined as an acute infection of the middle ear and must be differentiated from otitis media with effusion (OME). Not all patients with effusions of the middle ear need antibiotic therapy and associated signs and symptoms of an acute infection must be sought.

Symptoms
- Irritability/pain ++++
- Poor feeding +++
- Ear tugging +++
- Vomiting +

Signs
- Otalgia (in older children) ++++
- Fever +++
- Otorrhea +
- Conductive hearing loss (in older children)

Workup
The diagnosis of AOM is clinical and is best made by pneu-matic otoscopy or tympanometry. Findings in AOM include an middle ear effusion with decreased mobility of the tympanic membrane; a erythematous, bulging, and/or opaque tym-panic membrane with loss of the normal landmarks; and/or otorrhea present in the ear canal (Fig. 22-2). Fever and ear pain increase the likelihood of AOM.

Comments and Treatment Considerations
In patients with AOM, bacterial pathogens can be isolated from the middle ear fluid in approximately 60% of patients and viruses can be cultured or detected by antigens in up to 40% of patients. The organisms that inhabit the nasopharynx are the same ones that cause otitis media. *Streptococcus pneumoniae*

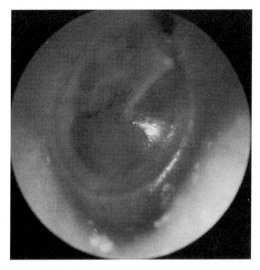

Fig. 22-2   Otoscopic appearance in otitis media with effusion. The handle and short process of the malleus are brought into relief as a result of retraction of the eardrum.

infection is the most common cause, responsible for approximately 40% of all bacterial causes of otitis media. *Haemophilus influenzae* (mostly nontypeable strains) and *Moraxella (Branhamella) catarrhalis* are the next most likely causative organisms, responsible for approximately 25% and 15% of bacterial cases, respectively. The remaining 20% of bacterial causes include group A *Streptococcus*, *Staphylococcus aureus*, *Pseudomonas aeruginosa*, and *Mycoplasma pneumoniae*. The most commonly isolated virus is respiratory syncytial virus (RSV), followed by rhinovirus, adenovirus, parainfluenza virus, coronavirus, influenzavirus, and enterovirus.

Up to 80% of cases of otitis media will resolve without treatment and the most recent recommendations support the judicious use of antibiotics, which in the past have been the mainstay of therapy. Empiric antibiotic therapy is still recommended for suspected AOM in infants 2 to 6 months of age. However, symptomatic treatment with analgesics and reevaluation of patient in 24 hours for children 6 months-2 years with continued fever is warranted before initiating antibiotics in patients without severe illness. Symptomatic treatment should be continued for 72 hours while observing for additional signs of AOM before beginning antibiotics in children older than 2 years (this is often termed "watchful waiting").

The choice of antibiotic should be guided by the distribution of the bacterial pathogens encountered in your area and knowledge of their susceptibility patterns. High-dose amoxicillin 80 to 100 mg/kg/day PO divided tid is the recommended antibiotic of choice. If the patient fails treatment despite adequate dosing of amoxicillin, the second-line agent of choice is amoxicillin–clavulanic acid (Augmentin), which provides coverage against β-lactamase–producing organisms, such as *H. influenzae*. However, amoxicillin–clavulanic acid will not provide additional benefit over high-dose amoxicillin in a patient with resistant *S. pneumoniae*. Third-line agents include azithromycin or second- and third-generation cephalosporins (including cefuroxime, ceftriaxone, cefpodoxime, cefdinir, and cefprozil, among others). Pediazole and Bactrim are generally avoided secondary to increasing resistance patterns and side effects. For penicillin-allergic patients (those with true type I hypersensitivity) azithromycin 30 mg/kg PO (max 1500 mg) as a single dose becomes the first-line agent. Second-line agents for the penicillin-allergic patients may include clindamycin or a fluoroquinolone.

Supportive measures include the use of systemic antipyretics/analgesics (acetaminophen and ibuprofen) and topical analgesics (benzocaine/antipyrine drops). A 3-week follow-up visit with the primary care provider to assess for persistent effusion should be considered in patients with recurrent infections.

 ## *CORNEAL ABRASION*

Corneal abrasions are a common cause of irritability, which if not considered are overlooked (see Chapter 12, Eye Pain and Redness).

�֎ *HAIR-THREAD TOURNIQUET SYNDROME*

A hair, thread, or similar fiber can become wrapped circumfer-
entially around a digit (Fig. 22-3), the penis, or even the clitoris
of an infant, causing constriction, edema, erythema, and extreme
pain. If left untreated, it may result in ischemic necrosis and
amputation of the involved appendage. Hair or loose thread is
most prone to wrap around an appendage when the appendage
is confined in a tight-fitting garment, such as mittens or socks.

In a review by Barton et al (1988) of 66 cases of hair-thread
tourniquets from the medical literature, 43% involved toes, and
33% involved the external genitalia, and 24% involved fingers.

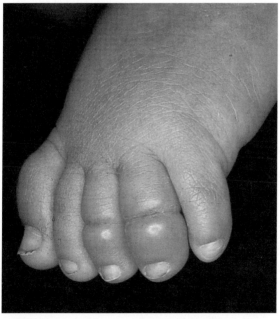

Fig. 22-3   Hair tourniquet syndrome. The mild erythema and
edema of the third and fourth toes are the result of constriction
by hairs that accidentally became wrapped around them. (From
Gantner JC, Zitelli B: *Common and chronic symptoms in pediatrics,* St. Louis, 1997, Mosby. Courtesy Dr. Thomas J. Daley,
Bronx-Lebanon Hospital, Bronx, New York.)

The median ages at involvement for the toe, finger, and penis were 12 weeks, 3 weeks, and 2 years, respectively. Hair was the cause of constriction in 79% of infants with toe involvement and 95% of cases with genitalia involvement, whereas thread was responsible for 80% of the cases involving fingers.

Symptoms
- Irritability ++++
- Inconsolable crying +++
- Pain of the digit, penis, or clitoris +++

Signs
- Early signs include erythema and edema of the affected appendage
- Late signs include ecchymosis and ischemic necrosis of the affected appendage
- The constricting hair or fibers can become embedded in and obscured by the surrounding edematous tissue, making it difficult or impossible to discern

Workup
- High index of suspicion and thorough physical examination of the digits and external genitalia.

Comments and Treatment Considerations
Prompt recognition of the tourniquet effect and removal of the offending constricting agent are critical to prevent damage to or loss of the involved appendage. Fine-toothed forceps and microscissors facilitate removal of the embedded constricting agent. Examination with the child under sedation may be required. Most cases reported in the literature seem to be accidental, although child abuse must be considered, especially with involvement of the genitalia.

 TEETHING

Teething refers to the combination of behaviors observed in infants (most commonly between the ages of 4 and 18 months)

secondary to the inflammation and sensitivity that sometimes occur as teeth penetrate the gums. Eruption of primary teeth begins with the central incisors and generally progresses laterally. The mean ages for eruption of the various primary teeth are as follows: central incisors, 6 months; lateral incisors, 9 months; canines, 18 months; first molars, 12 months; and second molars, 25 months.

The effect of teething on infant health and behavior has been debated for thousands of years, and traditional beliefs on this issue have still not been supplanted by reproducible and widely accepted scientific findings. Over the years many symptoms have been attributed to teething in infants. Fortunately, there is little evidence that serious systemic disturbances result from teething.

In a recent large prospective study of 125 healthy infants aged 4 to 12 months designed to ascertain signs and symptoms attributed to teething, Macknin et al. (2000) collected daily symptom data for 19,422 child-days and 475 tooth eruptions. Although many signs and symptoms were statistically correlated with teething, none occurred in >35% of teething infants, and no symptom cluster could reliably predict the imminent emergence of a tooth. Nevertheless, the following symptoms and signs were statistically associated with teething.

Symptoms
- Mild irritability and crying +++
- Mouthing, biting, sucking, and gum-rubbing behaviors ++++
- Drooling and increased salivation ++++
- Wakefulness ++
- Ear rubbing ++
- Decreased appetite for solid foods ++

Signs
- Perioral facial erythema and/or rash ++
- Mild temperature elevation of ≤100° F

Workup
- Careful inspection of the gums and exclusion of other causes of irritability.

Comments and Treatment Considerations
Instruct parents to try gently rubbing or massaging the gums with their fingers. A blunt firm object for the infant to bite on such as a teething ring usually provides relief. Topical anesthetic gels are not necessary or useful, because they wash out of the baby's mouth within minutes. They may be associated with potential toxicity (such as methemoglobinemia) from parental overuse and frequent reapplication.

If the child has a fever >100° F or seems particularly miserable, teething is unlikely the sole cause. In other words before attributing any signs or symptoms of a potentially serious illness to teething, all other possible causes must be ruled out.

 COLIC

Excessive inconsolable crying in an infant is often attributed to colic. Although much has been written on infant colic, there is no universally accepted definition of colic. *Colic* may be best defined as crying during the first 3 to 4 months of life for ≥3 hours per day, on ≥3 days per week in infants who are not suffering from other conditions that may cause prolonged crying such as organic disease, hunger, or neglect. The general pattern of colic begins with inconsolable crying at 2 to 4 weeks of age, peaking at 6 to 8 weeks of age and resolving by approximately 4 months of age.

The occurrence rate of colic varies greatly in the literature (from 4% to 25%), depending on the method of study and the definition of *colic* used. Although there are numerous theories, there is no well-established etiology for infant colic. Most developmental specialists attribute colic to a part of the normal developmental process of infants who are perceived as somewhat temperamental. In other words, colic may best be viewed as a clinical manifestation of normal emotional development in which an infant has a diminished capacity to regulate the duration of crying. On the other hand, most parents incorrectly attribute a colicky infant's crying as a response to pain or gastrointestinal symptoms such as "gas" or "cramps."

Symptoms
- Excessive crying
- Difficulty consoling
- Overwhelmed and exhausted parents

Signs
- Crying associated with facial flushing and grimacing, tense abdomen, arched back, clenched fists, and flexed extremities that typically occurs in the late afternoons and evenings
- Paroxysmal crying that is higher pitched, begins suddenly, and has a rapid crescendo

Workup
Organic disease accounts for fewer than 5% of infants presenting with colic syndrome. Unfortunately, there is no reliable way for diagnosing an infant's crying as colic. Only after all emergent and potentially serious diagnoses have been adequately considered and eliminated can a diagnosis of infant colic be entertained. The infant must have a normal physical examination, normal neurologic development, and normal growth patterns.

Comments and Treatment Considerations
Although many physicians manage infant colic by prescribing a succession of medications (such as simethicone, ranitidine, antispasmodics, and sedatives) and nonmedical interventions (such as formula changes, fiber supplementation, early introduction of solids, and frequent burping), none of these treatments has been rigorously shown in the medical literature to be both safe and effective. This approach may be useful for frantic parents who feel that "something needs to be done" to calm their distressed infant; however, this same approach incorrectly suggests to these same parents that "something is wrong" with their infant that requires treatment.

Simple soothing maneuvers for the infant that are promptly initiated (such as rhythmic rocking, wind-up swings, patting the infant's back, back-and-forth movements in a stroller, long car rides, secure swaddling, monotonous noise, and nonnutritive sucking) may be helpful. A caring, understanding, supportive, and nonjudgmental approach to frantic parents that builds rapport is the *sine qua non* for successful management of infant colic.

Most of all, parents need reassurance that their infant is healthy and normal, and that colic is a temporary benign pattern of behavior that is time limited and disappears by 4 months of age. There is light at the end of the tunnel!

REFERENCES

American Academy of Pediatrics, Committee on Drugs: Neonatal drug withdrawal, *Pediatrics* 101(6):1079, 1998.

Barr RG: Colic and crying syndromes in infants, *Pediatrics* 102:1282, 1998.

Barton DJ, Sloan GM, Nichter LS, Reinisch JF: Hair-thread tourniquet syndrome, *Pediatrics* 82:925, 1988.

Berman S: Otitis media in children, *N Engl J Med* 332:1560, 1995.

Byington CL: Diagnosis and management of otitis media with effusion, *Pediatr Ann* 27:96, 1998.

Chiriboga CA: Neurological correlates of fetal cocaine exposure, *Ann N Y Acad Sci* 846:109, 1998.

Conners G: Index of suspicion. Case 2: hair tourniquet, *Pediatr Rev* 18:283, 1997.

Conrad D: Should acute otitis media ever be treated with antibiotics? *Pediatr Ann* 27:66, 1998.

Coyle MG, Ferguson A, Lagasse L, et al: Diluted tincture of opium (DTO) and phenobarbital versus DTO alone for neonatal opiate withdrawal in term infants, *J Pediatr* 140(5):561, 2002.

Dowell SF et al: Acute otitis media: management and surveillance in an era of pneumococcal resistance: a report from the drug-resistant *Streptococcus pneumoniae* therapeutic working group, *Pediatr Infect Dis J* 18:1, 1999.

Fleisher DR: Coping with colic, *Contemp Pediatr* 15:144, 1998.

Frank DA, Augustyn M, Knight WG, et al: Growth, development, and behavior in early childhood following prenatal cocaine exposure: a systematic review, *JAMA* 285:1613, 2001.

Glatt SJ, Bolanos CA, Trksak GH, Jackson D: Effects of prenatal cocaine exposure on dopamine system development: a meta-analysis, *Neurotoxicol Teratol* 22:617, 2000.

Heikkinen T, Thint M, Chonmaitree T: Prevalence of various respiratory viruses in the middle ear during acute otitis media, *N Engl J Med* 340:260, 1999.

Hoberman A, Paradise JL: Acute otitis media: diagnosis and management in the year 2000, *Pediatr Ann* 29:609, 2000.

Keller RW, Snyder-Keller A: Prenatal cocaine exposure, *Ann N Y Acad Sci* 909:217, 2000.

Kozyrskyj AL et al: Treatment of acute otitis media with a shortened course of antibiotics: a meta analysis, *JAMA* 279:1736, 1998.

Lehtonen LA, Rautava PT: Infantile colic: natural history and treatment, *Curr Probl Pediatr* 26:79, 1996.

Macknin ML, Piedmonte M, Jacobs J, Skibinski C: Symptoms associated with infant teething: a prospective study, *Pediatrics* 105:747, 2000.

Maxson S, Yamauchi T: Acute otitis media, *Pediatr Rev* 17:191, 1996.

Merenstein GB, Gardner SL: *Handbook of neonatal intensive care*, St. Louis, 2002, Mosby.

Rich MA, Keating MA: Hair tourniquet syndrome of the clitoris, *J Urol* 162:190, 1999.

Osborn DA, Jeffery HE, Cole MJ: Sedative for opiate withdrawal in newborn infants, *Cochrane Database Syst Rev* (3):CD002053, 2002.

Osborn DA, Cole MJ, Jeffery HE: Opiate treatment for opiate withdrawal in newborn infants, *Cochrane Database Syst Rev* (3):CD002059, 2003.

Rosenfeld JA, Clarity G: Acute otitis media in children, *Primary Care Clin Office Pract* 23:677, 1996.

Shelov SP, editor: Teething. In *American Academy of Pediatrics: caring for your baby and young child: birth to age 5*, New York, 1993, Bantam Books.

Sylwestrzak MS, Fischer BF, Fischer H: Recurrent clitoral tourniquet syndrome, *Pediatrics* 105:866, 2000.

Thomas CL, editor: Irritability. In *Taber's cyclopedic medical dictionary*, 17 ed, Philadelphia, 1993, FA Davis Company.

Wake M, Hesketh K, Lucas J: Teething and tooth eruption in infants: a cohort study, *Pediatrics* 106:1374, 2000.

Wang M, Schott J, Tunnessen WW: Picture of the month: hair-thread tourniquet syndrome, *Arch Pediatr Adolesc Med* 155:515, 2001.

CHAPTER 23

Jaundice

MICHAEL W. SHANNON

Jaundice is a yellow discoloration of the skin produced by accumulation of the bile acid bilirubin (hyperbilirubinemia) and is usually accompanied by *icterus*, a yellow discoloration of the sclera. Jaundice is invariably caused by one of two processes: impaired elimination or increased production of bilirubin. Bilirubin is normally produced by the hepatocytes and then is conjugated with a glucuronide molecule. From the hepatocytes, bilirubin is secreted into the bile canaliculi, then into the cystic duct, and then is stored in the gallbladder. From the gallbladder it is secreted into the duodenum with partial reabsorption in the distal ileum. Abnormalities in any step of this pathway can lead to hyperbilirubinemia and jaundice. Similarly, increases in the production of bilirubin at a rate exceeding the capacity for excretion can also cause jaundice.

Jaundice in children must be distinguished from *carotenemia*, the accumulation of carotene and other vitamin A congeners in the skin, acquired from the excess consumption of carotene-containing foods, such as squash, pumpkins, and carrots. Carotenemia is distinguished from jaundice by the absence of icterus and pruritus and when in doubt a bilirubin level. Causes of jaundice should be differentiated by the presence of *direct* (conjugated) or *indirect* (unconjugated) hyperbilirubinemia (Table 23-1).

Almost all cases of hyperbilirubinemia require an evaluation seeking an underlying cause; however, infants younger than 1 week who may be presenting for the first time with significant unconjugated hyperbilirubinemia may be life-threateningly ill and require prompt evaluation and therapy. Additionally, an older patient may be acutely ill, with jaundice as an indicator of overwhelming liver failure resulting from a life-threatening

Table 23-1 Common Causes of Direct (Conjugated) versus Indirect (Unconjugated) Hyperbilirubinemia

Direct (conjugated) hyperbilirubinemia
- Biliary tract disease
  - Cholelithiasis (gallstones)
  - Cholangitis
    - Extrahepatic mass, such as tumor
    - Choledochal cyst
  - Cholestasis
    - Cystic fibrosis
- Biliary atresia
- Bile duct stenosis
  - Pancreatitis
- Alagille syndrome

Indirect (unconjugated) hyperbilirubinemia
- "Physiologic"
- Immune hemolysis, for example, Rh incompatibility
- Crigler-Najjar syndrome
- Gilbert's disease
- Hepatitis

infection, coagulopathy, or congenital disease. However, many patients will be relatively well appearing, requiring an initial evaluation looking for a number of potential etiologies based on whether they have a conjugated or nonconjugated hyperbilirubinemia. Newborns are particularly challenging and are discussed at the end of this chapter.

DIRECT (CONJUGATED) HYPERBILIRUBINEMIA

BILIARY TRACT DISEASE

The biliary tract can be obstructed by processes including precipitation of bile acids producing cholelithiasis (gallstones), extrinsic duct compression by tumor or structural defects such as a choledochal cyst (a congenital anomaly characterized by cystic dilatation of the biliary tract), and intrinsic biliary tract inflammation resulting in duct obstruction and cholestatic jaundice. All three etiologies of biliary tract disease present with similar signs and symptoms usually requiring an imaging study for definitive diagnosis.

Symptoms

- Right upper quadrant (RUQ) pain, which may be intermittent (biliary colic) and worse after eating, especially in patients with gallstones; pain is also common with choledochal cysts
- Acholic stools most common with significant obstruction and decreased excretion of bilirubin into the gastrointestinal system
- Fever is common with choledochal cysts and in any infectious causes of cholangitis or cholecystitis
- Nausea and vomiting

Signs

- Pain on palpation of RUQ
- Jaundice
- Hepatomegaly
- Fever

Workup

- Abdominal US and/or radionuclide imaging are highly sensitive at diagnosing most disorders of the biliary tract, but radionuclide imaging is more sensitive for diagnosis of obstruction. Commonly, US is obtained first and is used to diagnose or rule out most anatomic etiologies. When doubt remains, a radionuclide study may be obtained. Some infants may require 5 days of phenobarbital before a radionuclide study to increase liver activity.
- Alkaline phosphatase, 5-nucleotidase, and gamma-glutamyltransferase (GGT) are enzymes whose levels increase with obstruction and are more specific to biliary tract than hepatocyte function.

- Total and direct bilirubin, because significantly increased conjugated bilirubin (>20%) reliably occurs with diseases of the biliary tract.
- Urine dipstick for urobilinogen because urinary urobilinogen reflects bilirubin metabolism by gut flora; the presence of jaundice without urinary urobilinogen is diagnostic of decreased secretion of bilirubin into the gut, the major characteristic of biliary tract disease.
- Serum transaminases.

Comments and Treatment Considerations

Surgical consultation is usually required and intervention may be indicated. Choledochal cysts typically present during the first months of life with jaundice, direct hyperbilirubinemia, and acholic (pale and pasty) stools. Epigastric pain and fever may result from recurrent cholangitis. Up to 20% of children will have the triad of pain, jaundice, and a palpable abdominal mass. Gallstone formation is a complication of sickle cell disease because of the excess production of bilirubin associated with this disease. Cholestatic jaundice, which is characterized by an elevation in serum alkaline phosphatase and GGT, is most commonly caused by medications including phenothiazines and erythromycin estolate. Cystic fibrosis can also be associated with bile inspissation and/or pancreatitis, both of which can impair biliary excretion into the gut.

 HEMOLYSIS

Bilirubin is the natural product of red blood cell destruction. Therefore any condition associated with the accelerated destruction of erythrocytes can produce hyperbilirubinemia and jaundice. A patient with an acute hemolytic crisis may exhibit signs of cardiac failure or shock (see Chapter 28, Pallor).

POISONING (DRUGS AND TOXINS)

A number of drugs and toxins can produce jaundice by causing decreased elimination of bilirubin or increased destruction of erythrocytes. Of all drug-related etiologies of jaundice, acetaminophen hepatotoxicity is the most important to recognize because it is commonly ingested and an effective antidote is available (*N*-acetylcysteine), although its efficacy is time dependent (see Chapter 35, Toxic Ingestion, Approach To, for a detailed discussion of specific ingestions). Other common hepatotoxins causing jaundice are found in Table 23-2.

Symptoms
- Admission or suspicion of ingestion of known hepatotoxin
- History of psychiatric disorder or suicidal gesture

Table 23-2   Common Hepatotoxic Drugs

Primary hepatotoxins
   Acetaminophen
   Amiodarone
   Antiretroviral agents
   Ethanol
   Halothane
   Hepatotoxic mushrooms
   Herbs, such as pyrrolizidine alkaloids ("herbal hepatitis")
   Iron
   Isoniazid
   Phenytoin
   Valproic acid
   Tetracyclines
   Vitamin A
Drugs that commonly produce cholestatic jaundice
   Phenothiazines
   Erythromycin

Signs
- RUQ tenderness
- Jaundice
- Evidence of coagulopathy such as oozing at puncture sites or easy bleeding or bruising
- CNS changes indicative of hepatic encephalopathy, which is caused in part by impairment of the urea cycle with resulting hyperammonemia
- Fulminant liver failure or hepatorenal syndrome

Workup
- Total and direct bilirubin, hepatic transaminases, alkaline phosphatase.
- PT and PTT because hepatocyte injury impairs the production of clotting proteins.
- Blood ammonia level, because hepatic encephalopathy is caused in part by impairment of the urea cycle with resulting hyperammonemia.
- Drug levels, such as phenytoin and valproate.

Comments and Treatment Considerations

For most drug ingestions or overdoses, currently recommended management strategies include empiric administration of activated charcoal (see Chapter 35, Toxic Ingestion, Approach To). When in doubt, consult your local poison center. Clinically significant coagulopathy, manifested as oozing from puncture sites, hematemesis, or lower gastrointestinal tract bleeding, may require administration of fresh frozen plasma.

Acetaminophen and mushroom poisoning present with vomiting, which can be intractable, followed by RUQ pain. Vomiting may be present shortly after ingestion, but abdominal pain and jaundice usually are delayed in presentation for 2 to 5 days based on the severity of the ingestion. If it progresses, lethargy and other signs of hepatic encephalopathy can appear, along with easy bruising. Therapy with the acetaminophen antidote *N*-acetylcysteine should be instituted for any patient with a toxic ingestion of acetaminophen and strongly considered for any suspected ingestion while awaiting laboratory confirmation (see Chapter 35, Toxic Ingestion, Approach To).

 ## HEPATITIS

There are infectious, metabolic, drug, and toxic etiologies that can cause hepatocellular inflammation and resultant hepatitis. Infectious causes are the most common and patients can have a range of symptoms from as minor as asymptomatic transaminase elevations to fulminant hepatic failure.

Infectious hepatitis is usually viral in origin. The family of hepatitis viruses is large and includes more than six members. These viruses all can produce hepatocyte injury, which can be extensive. In addition to the hepatitis viruses, which specifically and exclusively infect hepatocytes, a number of other viruses can infect the liver and other organs (Table 23-3).

The hepatitis viruses, despite their similarities, have differing sources and clinical courses, as follows:

- *Hepatitis A* is a self-limited disease most commonly associated with ingestion of contaminated food or contact with infected individuals, for example, by sharing kitchenware. Outbreaks among children in day care centers can occur. Hepatitis A typically produces a mild disease with >80% of cases being asymptomatic.
- *Hepatitis B* is transmitted parenterally (e.g., needle punctures), vertically (from mother to newborn), and sexually. Chronic hepatitis B virus (HBV) infection can occur in as many as 90% of children infected perinatally.
- *Hepatitis C*, formerly known as *non-A, non-B hepatitis*, is primarily acquired parenterally, for example, through blood transfusions. Current estimates are that as many as 20% of individuals who received blood transfusions before 1992 are infected with hepatitis C. Persistent infection occurs in 75% to 85% of those infected with hepatitis C.
- *Hepatitis D through G* virus infections are uncommon in children: Their sources and epidemiologic patterns have not been well defined in the pediatric population.

Table 23-3   Causes of Hepatitis

Infectious
    Hepatitis A
    Hepatitis B
    Hepatitis C
    Hepatitis D, E, F, G*
    Epstein-Barr virus
    Herpesvirus
    Adenovirus
    Toxoplasma
    Syphilis
Metabolic
    Wilson's disease
    α_1-Antitrypsin deficiency
Drugs and toxins
    Acetaminophen
    Ethanol
    Iron
    Isoniazid
    Hepatotoxic mushrooms, such as *Amanita phalloides*

*Relatively uncommon in children.

- *Neonatal hepatitis* is often noninfectious in origin, resulting from congenital disorders such as homozygous α_1-antitrypsin deficiency. Infectious etiologies specific to the newborn include the congenital TORCH viruses: *t*oxoplasmosis, *r*ubella, *c*ytomegalovirus, and *h*erpes simplex.

Symptoms
- Malaise, fatigue
- Myalgias
- Nausea, vomiting
- Change in sense of smell or taste
- Diarrhea (may have pale stools)

Signs
- Jaundice
- RUQ pain

Workup

- Hepatic aminotransferases, alkaline phosphatase, total and direct bilirubin.
- CBC.
- Hepatitis serology (hepatitis viruses A, B, or C).
- Monospot or EBV titers.
- PT and PTT because hepatocyte injury impairs the production of clotting proteins.
- Blood ammonia because hepatic encephalopathy is caused in part by impairment of the urea cycle with resulting hyperammonemia.

Comments and Treatment Considerations

The diagnosis of a specific hepatitis virus is made on the basis of serologic testing. Therapy for any of the hepatitis infections is supportive, with the major concern for development of chronic infection that may lead to permanent liver damage. Hepatitis A is generally self-limited, although chronic cases occur. Chronic hepatitis B infection occurs in as many as 90% of infants infected perinatally and 2% to 6% of older children. Persistent hepatitis C infection occurs in 75% to 85% of infected persons, and of these, 60% to 70% develop chronic hepatitis. Gastroenterology consultation should be sought for severe cases.

Immunoglobulin therapy is available after exposure for hepatitis A and B (particularly for newborns with a maternal history positive for Hepatitis B), in addition to prophylactic vaccine. Hepatitis A postexposure prophylaxis is provided by giving immunoglobulin, dosed at 0.02 ml/kg intramuscularly (IM) × one dose given as soon as possible, within 2 weeks of exposure. Hepatitis B immune globulin (HBIG) for perinatal postexposure is dosed at 0.5 ml/dose and ideally given within 12 hours of birth. For percutaneous or sexual exposure, HBIG is dosed at 0.06 ml/kg IM × 1 dose (max 5 ml/dose) within 24 hours of percutaneous exposure and within 2 weeks of sexual contact. Routine hepatitis A vaccine is recommended for populations living in specific states/regions and at-risk persons. Current recommendations in the United States are for all children to be routinely vaccinated against hepatitis B in a three-shot series as young children, usually initiated at birth and followed by vaccinations at 1 and 6 months.

The diagnosis of EBV infection can occasionally be made by the presence of a positive rapid Monospot test. However, the Monospot test has a low sensitivity in the pediatric age-group and its results are rarely positive in children younger than 5 years who have EBV infection. EBV titers are sensitive but take longer to obtain results. Treatment is primarily supportive (see Chapter 39, Weakness/Fatigue).

METABOLIC, IMMUNE, AND IDIOPATHIC

Metabolic diseases associated with jaundice may first appear in the childhood years. These diseases represent a heterogeneous group of disorders that usually require pediatric specialists and highly specific testing for diagnosis. Some of the more common "rare" disorders include the following:

- *Wilson's disease* is a disorder of copper metabolism. Its clinical presentation ranges from the identification of asymptomatic elevations in hepatic transaminases to jaundice with the appearance of neuropsychiatric illness in adolescents.
- *Enzyme defects* associated with jaundice include α_1-antitrypsin deficiency, galactosemia, and tyrosinemia.
- *Infiltrative diseases* include Gaucher's and glycogen storage diseases. These may present with hepatomegaly and jaundice.
- *Immune-mediated diseases,* including systemic lupus erythematosus, occasionally appear in the pediatric age-group.
- *Idiopathic fulminant hepatic failure* (FHF) can appear at any age in childhood and is a diagnosis of exclusion. Children with FHF show evidence of severe hepatic dysfunction including elevated hepatic transaminases, serum bilirubin, coagulopathy resulting from impaired production of clotting factors, and elevated serum ammonia level.

Symptoms

- Lethargy
- Malaise, fatigue
- Easy bruising

Signs

- Hepatomegaly
- Bleeding diatheses
- Hyperammonemia
- Hepatic coma

Workup

- CBC, hepatic transaminases, gamma-glutamyltransferase, alkaline phosphatase.
- PT, PTT, GGT.
- Blood ammonia.
- Hepatitis serologies.
- Consider serum copper, ceruloplasmin, α_1-antitrypsin.

Comments and Treatment Considerations

Care is primarily supportive with referral to pediatric specialists for further management options.

 ## *DISORDERS OF BILIRUBIN METABOLISM*

Numerous disorders of bilirubin metabolism caused by genetic abnormalities are characterized by the appearance of jaundice. Again, these disorders are relatively rare and usually require pediatric specialists and highly specific testing for diagnosis. These include the following:

- *Gilbert's syndrome*, a defect of bilirubin excretion producing low-grade indirect hyperbilirubinemia
- *Crigler-Najjar syndrome*, which can present with severe hyperbilirubinemia and kernicterus in the first few days of life

Symptoms

- Asymptomatic jaundice or icterus

Signs
- Indirect hyperbilirubinemia
- Normal hepatic transaminases

Workup
- Total and direct bilirubin.
- Hepatic transaminases, alkaline phosphatase.
- Coombs' test.

Comments and Treatment Considerations
Care is primarily supportive with referral to pediatric specialists for further management options.

 NEONATAL

Newborns with jaundice represent a unique subset of patients. Common causes of neonatal hyperbilirubinemia are listed in Table 23-4. Full-term infants who are clinically jaundiced at ≤24 hours after birth are not considered healthy and require transfer to a neonatal care unit for further evaluation of congenital liver disease, hemolysis, and systemic infection.

In this section, biliary atresia and indirect hyperbilirubinemia of the newborn are discussed. Please see earlier sections in this chapter for evaluation of other possible etiologies of jaundice not specific to the newborn.

Table 23-4   Common Causes of Neonatal Hyperbilirubinemia

Physiologic	Pathologic
Breast-feeding	Birth trauma with cephalohematoma
Prematurity	Rh incompatibility
Congenital	ABP incompatibility
Biliary atresia	G6PD deficiency
	Infection, such as urinary tract infection
	Polycythemia

DIRECT HYPERBILIRUBINEMIA

Although rare, biliary atresia is the most important etiology of pathologic neonatal jaundice in the newborn with hepatomegaly, direct hyperbilirubinemia with a bilirubin level >2.5 mg/dl, and severe jaundice. Diagnosis is made by ultrasound and/or radionuclide imaging. These patients should be immediately referred to a pediatric surgeon for recommendations for evaluation and for definitive surgical correction (*Kasai procedure*).

INDIRECT HYPERBILIRUBINEMIA

The most common cause of jaundice across the pediatric age-group is neonatal hyperbilirubinemia. Also termed *physiologic jaundice*, the cause of neonatal hyperbilirubinemia is the combination of shortened fetal red blood cell life span (particularly in preterm infants) and an impaired ability to excrete bilirubin. Neonatal jaundice is more common in breast-fed babies and occurs in the first few days of life in full-term infants and within the first week of life in premature infants. Serum bilirubin concentrations >17 mg/dl are not considered physiologic and require further evaluation.

Pathologic hyperbilirubinemia resulting from any of the causes listed in Table 23-4 must be diagnosed and differentiated from the physiologic causes of hyperbilirubinemia. Initial workup and management is identical, with the exception that any systemic infections identified require antibiotic therapy (see Chapter 14, Fever).

Symptoms
- Jaundice, icterus
- Lethargy, poor feeding

Signs
- Signs of sepsis, for example, fever

Workup
- Total and direct bilirubin level.
- Maternal and infant blood type (to identify ABO or Rh incompatibility).

- Coombs' test.
- Consider CBC count, blood culture, LP for signs of sepsis or concerning risk factors.

Comments and Treatment Consideration

Any child with signs of systemic infection should immediately be started on empiric antibiotics and transferred to a neonatal intensive care unit. Ceftriaxone should be avoided in neonates with hyperbilirubinemia, because the drug can displace bilirubin from albumin-binding sites.

Pathologic neonatal hyperbilirubinemia is often benign, although extreme elevations in bilirubin can cause *kernicterus*, a condition characterized by a range of neurotoxic effects varying from deafness to devastating neurologic injury. The serum bilirubin concentration at which kernicterus occurs is based on a number of factors including the peak serum bilirubin concentration, the infant's gestational age, and the presence of other conditions, such as shock or hypoalbuminemia. Although peak serum bilirubin concentration is not completely predictive of neurologic injury, the risk of CNS toxicity increases as serum bilirubin concentration rises to >20 mg/dl. Significant hyperbilirubinemia (bilirubin >15 mg/dl) is therefore treated initially by phototherapy and, if elevations are excessive, exchange transfusion. Supplemental fluids either orally or intravenously may be beneficial, particularly if there is evidence of dehydration or poor feeding.

Stable newborns with physiologic causes of hyperbilirubinemia do not develop concerning high levels of hyperbilirubinemia but may benefit from phototherapy, particularly while evaluation is being completed. See Table 23-5 for management suggestions for healthy newborn infants. Once bilirubin levels fall to a nonconcerning level, phototherapy is discontinued and a rebound bilirubin level is drawn 12 to 24 hours later. Consult neonatology for levels >20 mg/dl in full-term infants and levels >15 mg/dl in premature infants, particularly if the infant is not rapidly responding to initial phototherapy. Persistently elevated levels despite phototherapy are also cause for concern and warrant further evaluation for an underlying abnormality.

Table 23-5 Management of Hyperbilirubinemia in the Healthy Term Newborn

Total Serum Bilirubin Level, mg/dl (pmol/L)

Age, (hr)	Consider Phototherapy*	Phototherapy	Exchange Transfusion if Intensive Phototherapy Fails†	Exchange Transfusion and Intensive Phototherapy
≤24‡	—	—	—	—
25-48	≥12 (210)	≥15 (260)	≥20 (340)	≥25 (430)
49-72	≥15 (260)	≥18 (310)	≥25 (430)	≥30 (510)
> 72	≥17 (290)	≥20 (340)	≥25 (430)	≥30 (510)

*Phototherapy at these total serum bilirubin (TSB) levels is a clinical option; that is, the intervention is available and may be used on the basis of individual clinical judgment.

†Intensive phototherapy should produce a decline of TSB of 1-2 mg/dl within 4-6 hours and the TSB level should continue to fall and remain below the threshold level for exchange transfusion. If this does not occur, it is considered a failure of phototherapy.

‡Full-term infants who are clinically jaundiced at ≤24 hours after birth are not considered healthy and require further evaluation.

REFERENCES

AAP Subcommittee on Hyperbilirubinemia: Management of hyperbilirubinemia in the newborn infant 35 or more weeks of gestation, *Pediatrics* 114(1): 297-316, 2004.

AAP Provisional Committee for Quality Improvement and Subcommittee on Hyperbilirubinemia: *Pediatrics* 94(4), 1994.

Balistreri WF: Manifestations of liver disease. In *Nelson textbook of pediatrics*, 16th ed, Philadelphia, 2000, WB Saunders.

D'Agata ID, Balistreri WF: Evaluation of liver disease in the pediatric patient, *Pediatr Rev* 20:376-389, 1999.

Lee WM: Drug-induced hepatotoxicity, *N Engl J Med* 333:1118-1127, 1995.

McEvoy CF, Suchy FJ: Biliary tract disease in children, *Pediatr Clin North Am* 43:75-98, 1996.

Ryder SD, Beckingham IJ: Acute hepatitis, *Br Med J* 322(7279):151-153, 2001.

Sackey K: Hemolytic anemia: part 1, *Pediatr Rev* 20:152-159, 1999.

CHAPTER 24

Joint Pain and Swelling

MARISA BRETT-FLEEGLER

Joint disease may manifest as local or referred pain, limp, or refusal to walk. When evaluating joint disease the clinician should be mindful of the need to diagnose or exclude those conditions that require emergent intervention to prevent significant destruction to the joint and subsequent disability. Traumatic causes of joint pain are typically distinguished by history. This chapter focuses on the nontraumatic causes of joint pain. Recall, however, that children frequently have a history of minor trauma when presenting with nontraumatic conditions; thus a history of trauma in a child with joint pain or swelling should not preclude investigation for other etiologies.

TRAUMA

Traumatic causes of joint pain are typically distinguished by history and careful consideration of possible inflicted injury (see Chapter 2, Abuse/Rape; Chapter 25, Limp; and Chapter 15, Fractures Not to Miss).

SEPTIC ARTHRITIS

Septic or suppurative arthritis occurs when microbial pathogens, most commonly bacteria, proliferate within the articular capsule of a joint. Subsequent cytokine production and neutrophil chemotaxis lead to inflammation and damage to cartilage. The most common bacterial pathogens in septic arthritis are *Staphylococcus aureus*, group A *Streptococcus*, *Streptococcus pneumoniae*, and before immunization, *Haemophilus influenzae*. In neonates, *group B Streptococcus* and *Neisseria gonorrhoeae* are common pathogens and should be included in empiric coverage. *N. gonorrhoeae* and gram-negative organisms are a consideration in adolescents.

Septic arthritis occurs in all age-groups but is most common in infants and young children, with 50% of cases occurring in children younger than 2 years. Boys are more commonly affected than girls. Approximately 80% of cases occur in the lower extremities, most often developing in the knee and the hip. Because this disease has significant morbidity even when treated promptly, a suspected septic joint should be evaluated emergently.

Symptoms
- Pain
- Limp
- Inability/refusal to bear weight ++++
- Fever +++
- Chills +
- Arthralgia (pain may radiate to nearby areas, classically the knee or anterior thigh for an affected hip)
- Malaise
- Neonates
  - Septic appearance
  - Irritability
  - Poor feeding
  - Pseudoparalysis

Signs
- Decreased range of motion of joint
- Joint erythema
- Joint swelling
- Joint warmth
- A septic hip will be positioned in abduction, external rotation, and flexion

Workup
- Any patient with fever and evidence of a joint effusion by any imaging modality should undergo arthrocentesis to

examine the joint fluid. Joint fluid should be sent for cell count and differential, glucose and protein concentration, Gram stain, and culture.

- US will identify the presence of an effusion in the evaluation of a hip joint but will not differentiate between a septic hip and toxic synovitis.
- WBC, ESR, and CRP are nonspecific but if elevated may be helpful in supporting the diagnosis.
- Blood culture, in an attempt to identify organism.
- Plain radiographs are a good first step to assess for an effusion based on joint space enlargement. They may also rule out other diagnoses such as fractures, neoplasm, or in the hip, Legg-Calvé-Perthes (LCP) disease.
- Consider bone scan or MRI to identify osteomyelitis.
- Consider cervical or urethral cultures for gonorrhea in sexually active adolescents.

Comments and Treatment Considerations

Neither laboratory values nor clinical symptoms are specific for septic arthritis. The diagnosis should be ruled out by arthrocentesis in any patient in whom it is suspected. Cultures are positive in only 50% to 80%, likely because of the intrinsic bacteriostatic properties of the synovial fluid. Fluid WBC counts >100,000 cells/mm^3 are considered clear evidence of infection, and counts >50,000 cells/mm^3 indicate probable evidence of infection. However, septic arthritis can also present with much lower counts. A polymorphonuclear predominance is also suggestive of infection.

Treatment of septic arthritis includes joint immobilization, fluid drainage, and parenteral antibiotics. Pediatric orthopedic consultation is indicated. Surgical drainage is required in many cases, including all those involving the hip, most involving the shoulder, severe infections, those failing parenteral antibiotic therapy, and most cases in infants and young children. Arthroscopic drainage may be an option for some patients.

Empiric antibiotic coverage should include an antistaphylococcal agent such as a β-lactamase–resistant penicillin or first-generation cephalosporin; additional gram-negative coverage is indicated in neonates and adolescents. Patients with sickle cell disease are a special group and are at high risk for salmonella osteomyelitis but do not appear to have a higher incidence of septic arthritis caused by salmonella. Before widespread vaccination, antibiotic therapy also needed to include *H. influenzae* coverage. Additional antimicrobial coverage should be tailored to the individual case.

First-line treatment options include the following:

Cefazolin 100 to 150 mg/kg/day IV divided q8h (max 6 g/day)
OR
Oxacillin 150 to 200 mg/kg/day IV divided q4-6h (max 12 g/day)
OR
Nafcillin 100 to 200 mg/kg/day IV divided q4-6h (max 12 g/day)

Duration of antibiotic therapy is at least 3 to 4 weeks. Conversion to oral therapy is based on the individual pathology and patient response, with strict attention to compliance issues. Sequelae of septic arthritis may include limited motion, limb length discrepancy, pain, and degenerative arthritis even with appropriate therapy. The hip is particularly prone to sequelae.

 LEGG-CALVÉ-PERTHES DISEASE

Legg-Calvé-Perthes (LCP) disease is an avascular necrosis of the femoral head, often followed by collapse, remodeling, and disability. It occurs in children aged 2 to 13 years, but most cases occur in children between 4 and 8 years of age. LCP disease is more common in boys and is bilateral in approximately 10% of cases. Children may be short or overweight and have delayed skeletal maturation. Steroid use is a risk factor. Other proposed etiologies include endocrine abnormalities and coagulation disorders that could impede blood flow to the femoral head.

Symptoms
- Hip pain, often of insidious onset
- Limp
- Knee, medial thigh pain

Signs
- Pain on range of motion
- Decreased hip abduction and internal rotation
- Thigh, calf, and/or buttock atrophy in chronic cases
- Leg length discrepancy

Workup
- WBC, ESR, and CRP are usually normal and may be performed as an adjunct in evaluating other conditions.
- Radiographs (anteroposterior and frogleg) initially show no abnormalities then reveal a small osteopenic femoral head with a widened joint space; later changes are subchondral fragmentation, reossification, and ultimately healing, with or without deformity. The degree of femoral head involvement seen on plain film has prognostic significance.
- Bone scan or MRI may be useful in making the diagnosis.

Comments and Treatment Considerations
The goal of treatment is to return normal range of motion via femoral head containment. This is accomplished by keeping the femoral head within the acetabulum and avoiding subluxation or extrusion. Pediatric orthopedic consultation is indicated. NSAIDs, activity restriction, physical therapy, crutches, and bracing are the mainstays of therapy. Operative management is indicated in severe cases.

 ## SLIPPED CAPITAL FEMORAL EPIPHYSIS

Slipped capital femoral epiphysis (SCFE) is a displacement of the normal relationship between the femoral head and femoral neck through the growth plate. SCFE is most common in early adolescence, especially during the growth spurt, occurs more than twice as often in males as in females, and is more common in obese children and African Americans. During early adolescence the geometry of proximal femur contributes to increased shear force across the physis. Children with endocrine abnormalities, particularly hypothyroidism, are at greater risk of SCFE, but it is most frequently found in children without underlying abnormalities. SCFE is considered "acute" when symptoms have been present for <3 weeks and is considered "chronic" thereafter. It may present in the setting of minor trauma that represents an acute on chronic slip.

Symptoms
- Hip pain, often chronic, worsened by activity ++
- Anteromedial groin, thigh and/or knee pain
- Limp, often chronic

Signs
- Hip found in flexion and external rotation
- Pain on range of motion, especially flexion, internal rotation, abduction, and straight-leg raise
- Anterior hip tenderness
- Limb length discrepancy

Workup
- Anteroposterior and frogleg radiographs to look for epiphyseal displacement. Always obtain bilateral views of the hips for comparison. In a pre-slip condition early changes such as increased physeal thickness, irregularity, and changes in the femoral metaphysis may be seen. Displacement is obvious in some cases, although mild slips may be detected by drawing Klein's line along the superior margin of the femoral neck cortex on the anteroposterior views. Klein's line normally intersects the epiphysis but will not do so in a slip (Figs. 24-1 and 24-2).

Comments and Treatment Considerations
SCFE requires urgent surgical correction and consultation with a pediatric orthopedist. Definitive management typically involves the placement of screws through the femoral neck into the epiphysis to prevent further displacement. The epiphysis is rarely realigned.

The most common complications are chondrolysis (a narrowing of the joint space as a result of the loss of articular cartilage) and avascular necrosis of the epiphysis. Femur remodeling usually occurs after closure of the physis. The sequelae of

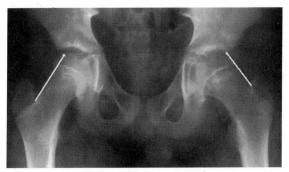

Fig. 24-1 Anteroposterior view of the pelvis showing slipped capital femoral epiphysis on the left. Arrows are drawn along the superior border of the femoral neck (Klein's line) and intersect a portion of the epiphysis on the right but do not on the left. (From Perron AD: *Am J Emerg Med* 20(5):484-487, 2002.)

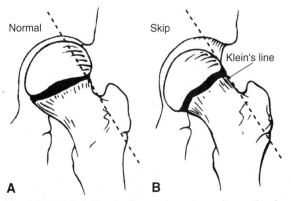

Fig. 24-2 Klein's line is drawn along the radiographic border of the neck of the femur. **A,** Normal Klein's line; **B,** Klein's line in slipped capital femoral epiphysis. (From Perron AD: *Am J Emerg Med* 20(5):484-487, 2002.)

degenerative arthrosis occur in proportion to the severity of the slip, the degree of deformity, and presence of complications.

TOXIC SYNOVITIS

Toxic or transient synovitis is a self-limited benign inflammation of the hip. It occurs in children from toddlers to preadolescents and peaks between 3 and 6 years of age. Males are affected at least two times more often than females. It is thought to be a postviral inflammation, usually following an upper respiratory tract illness. The primary objective in the evaluation of toxic synovitis is the exclusion of other more serious diagnoses, particularly septic arthritis (see earlier section).

Symptoms
- Hip pain (may be referred to anterior thigh or medial knee)
- Limp/inability to bear weight
- Fever (usually low grade) +
- Nontoxic appearance

Signs
- Hip held in flexion, external rotation, abduction
- Mild pain with range of motion

Workup
- As in the evaluation of septic arthritis, plain radiographs are useful to rule out other diagnoses. They may reveal an effusion suggestive of either a septic hip or a toxic synovitis.
- Ultrasound is indicated to assess for the presence of effusion.
- Serum WBC, ESR, and/or CRP to help assess suspicion for a septic hip.
- Consider sending a blood culture if concerned for a possibly septic joint (see earlier section).
- Arthrocentesis may be needed to rule out a septic hip. This will require ultrasonic guidance. In cases with large effusions aspiration may be therapeutic by relieving pressure compromising epiphyseal blood flow.

Comments and Treatment Considerations

If there is any suspicion of a possible septic arthritis, joint aspiration is mandatory. Treatment of a toxic synovitis consists of supportive care with NSAIDs, such as ibuprofen dosed at 10 mg/kg/dose (max 800 mg/dose) PO q8h, and rest. Patients are initially non–weight bearing and should gradually return to activity, with unrestricted activity only when pain has resolved. Traction is now believed to be potentially harmful and is not indicated. Most cases resolve within 2 weeks, but symptoms can persist for several weeks. If symptoms persist or worsen, the suspicion of LCP disease should be raised.

 RHEUMATOLOGIC

Various rheumatologic conditions may cause joint pain and swelling. They are often distinguished by multi-articular involvement. The clinician should always be alert for historical and clinical clues that suggest any of these conditions, including Kawasaki disease, Henoch-Schönlein purpura, acute rheumatic fever, systemic lupus erythematosus, inflammatory bowel disease, and serum sickness (see Chapter 14, Fever; Chapter 25, Limp; and Chapter 29, Rash). Additionally, a wide variety of infectious diseases, which should be readily distinguished by their clinical course, present concomitantly with or precede a sterile reactive arthritis. These include *Chlamydia*, *Yersinia*, *Salmonella*, *Shigella*, *Mycoplasma*, and *Campylobacter* infection and viruses including hepatitis A and B, rubella, human immunodeficiency virus, mumps, parvovirus B19, enteroviruses, and herpesviruses.

JUVENILE RHEUMATOID ARTHRITIS

Juvenile rheumatoid arthritis (JRA) describes a chronic synovial inflammation that has multiple subtypes. Characteristically, joints are painful, swollen, and stiff; have limited range of motion; and are occasionally mildly warm and erythematous (see Chapter 25, Limp).

LYME DISEASE

The arthritis of Lyme disease, caused by the spirochete *Borrelia burgdorferi*, occurs in the second and third stages of the disease. The second stage of Lyme disease, early disseminated disease, occurs weeks after the tick bite and includes generalized arthralgias, other systemic symptoms, and organ system–specific manifestations such as cranial nerve palsies, meningitis, and rarely carditis. The third stage of Lyme disease, late disease, occurring months after the first stage, is an oligoarthritis, most commonly involving the knee. Central nervous system symptoms may also be seen in late-stage disease. The arthritis of Lyme disease may become chronic and recur over months to years. Treatment with antibiotics is recommended (see Chapter 29, Rash).

REFERENCES

American Academy of Pediatrics: Lyme disease. In Pickering LK, editor: *2000 red book: report of the Committee on Infectious Diseases*, 25th ed, Elk Grove Village, Ill, 2000, American Academy of Pediatrics.

Bachman D, Santora S: Orthopedic trauma. In Fleisher GR, Ludwig S, Henretig FM, et al, editors: *Textbook of pediatric emergency*, Philadelphia, 2000, Lippincott Williams & Wilkins.

Do TT: Transient synovitis as a cause of painful limps in children, *Curr Opin Pediatr* 12:48-51, 2000.

Giannini EH, Cawkwell GD: Drug treatment in children with juvenile rheumatoid arthritis, *Pediatr Clin North Am* 42(5):1099-1125, 1995.

Joffe MD, Loiselle J: Orthopedic emergencies. In Fleisher GR, Ludwig S, Henretig FM, et al, editors: *Textbook of pediatric emergency*, Philadelphia, 2000, Lippincott Williams & Wilkins.

Kermond S, Fink M, Graham K, et al: A randomized clinical trial: should the child with transient synovitis of the hip be treated with nonsteroidal anti-inflammatory drugs? *Ann Emerg Med* 40(3), 2002.

Kim MK, Karpas A: Orthopedic emergencies: the limping child, *Clin Pediatr Emerg Med* 3(2): 129-137.

Kocher MS, Zurakowski D, et al: Differentiating between septic arthritis and transient synovitis of the hip in children: an evidence-based clinical prediction algorithm, *J Bone Joint Surg* 81-A(12):1662-1670, 1999.

Koop S, Quanbeck D: Three common causes of childhood hip pain, *Pediatr Clin North Am* 43(5):1053-1066, 1996.

Kost S: Limp. In Fleisher GR, Ludwig S, Henretig FM, et al, editors: *Textbook of pediatric emergency*, Philadelphia, 2000, Lippincott Williams & Wilkins.

Luhmann JD, Luhmann SJ: Etiology of septic arthritis in children: an update for the 1990s, *Pediatr Emerg Care* 15(1):1662-1670, 1999.

Reynolds RR: Diagnosis and treatment of slipped capital femoral epiphysis, *Curr Opin Pediatr* 11:80-83, 1998.

Roy DR: Current concept in Legg-Calvé-Perthes disease, *Pediatr Ann* 28(12):748-752, 1999.

Scarfone RJ: Joint pain. In Fleisher GR, Ludwig S, Henretig FM, et al, editors: *Textbook of pediatric emergency*, Philadelphia, 2000, Lippincott Williams & Wilkins.

Schaller JG: Juvenile rheumatoid arthritis, *Pediatr Rev* 18(10):337-349, 1997.

Sonnen GM, Henry NK: Pediatric bone and joint infections: diagnosis and antimicrobial management, *Pediatr Clin North Am* 43(4):933-947, 1996.

Steere AC: Lyme disease, *N Engl J Med* 345(2):115-125, 2001.

Sundel RJL: Rheumatologic emergencies. In Fleisher GR, Ludwig S, Henretig FM, et al, editors: *Textbook of pediatric emergency*, Philadelphia, 2000, Lippincott Williams & Wilkins.

Wagner DC: Musculoskeletal infections in adolescents, *Adolesc Med State Art Rev* 11(2):375-400.

Wall EJ: Legg-Calve-Perthes' disease, *Current Opin in Pediatr* 11:76-79.

Zawin JK, Hoffer FA, et al: Joint effusion in children with an irritable hip: US diagnosis and aspiration, *Radiology* 187:459-463, 1993.

CHAPTER 25

Limp

THERESA MOORE BECKER

Evaluation of a child with an acute limp poses a diagnostic challenge. In general, a limp is an abnormal gait that is due to pain, weakness, or deformity. The etiologies are numerous, with the primary challenge being to localize the site of discomfort. One must consider all joints and structures that contribute to a normal gait from the pelvis and hip to the feet, as well as referred pain from the back or abdomen. The most common (and emergent) etiologies are infection and trauma, although inflammation, malignancy, and arthritis must also be considered. Neurologic conditions are an unusual cause of gait disturbance in otherwise normal children and are not discussed in this chapter (see Chapter 39, Weakness/Fatigue). Often the history and physical examination, with an age-directed focus, help establish a presumptive diagnosis. When in doubt, it is sometimes necessary to obtain radiographs of the pelvis and/or lower extremity.

 ## SEPTIC ARTHRITIS

Septic arthritis is a medical emergency. The diagnosis must be ruled out in patients with an acutely painful joint. Delay in diagnosis and treatment can lead to destruction of the joint (see Chapter 24, Joint Pain and Swelling).

 ## OSTEOMYELITIS

Osteomyelitis is an infection of the bone. Osteomyelitis typically involves a single long bone (>90% in one series).

In children, two-thirds of cases involve the femur, tibia, and fibula. As a result, children often present with a limp. Bacterial osteomyelitis is the result of either hematogenous spread secondary to bacteremia, direct inoculation after trauma, or local invasion of a contiguous infection. The sluggish blood flow predisposes bacterial seeding at the metaphyseal-epiphyseal junction, either after bacteremia or trauma. As the bacteria proliferate and cause a host inflammatory response, the resulting pressure causes extension of the infection into the bony cortex. The relatively thick periosteum usually localizes the disease to that single point, so multifocal osteomyelitis is relatively uncommon (<7% of cases). In newborns the purulent fluid may rupture through the thinner periosteum and spread into the adjacent tissue, resulting in contiguous septic arthritis in 50% to 70% of cases.

The most common pathogen responsible for bacterial osteomyelitis is *Staphylococcus aureus* (which accounts for 67% to 89% of cases) followed by *streptococci*, *Staphylococcus non-aureus*, and various gram-negative rods. In neonates, group B *streptococcus* is the second most common bacterial pathogen.

Symptoms
- Pain, especially with movement
- Fever
- Limp
- "Pseudoparalysis" (refusal to move affected limb)

Signs
- Point tenderness ++++
- Fever ++++
- Localized erythema or warmth ++

Workup
- WBC elevation +++.
- ESR or CRP elevation +++++.
- Blood culture ++/+++.
- Bone culture +++.

- Plain radiograph findings are negative early in the course but may show soft-tissue involvement after a few days; periosteal reaction or lytic lesions within the cortex appear 10 to 21 days into the disease course.
- Bone scan (sensitivity ~90%).
- MRI (sensitivity 88% to 100%, specificity 75% to 100%).

Comments and Treatment Considerations

Bone scans and MRI are helpful in the diagnosis of osteomyelitis when physical examination and plain radiograph findings are inconclusive. Bone scans have the advantage of identifying the possibility of multifocal disease, as well as scanning the entire body when there are no localizing signs. MRI is both more sensitive and specific but requires some localization of disease, as well as possible need for sedation in the infant or young pediatric patient. Evaluation for osteomyelitis should be considered in any patient with *S. aureus* bacteremia. Once the diagnosis is made, orthopedics should be consulted for possible surgical debridement.

Medical treatment of bacterial osteomyelitis should include antibiotics with excellent gram-positive coverage. First-line treatment options include the following:

Cefazolin 150 mg/kg/day IV divided q8h (max 6 g/day)
OR
Oxacillin 150 or 200 mg/kg/day IV divided q4-6h (max 12 g/day)
OR
Nafcillin 100 to 200 mg/kg/day IV divided q4-6h (max 12 g/day)

If methicillin-resistant strains of *S. aureus* are identified or strongly suspected, treatment with vancomycin 45 to 60 mg/kg/day IV divided q6-8h (initial max 2 g/day, titrate based on trough levels) and infectious disease consultation should be initiated.

The duration of total antibiotic therapy is typically 4 to 6 weeks. Timing of conversion to oral therapy is controversial, but most experts base their decision on clinical response (improvement of pain, resolution, or improvement of fever) or falling chemical markers of inflammation (ESR or CRP).

TRAUMA

Major fractures with displacement are apparent clinically and prevent children from walking. Trauma of lesser magnitude can produce a pathologic lesion that is less apparent clinically and requires a high index of suspicion and appropriate radiographs to establish the diagnosis. Diagnoses to consider include stress fractures, toddler's fractures, sprains, strains, contusions, child abuse, spondylodesis, and herniated disk (see Chapter 15, Fractures Not to Miss).

ABDOMINAL PAIN

Patients with abdominal pain, particularly appendicitis, may limp (see Chapter 1, Abdominal Pain).

HEMOPHILIA

Limping may occur secondary to the hemarthroses associated with hemophilia. In severe disease, this common complication may occur in the absence of known trauma. Large joints such as the knee are typically affected (see Chapter 6, Bleeding and Bruising).

MALIGNANCY (NEOPLASMS)

Benign and malignant neoplasms may produce limping caused by pain that is due to the lesion itself or to a pathologic stress fracture in the surrounding bone. Often the diagnosis is made when a radiograph is obtained to rule out fracture/effusion or when a hematologic abnormality is found during evaluation for possible septic joint.

The differential diagnosis includes malignant and benign bone tumors, as well as leukemia. Osteosarcoma is the most common malignant bone tumor of children and Ewing's sarcoma is the second. Both osteosarcoma and Ewing's sarcoma are usually diagnosed in the second decade of life but may occur at any age. Osteosarcoma most commonly affects the distal femur, the proximal tibia, and the proximal humerus. Ewing's sarcoma most often develops in the axial skeleton, particularly in the pelvis, although the humerus and femur may also be involved. Leukemia is the most common childhood malignancy and bone pain is the presenting symptom in 25% of patients (see Chapter 6, Bleeding and Bruising).

Symptoms

- Bone pain (noted to cause night-time wakening in acute leukemia)
- Local swelling
- Fever and malaise
- Joint pain

Signs

- Bleeding manifestations
- Organomegaly
- Lymphadenopathy
- Soft-tissue mass

Workup

- Plain radiograph of the site of localized pain.
- CBC with platelet count and differential looking for abnormal WBC count, thrombocytopenia, anemia, and blastocytes on smear.

Comments and Treatment Considerations

In many instances confirmation of the diagnosis is not made in the ED. A bone marrow biopsy is needed to definitively diagnose leukemia and a tissue biopsy is required to diagnose osteosarcoma or Ewing's sarcoma. Appropriate consultation and follow-up are required.

KAWASAKI SYNDROME

Arthritis is an associated feature in 30% of patients diagnosed with Kawasaki syndrome. Onset of arthritis is more common in the second week of illness, and large weight-bearing joints such as the knee and ankles are affected most often (see Chapter 14, Fever).

SLIPPED CAPITAL FEMORAL EPIPHYSIS

Slipped capital femoral epiphysis is the most common hip problem in adolescence. There is an increased incidence among obese, active males. The most common features are groin, hip, or knee pain causing a limp that is characterized by an externally rotated leg and a Trendelenburg gait (see Chapter 24, Joint Pain and Swelling).

TOXIC SYNOVITIS (ACUTE TRANSIENT SYNOVITIS)

Toxic synovitis of the hip or knee may cause a limp. This diagnosis may be difficult to distinguish from septic arthritis (see Chapter 24, Joint Pain and Swelling).

LYME DISEASE

Arthritis is the classic manifestation of late Lyme disease (third stage), occurring in about 7% of affected children. Myalgias and arthralgias that may manifest as a limp are also noted in early localized disease during the first stage (see Chapter 29, Rash).

HENOCH-SCHÖNLEIN PURPURA

A transient arthritis may be the initial manifestation of Henoch-Schönlein purpura (HSP), making it difficult to diagnose until the characteristic rash appears. Knee and ankle joints are commonly involved. Polyarthritis, colicky abdominal pain, and nephritis are also seen (see Chapter 6, Bleeding and Bruising).

 ## ACUTE RHEUMATIC FEVER

The joint swelling and pain associated with acute rheumatic fever may present as a limp secondary to limitation of motion (see Chapter 24, Fever).

 ## RHEUMATOLOGIC

Arthritis is defined as swelling within a joint or limitation of joint movement, accompanied by joint pain or tenderness. Common rheumatologic diagnoses in the pediatric population that cause an arthritic type pain include juvenile rheumatoid arthritis (JRA), systemic lupus erythematosus (SLE), and juvenile dermatomyositis (JDM). These diseases all commonly cause pain in a lower extremity joint or early morning stiffness, both of which may cause limping. Seldom is the specific diagnosis of a rheumatologic disease emergent, but excluding other conditions such as infection is required. Only after joint, limb, and life-threatening conditions are excluded should referral to a rheumatologist be considered.

JUVENILE RHEUMATOID ARTHRITIS

The American College of Rheumatology criteria for diagnosing JRA is persistent unexplained arthritis of one or more joints lasting >6 weeks in a child younger than 16 years not explained by any other etiology. Symptoms are caused by persistent inflammation of synovium. Based on clinical presentations there are three types: pauciarticular (four or fewer joints affected over the first 6 months); polyarticular (five or more joints affected); and systemic (occurrence of fever and other systemic symptoms). Rarely systemic disease can present with a disseminated intravascular coagulation (DIC) type of picture with leukopenia, thrombocytopenia, profound anemia, elevated

D-dimer, and decreased fibrinogen known as *macrophage activation syndrome*.

Symptoms
- Joint pain
- Morning stiffness lasting at least 15 minutes (often affects the child's ability to perform routine morning activities such as toileting, bathing, and dressing)

Signs
- Fever
- Arthritic pain
- Warmth, erythema, and/or swelling of one or more joints
- Systemic symptoms
  - Generalized lymphadenopathy
  - Hepatomegaly or splenomegaly
  - Progressive fatigue and malaise
  - Salmon-pink evanescent maculopapular rash
  - Uveitis
  - Serositis—pericardial, pleural, or peritoneal

Workup
- Plain films—especially if complaints isolated to one joint to rule out other possible etiologies, as well as to look for destructive lesions in long-standing disease.
- Leukocytosis >40,000 and thrombocytosis >1 million may be seen in the systemic type but may be normal in other types.
- ESR and CRP are usually elevated.
- Antinuclear antibody (ANA) positive ++++.
- Rheumatoid factor and anti-DNA usually negative.
- UA.
- Chemistry screen for renal and liver function tests.

Comments and Treatment Considerations
The mainstay of therapy is directed at preventing joint destruction with NSAIDs and remittent agents such as hydroxychloroquine, sulfasalazine, methotrexate, and cyclosporine. Appropriate consultation to establish the diagnosis and develop a treatment plan is required.

SYSTEMIC LUPUS ERYTHEMATOSUS

SLE is an autoimmune disease in which a patient develops numerous autoantibodies, causing the multitude of systemic symptoms associated with the disease. The mean age at presentation is 12 to 13 years, although disease may present at any age. Arthritis, dermatitis, and nephritis are the most common manifestations, but any organ system may be affected.

Symptoms
- Fatigue
- Arthralgias

Signs
- Fever ++++
- Anorexia +++
- Arthritis +++
- Skin rash (malar/butterfly or discoid rash) +++
- Renal involvement (glomerulonephritis, nephrotic syndrome, hypertension, renal failure) +++
- Pericarditis
- Neurologic manifestations (stroke, seizures, chorea, pseudotumor cerebri, and headaches) ++
- Pulmonary involvement, such as pleuritic pain or pulmonary hemorrhage

Workup
- ANA positive +++++.
- CBC showing anemia, thrombocytopenia, and leukopenia.
- UA looking for urinary protein >0.5 g/dl or cellular casts. Albumin, BUN, and SCr to assess renal involvement.
- Autoantibodies:
  - Anti–double-stranded DNA +++
  - Anti-Sm and anti–70-kd ribonucleoprotein antibodies +++
  - Antiphospholipid antibodies +++
  - Anti-Ro and/or anti-La antibodies ++
  - Rheumatoid factor positive +
  - Anti-ribosomal P +
  - ESR and CRP

- Direct Coombs' test result is often positive.
- Thyroid function tests.
- Complement levels.
- Renal biopsy if significant renal involvement.

Comments and Treatment Considerations

The World Health Organization divides SLE into a number of morphologic classifications based on the clinical, laboratory, and pathologic findings in a given patient. Consultation with rheumatology and nephrology is often necessary for classification and the development of a treatment plan. Long-term morbidity and mortality is high, particularly within some classifications, and is beyond the scope of this discussion. The mainstay of therapy is corticosteroids with or without other immunosuppressive agents.

JUVENILE DERMATOMYOSITIS

JDM is a systemic connective tissue disease characterized by chronic skeletal muscle and cutaneous inflammation of unknown cause affecting multiple organ systems. The pathogenesis is unknown but is thought to involve chronic immune activation in genetically susceptible individuals after exposure to specific environmental triggers. Symptoms may overlap other rheumatologic disorders.

Symptoms
- Fatigue
- Low-grade fever
- Weight loss
- Irritability

Signs
- Heliotrope rash (purple rash over the eyelids)
- Facial edema and eyelid telangiectasia +++
- Gottron's papules (erythematous plaques over extensor surfaces particularly small joints of the hands, but elbows, knees, and ankles are commonly affected) (Fig. 25-1)
- Proximal muscle weakness manifested by difficulty combing hair or climbing stairs; may see the inability to rise from floor without "climbing up the body" (Gowers' sign)

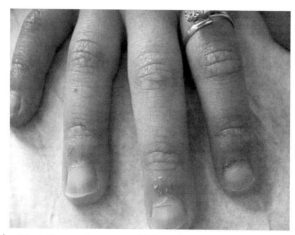

Fig. 25-1 Gottron's papules. This pathognomonic juvenile dermatomyositis rash, here overlying the knuckles, is papulosquamous and may be present over the extensor surfaces of many joints.

- Involvement of striated and smooth muscle of the gastrointestinal tract may cause hoarseness or difficulty handling secretions + + +
- Involvement of striated and smooth muscle of the respiratory system may lead to restrictive lung disease

Workup

The diagnostic system of Bohan and Peter requires the following:

- Characteristic heliotrope rash or Gottron's papules plus two of the following:
  - Symmetric proximal muscle weakness
  - Increased creatine kinase, aldolase, LDH, or transaminases
  - Characteristic electromyographic abnormalities
  - Characteristic muscle biopsy abnormalities

Comments and Treatment Considerations

Appropriate consultation is required. The mainstay of therapy is corticosteroids (often high "pulse" dose) with or without other immunosuppressive agents. Sun exposure often exacerbates the disease, and sunscreens or sun avoidance is recommended.

LEGG-CALVÉ-PERTHES

The child with Legg-Calvé-Perthes disease or idiopathic avascular necrosis of the femoral head presents with a limp of insidious onset and associated pain. The pain is usually in the groin area but may be referred to the thigh or knee (see Chapter 24, Joint Pain and Swelling).

OSGOOD-SCHLATTER DISEASE

Osgood-Schlatter disease is the result of repetitive microtrauma to the tibial tubercle. It presents during the adolescent growth spurt in boys between 13 and 14 years of age and in girls between 10 and 11 years of age. Limping may be noted after exercise and bilateral involvement is noted 30% of the time.

Symptoms
- Knee pain, localized to tibial tubercle
- Localized swelling of the tibial tubercle

Signs
- Tenderness to palpation
- Pain exacerbated by resisted knee extension

Workup
- Plain films of the knee, including a lateral view may show soft-tissue swelling over the tibial tubercle but more importantly can rule out other pathology (Fig. 25-2).

Comments and Treatment Considerations

Appropriate clinical management includes the use of antiinflammatory medications such as ibuprofen dosed at 10 mg/kg/dose

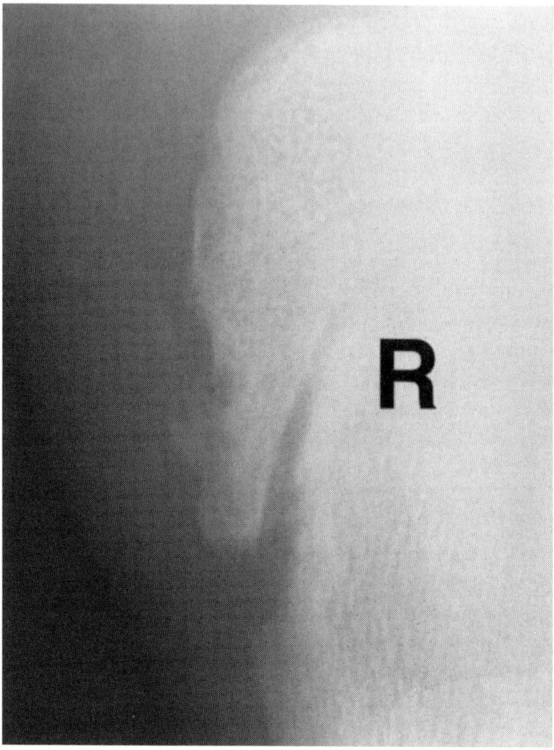

Fig. 25-2 Osgood-Schlatter disease changes. (From DeLee J, Drez D, Miller M: *DeLee and Drez's Orthopaedic Sports Medicine* 2nd ed, New York, 2003, Elsevier.)

(max 800 mg/dose) PO q6h as needed, restricted activities, quadriceps stretching, strengthening, and cross training.

FOOT: FOREIGN BODY

A foreign body, such as a splinter in the foot, may cause a painful limp in a young child. Entry may occur from stepping on the object or from a fall. The vast majority of foreign bodies can be identified and removed without difficulty.

Symptoms

- Antalgic gait or painful limp
- Direct visualization or palpation of a foreign body

Signs

- Puncture wound
- Local redness

Workup

- Standard radiograph will identify radiopaque foreign bodies such as most glass, metal, and gravel.
- Ultrasound for the identification of radiolucent foreign bodies ++++.
- CT or MRI scans may be helpful when foreign body has remained in long enough to cause a foreign body reaction.

Comments and Treatment Considerations:

Most foreign bodies should be removed because retention may lead to infectious and inflammatory complications. Consider orthopedic or surgery consultation for removal under fluoroscopy because nonpalpable nonvisible foreign bodies can be exceedingly difficult to remove in the ED. Administer tetanus prophylaxis as indicated (see Chapter 5, Bites, for tetanus prophylaxis recommendations).

 NEW SHOES

New shoes may cause tenderness on the bony prominences of the foot. Young children unable to articulate their resulting discomfort may come to the ED with a limp.

Symptoms

- Fussiness during ambulation (child's gait should be observed with and without shoes)

Signs

- Erythema/skin irritation noted on the foot
- Blister formation

Workup

- Radiographs are indicated only if diagnosis is not clear and possible subtle fracture is suspected (see Chapter 15, Fractures Not to Miss).

Comments and Treatment Considerations

The diagnosis is made clinically.

REFERENCES

Athreya BH: Vasculitis in children, *Pediatr Clin North Am* (5): 1239-1261, 1995.

Cohen AR: Hematologic emergencies. In Fleisher GR, Ludwig S, editors: *Textbook of pediatric emergency medicine*, 4th ed, Philadelphia, 2000, Lippincott Williams & Wilkins.

Dabney KW, Lipton G: Evaluation of limp in children, *Curr Opin Pediatr* 7(1):88-94, 1995.

Davids JR: Pediatric knee: clinical assessment and common disorders, *Pediatr Clin North Am* 43(5):1067-1090, 1996.

Feldman B: Musculoskeletal disorders. In Feldman W: *Evidence-based pediatrics*, New York, 2000, BC Decker.

Fischer SU, Beattie TF: The limping child: epidemiology, assessment and outcome, *J Bone Joint Surg (Br)* 81(6):1029-1034, 1999.

Himelstein BP, Dormans JP: Malignant bone tumors of childhood, *Pediatr Clin North Am* 43(4):967-984, 1996.

Jacobson JA, et al: Wooden foreign bodies in soft tissue: detection at US, *Radiology* 206(1):45-48, 1998.

Klein-Gitelman MS, Miller ML: Systemic lupus erythematosus. In Behrman RE, et al, editors: *Nelson textbook of pediatrics,* 16th ed, Philadelphia, 2000, WB Saunders.

Koop S, Quanbeck D: Three common causes of childhood hip pain, *Pediatr Clin North Am* 43(5):1053-1066, 1996.

Lowry DW: Arthritis. In Marx RM: *Rosen's emergency medicine: concepts and clinical practice*, 5th ed, St. Louis, 2002, Mosby.

Melish ME: Kawasaki syndrome, *Peds in Review* 17(5):52-62, 1996.

Miller ML, Cassidy JT: Juvenile rheumatoid arthritis. In Behrman RE, et al, editors: *Nelson textbook of pediatrics*, 16th ed, Philadelphia, 2000, WB Saunders.

Ostrov BE, Goldsmith DP, Athreya BH: Differentiation of systemic rheumatoid arthritis from acute leukemia near the onset of disease, *J Pediatr* 122(4):595-598, 1993.

Pachman LM: Juvenile dermatomyositis. In Behrman RE et al, editors: *Nelson textbook of pediatrics*, 16th ed, Philadelphia, 2000, WB Saunders.

Phillips WA: The child with a limp, *Orthop Clin North Am* 18(4): 489-501, 1987.

Rennebohm RM: Rheumatic diseases of childhood, *Pediatr Rev* 10(6):183-190, 1988.

Renshaw TS: The child who has a limp, *Pediatr Rev* 16(12):458-465, 1995.

Shapiro ED: Lyme disease, *Pediatr Rev* 19(5):147-154, 1998.

Silverman ED: Pediatric systemic lupus erythematosus. In Rudolph CD, Rudolph AM, editors: *Rudolph's pediatrics*, 21st ed, New York, 2003, McGraw-Hill.

Staheli LT: Shoes for children: a review, *Pediatrics* 88(2):371-375, 1991.

Staheli LT: Foreign body removal. In *Practice of pediatric orthopedics*, Philadelphia, 2001, Lippincott Williams & Wilkins.

Sundel RP: Rheumatologic emergencies. In Fleisher GR, Ludwig S, editors: *Textbook of pediatric emergency medicine*, 4th ed, Philadelphia, 2000, Lippincott Williams & Wilkins.

Taketomo CK, Hodding JK, Kraus DM, editors: *Pediatric dosage handbook,* 8th ed, Hudson, Ohio, 2001, Lexicomp.

Wallace CA, Sherry DD: Juvenile rheumatoid arthritis. In Rudolph CD, Rudolph AM, editors: *Rudolph's pediatrics*, 21st ed, New York, 2003, McGraw-Hill.

CHAPTER 26

Mouth and Throat Pain

CARA PIZZO

Sore throat and mouth pain are common pediatric complaints. A parent may tell you only that the child is not eating or drinking well or "does not seem right." It is then up to the physician to identify those serious or life-threatening disorders even though the visualization of the oropharynx in a child can be difficult. The most serious diagnoses to rule out include upper airway foreign body obstruction, epiglottitis (now increasingly rare as a result of *Haemophilus influenzae* and *Streptococcus pneumoniae* vaccines), retropharyngeal abscesses (RPAs), peritonsillar abscesses, caustic ingestions, acute pharyngitis, and serious oral/dental trauma or infections. All of these conditions can either cause life-threatening acute airway obstruction or lead to serious systemic infectious complications. The examination and assessment must initially focus on stabilization of the airway and then appropriate treatment of any infectious, inflammatory, or traumatic etiologies.

 ## FOREIGN BODY ASPIRATION

Throat pain may be associated with the aspiration of a foreign body even when the object is no longer present in the trachea or esophagus (see Chapter 30, Respiratory Distress).

 ## EPIGLOTTITIS

The clinician must consider the diagnosis of epiglottitis in any ill-appearing patient complaining of throat pain but with a normal-appearing posterior pharynx on examination. If a patient exhibits concerning signs and symptoms such as sitting forward, anxious-ness, and/or drooling, the patient may require immediate transfer to the operating room for further control of the airway. An anes-thesiologist should be consulted immediately (see Chapter 27, Neck Pain/Masses).

RETROPHARYNGEAL ABSCESS

In early childhood a potential space exists between the posterior pharyngeal wall and the prevertebral fascia. This space contains many lymph nodes that can enlarge and become infected. Typically, this potential space disappears during a child's third to fourth year of life. Most commonly a retropharyngeal abscess (RPA) develops as a complication of bacterial pharyngitis, although it can also occur from direct extension from infections such as vertebral osteomyelitis. If left untreated, an RPA may rupture and inflammatory and bacterial contents can track down fascial planes and result in fatal complications such as aspiration pneumonia, mediastinitis, carotid artery erosion, jugular venous thrombosis, and epidural abscess.

Symptoms
- Fever ++++
- Sore throat ++++
- Neck pain ++
- Dysphagia
- Poor oral intake +++
- Noisy breathing

Signs
- Nuchal rigidity +++
- Torticollis ++
- "Hot potato" voice ++
- Stridor
- Trismus ++
- Respiratory distress
- Drooling ++
- Cervical adenopathy
- Dyspnea

Workup

- Lateral neck radiographs with the neck in neutral position may reveal widening of the prevertebral soft-tissue structures. An abscess should be suspected if the soft-tissue space is more than one half of the adjacent vertebral body (Fig. 26-1).
- Contrast CT scan is the study of choice and can differentiate between retropharyngeal cellulitis and abscess.
- CBC and blood culture are generally not helpful.

Comments and Treatment Considerations

Children with an RPA often have both a sore throat and neck pain and frequently undergo LP to rule out meningitis. RPA should be considered as a diagnosis in anyone with these complaints and a negative LP finding. Consultation with an otolaryngologist is essential because surgical drainage may be necessary. In the meantime, antibiotic treatment should be initiated to cover oral flora. Ampicillin-sulbactam (Unasyn) dosed at 200 mg of ampicillin component/kg/day IV divided q6h (max 8 g ampicillin component/kg/day) or clindamycin 30 mg/kg/day IV divided q6-8h (max 4.8 g/day) are good

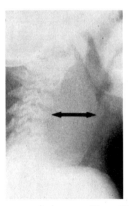

Fig. 26-1 Retropharyngeal abscess. (From Dhillon RS, East CA: *Ear, nose, and throat and head and neck surgery,* 2nd ed, New York, 1999, Churchill Livingstone.)

empiric antibiotic choices. A CXR should be performed to rule out mediastinal extension in any patient with significant chest pain, signs of respiratory distress after drainage, or worsening course despite therapy.

PERITONSILLAR ABSCESSES

Peritonsillar abscess is almost always a complication of bacterial pharyngitis; it typically occurs in older children and adolescents. This diagnosis can be made by direct inspection of the oropharynx.

Symptoms
- Severe sore throat, often on one side more than the other ++++
- Difficulty swallowing +++
- Fever ++
- Pain radiating to the ear

Signs
- Visible redness/fullness in posterior pharynx
- Deviation of uvula or other soft-tissue structures ++++
- Drooling or difficulty handling saliva ++
- "Hot potato" voice ++
- Trismus ++
- Foul odor to breath
- Bulge in soft palate fluctuant to palpation

Comments and Treatment Considerations
Patients with a peritonsillar abscess should undergo needle aspiration or incision and drainage (I/D) performed either by an experienced emergency medicine physician or by an otolaryngologist. Adequate suction must be available to prevent aspiration of pus. Needle aspiration without I/D has been shown to be effective and safe. Younger, uncooperative patients may need to have this procedure performed under general anesthesia. Antibiotic therapy should be started, directed toward oral flora (see earlier recommendations for RPA).

CAUSTIC INGESTIONS

When ingested, caustic substances can cause severe local irritation and erosion. Vomiting should never be induced (see Chapter 35, Toxic Ingestion, Approach To).

ACUTE PHARYNGITIS

Pharyngitis is most common in the 4- to 7-year-old age-group but continues throughout later childhood and adulthood. It is uncommon in the child younger than 1 year. Viral syndromes cause most cases but can be impossible to differentiate clinically from bacterial causes. Group A *Streptococcus* infection is the most common bacterial pathogen. Because it is impossible to routinely clinically differentiate pharyngitis caused by group A *Streptococcus* from other etiologies by clinical examination and given its prevalence and possible serious sequelae, rapid testing or culture should generally be obtained with appropriate antibiotic treatment prescribed for positive results. Incidence peaks in the late winter to early spring months.

Symptoms
- Sore throat +++++
- Fever +++
- Malaise
- Anorexia
- Rhinitis (much more likely to be viral in origin)
- Cough, conjunctivitis, and hoarseness (much more likely to be viral in origin)
- Headache and abdominal pain, especially with streptococcal infection in younger patients

Signs
- Ulcerative lesions on the palate, tonsils, or pharyngeal wall +++
- Tender cervical adenopathy
- Tonsillar exudates ++
- Palatal petechiae ++
- Exanthem (viral) or scarlatiniform rash (streptococcal infection)

Workup

- Rapid streptococcal antigen test (rapid antigen detection) is highly specific (95%), but the sensitivity generally ranges between 75% and 80%, in part because performance is operator dependent. Common practice is to obtain a rapid test, and if the results are positive, treat; if test results are negative, await culture results.
- Throat culture remains the gold standard for diagnosis of streptococcal pharyngitis.
- Monospot test if mononucleosis is being considered. A significant rate of false-negative results occurs in children younger than 5 years. In children younger than 5 years, consider Epstein-Barr virus titers.
- Gonococcal pharyngitis should also be considered in the sexually active patient or victim of sexual abuse.

Comments and Treatment Considerations

Many children may be carriers of group A *Streptococcus*; however, those with a positive culture result should still be treated because of risks of serious sequelae such as rheumatic fever. Although penicillin remains the drug of choice for treating group A streptococcal pharyngitis, amoxicillin is often chosen because it is more palatable. The dose of amoxicillin is usually 25 to 50 mg/kg/day divided q8-12h (max 500 mg/dose) for 10 days. Patients who are unlikely to be compliant with oral therapy should receive benzathine penicillin G 600,000 units IM × one dose if <27 kg, 1,200,000 units IM × one dose if >27 kg. Erythromycin base at 40 mg/kg/day PO divided bid to qid (max 2 g/day) or one of its derivatives such as azithromycin 10 mg/kg/day (max 500 mg/dose) PO q day × 1 day then 5 mg/kg/day (max 250 mg/dose) PO q day × 4 days may be substituted in the penicillin-allergic patient. Recurrent streptococcal pharyngitis may require a first-generation cephalosporin or clindamycin. Gonococcal infection should be treated in the same manner as genital disease (see Chapter 2, Abuse/Rape) and social services consulted as appropriate.

ORAL AND DENTAL INFECTIONS

Dental infections are a relatively common pediatric complaint. Initial treatment is frequently directed at providing antibiotic coverage and adequate pain relief until dental consultation can be obtained. Dental infections may track along fascial planes in the head and neck and potentially produce significant illness.

DENTOALVEOLAR ABSCESS
A dentoalveolar abscess forms at the base of an infected tooth.

Symptoms
- Pain
- Swelling
- Fever

Signs
- Tooth pain to percussion
- Mobility of tooth in the socket
- Erythematous or swollen soft tissues
- Pustular lesions on the gingival (fistulous tracts)
- Lymphadenopathy
- Facial cellulitis

Comments and Treatment Considerations
Definitive care requires dental consultation for abscess incision and drainage. Less severe cases may be treated with antibiotics covering oral flora such as penicillin VK dosed at 25 to 50 mg/kg/day PO divided q6-8h or 250 mg PO q6-8h. If the patient is allergic to penicillin, clindamycin can be used at a dose of 10 to 30 mg/kg/day PO divided q6-8h with referral within 48 hours to dentistry.

PERICORONITIS
Pericoronitis is a localized infection surrounding an erupting tooth and more typically occurs with molar teeth.

Symptoms
- Pain
- Fever

- Inability to completely close mouth
- Difficulty swallowing

Signs
- Erythema and edema in the surrounding gingiva
- Lymphadenopathy
- Trismus
- Visualization or palpation of cusps of erupting tooth

Comments and Treatment Considerations
Supportive treatment with local curettage, oral rinses, and heat. Consider dental referral. Antibiotics are needed if facial swelling or systemic symptoms exist and should be continued until the tooth has erupted.

GINGIVOSTOMATITIS
Stomatitis is an infection of the mouth, typically caused by herpes simplex or the coxsackie viruses. Thrush is a fungal infection caused by *Candida albicans* and typically occurs in infants or in immunosuppressed patients. Viral lesions can appear as vesicles, plaques, and ulcerations, whereas thrush appears as white plaques that often bleed when scraped (i.e., they cannot be "washed" off).

Symptoms
- Pain
- Irritability
- Decreased oral intake
- Fever
- Headache
- Nausea
- Bleeding gums

Signs
- Vesicles, ulcers, or plaques on lips, gums, oral mucosa, and/or tongue (Fig. 26-2)
- Erythematous, inflamed gingiva
- Lymphadenopathy
- Rash particularly on hands and feet but may also involve trunk (seen with coxsackie)

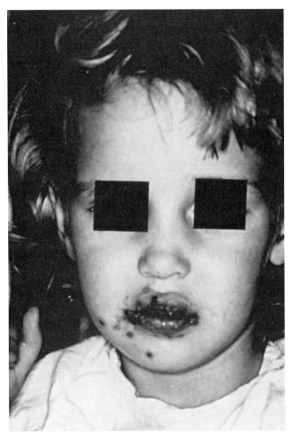

Fig. 26-2 Primary herpes simplex virus gingivostomatitis in a child, extending to involve the cheek, chin, and perioral skin. (From Mandell G, Bennett J, Dolin R: *Principles and practice of infectious diseases*, 5th ed, New York, 2000, Churchill Livingstone.)

Workup

- Direct fluorescent antibody staining, enzyme immunoassay, polymerase chain reaction, and culture of oral lesions can identify herpes but are seldom indicated except in an immunocompromised host.

- Tzanck preparation has low sensitivity and is no longer recommended.

Comments and Treatment Considerations

Treatment is supportive with the primary goal of preventing dehydration. Pain relief with topical anesthesia may be obtained with lidocaine rinses or mouthwashes with Maalox and diphenhydramine in a 1:1 mixture. Lidocaine toxicity can occur if large amounts are ingested or absorbed; therefore, ensure that excessive doses or frequencies are avoided. Some children may require admission for dehydration secondary to their refusal to drink. The rare child may require acetaminophen with codeine elixir for pain control. Oral acyclovir therapy may shorten the duration of symptoms for lesions caused by herpes, especially if treatment is initiated promptly. Acyclovir is commonly dosed at 30 mg/kg/day PO divided tid (max 800 mg/dose). Topical acyclovir is ineffective. Immunocompromised patients require admission for system intravenous therapy (see Chapter 21, Immunocompromised Patients: Special Considerations).

ACUTE NECROTIZING ULCERATIVE GINGIVITIS

Acute necrotizing ulcerative gingivitis is an infection of the gingiva caused by an increase in the fusiform bacillus in the mouth, an organism that is part of the normal oral flora.

Symptoms

- Soreness and point tenderness of the gingival mucosa
- Sensation of food being stuck between teeth
- Metallic taste in mouth
- Bleeding gums

Signs

- Foul odor to breath
- Hyperemic gingivae
- Pain with probing of the gingivae
- "Punched out" areas of the gingival mucosa between the teeth
- Occasionally grey necrotic pseudomembrane covering the gingivae

Comments and Treatment Considerations

Oral hygiene should be emphasized with 1:1 water/hydrogen peroxide rinses. Penicillin or clindamycin (see the section on Dentoalveolar Abscess, earlier in this chapter, for dosing) for 1 week should be prescribed with follow-up referral to dentistry.

TRAUMA TO THE MOUTH

Children may come to an acute care facility with mouth trauma most commonly to the teeth, mucosa, palate, or jaw.

DENTAL INJURIES

Permanent teeth that are completely avulsed should be replaced as soon as possible to improve long-term survival of the tooth. Tooth fractures may include the enamel, dentin, pulp, or nerve (Fig. 26-3). Pulp exposure results in an increased likelihood of bacterial infection and pulp necrosis and therefore requires immediate attention. When the periodontal structures are involved in trauma, a tooth may become concussed, subluxed, intruded, or completely avulsed. It is important to note whether the tooth is a primary or secondary tooth because primary teeth do not usually need to be salvaged.

DENTAL FRACTURES WITH PULP EXPOSURES
Symptoms
- Pain, particularly with exposure to air, heat, and cold ++++

Signs
- Central small red spot evident on fractured tooth

PERIODONTAL TRAUMA

Symptoms
- Pain
- Feeling of tooth misplaced

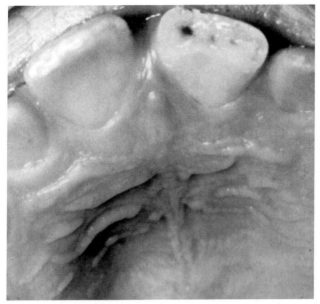

Fig. 26-3 Crown fracture exposing the pulp. (From Pinkham JR et al: *Pediatric dentistry,* 3rd ed, Philadelphia, 1999, WB Saunders.)

Signs
- Concussed—tooth tender to percussion, but not mobile
- Subluxed—tooth tender and has mild to moderate mobility
- Intruded—tooth pushed upward into socket
- Avulsed—tooth completely out of socket

Workup
- Only as indicated by associated trauma.

Comments and Treatment Considerations
If the tooth is completely avulsed, the best result will occur if it is placed back into the socket within ½ to 1 hour. The tooth may be gently cleansed in milk or normal saline. In an older patient, replace the tooth into the socket while awaiting emergent dental consultation. For a younger patient who is at risk of possible

aspiration if the tooth is replaced into the socket, the tooth can be transported in a container until the patient is brought to a dentist. Transporting the tooth in a dry medium can lead to a poor outcome. Ideally, the tooth should be transported in Hank's solution (a balanced pH cell culture media), which is available OTC as the "Save-a-Tooth" system. Otherwise, milk can be used. Dental consult is also required if pulp is exposed or if the tooth is significantly subluxed or intruded.

If there are symptoms suggestive of an aspirated foreign object, consider the possibility of tooth fragment aspiration.

MANDIBULAR FRACTURES

The mandible is among the most common facial bones fractured in children. Most fractures occur along the condyles, which is structurally the weakest part of the mandible.

Symptoms
- Pain with mouth opening +++
- Unable to open mouth +++
- Malocclusion

Signs
- Deviation of mandible to one side with mouth opening
- Malocclusion
- Depressed dental fragments
- Gingival lacerations
- Sublingual ecchymosis

Workup
- Mandibular x-rays, may require panoramic films.

Comments and Treatment Considerations

Dental or oromaxilofacial consult is necessary for definitive care. Some patients may require admission for intravenous fluid hydration and wiring.

PALATAL TRAUMA

Palatal trauma that occurs to the lateral aspects of the posterior pharynx is most concerning because of the possible injury to vascular structures in close proximity (e.g., the internal carotid artery, which lies within the cavernous sinus before it ascends to divide into the anterior and middle cerebral arteries). An injury to the central portion of the palate is unlikely to result in serious vascular or neural damage. Simple lacerations and puncture wounds generally do not require repair.

Symptoms
- Pain
- Posterior pharyngeal fullness

Signs
- Continued bleeding
- Decreased carotid pulses
- Crepitus on neck examination
- Expanding neck hematoma

Workup
- Emergent otolaryngology consult with subsequent angiogram or neck exploration may be required, especially in any patient who has a significant mechanism of injury, is symptomatic, or has lateral trauma.

Comments and Treatment Considerations

Consider emergent airway intervention if vascular injury is suspected. One must exclude the possibility of a retained foreign body in any palatal puncture or laceration.

REFERENCES

Bisno AL, Gerber MA, Gwalteny JM, et al: Diagnosis and management of streptococcal pharyngitis: a practice guideline, *Clin Infect Dis* 25:574-583, 1997.

Brook I: Peritonsillar, retropharyngeal, and parapharyngeal abscesses. In *Principles and practice of pediatric infectious diseases*, New York, 1997, Churchill Livingstone.

Fleisher G: Infectious disease emergencies. In Fleisher GR, Ludwig S, editors: *Textbook of pediatric emergency medicine*, 4th ed, Philadelphia, 2000, Lippincott Williams & Wilkins.

Fleisher GR: Sore throat. In Fleisher GR, Ludwig S, editors: *Textbook of pediatric emergency medicine*, 4th ed, Philadelphia, 2000, Lippincott Williams & Wilkins.

Handler S, Potsic W: Otolaryngolic trauma. In Fleisher GR, Ludwig S, editors: *Textbook of pediatric emergency medicine*, 4th ed, Philadelphia, 2000, Lippincott Williams & Wilkins.

Lieu TA, Fleisher GR, Schwartz JS: Clinical evaluation of a latex agglutination test for Streptococcal pharyngitis: performance and impact on treatment rates, *Pediatr Infect Dis J* 7(12):847-854, 1988.

Nady M, Pizzuto M, Blackstrom J, Brodsky L: Deep neck infections in children: a new approach to diagnosis and treatment, *Laryngoscope* 107(12 pt 1):1627-1634, 1997.

Nelson L, Needleman H, Padwa B: Dental trauma. In Fleisher GR, Ludwig S, editors: *Textbook of pediatric emergency medicine*, 4th ed, Philadelphia, 2000, Lippincott Williams & Wilkins.

Nelson L, Shusterman S: Dental emergencies. In Fleisher GR, Ludwig S, editors: *Textbook of pediatric emergency medicine*, 4th ed, Philadelphia, 2000, Lippincott Williams & Wilkins.

Puhakka H, Svedstrom E, Kero P, et al: Tracheobronchial foreign bodies: a persistent problem in pediatric patients, *Am J Dis Child* 143(5): 543-545, 1989.

Schunk JE: Foreign body—ingestion/aspiration. In Fleisher GR, Ludwig S, editors: *Textbook of pediatric emergency medicine*, 4th ed, Philadelphia, 2000, Lippincott Williams & Wilkins.

Tanz RR, Shulman ST: Pharyngitis. In *Principles and practice of pediatric infectious diseases*, New York, 1997, Churchill Livingstone.

CHAPTER 27

Neck Pain/Masses

MARK I. NEUMAN

Neck pain is a common complaint among children presenting to the clinic or emergency department. Children with neck pain after known or presumed trauma must be properly immobilized until the possibility of a fracture or cervical spine injury can be excluded.

In the absence of trauma, a diagnosis of meningitis must be excluded. Evaluating an infant or young child clinically for meningitis can often be difficult, and thus many experts recommend obtaining spinal fluid in all febrile infants younger than 3 months of age.

Most neck masses in children are the result of lymph node swelling/hyperplasia, either from a primary head, neck, or throat infection or from infection within the lymph node itself. The presence of constitutional symptoms such as fatigue, night sweats, and weight loss warrants further evaluation for malignancy. Cystic hygroma, branchial cleft cyst, and hemangioma are other diagnoses to be considered in the evaluation of infants with a neck mass.

 ## TRAUMA

Although cervical spine injuries in children are relatively rare, improper management of a patient with an unstable injury may have catastrophic consequences (see Chapter 36, Trauma).

 ## MENINGITIS

A diagnosis of meningitis must be considered in all febrile children with neck pain, particularly on flexion (see Chapter 3, Altered Mental Status, and Chapter 14, Fever).

✳ *EPIGLOTTITIS*

Epiglottitis is the most acute life-threatening etiology of stridor. Supraglottic obstruction results from inflammation or edema of the epiglottis, aryepiglottic folds, and false vocal cords. *Haemophilus influenzae* type b accounted for 75% of cases before the introduction of the *H. influenzae* type b vaccine. Although the incidence of epiglottitis has decreased dramatically in children, it has remained relatively stable in adults. Other infectious etiologies in children include group A β-hemolytic streptococci, *Streptococcus pneumoniae*, *Staphylococcus aureus*, parainfluenza virus, respiratory syncytial virus, and varicella-zoster virus.

Symptoms
- Fever ++++
- Sudden onset (6 to 24 hours) of difficulty breathing ++++
- Audible stridor ++++
- Sore throat +++
- Drooling ++++
- Toxic appearance +++
- Dysphagia ++++

Signs
- Throat pain with normal posterior pharynx
- Anxious appearance, "sniffing position"—sitting upright with mouth open and jaw thrust forward
- Muffled "hot potato" voice ++++ or aphonia
- Stridor +++
- High fever
- Tachypnea and respiratory distress with marked retractions
- Tachycardia

Comments and Treatment Considerations

Epiglottitis is a clinical diagnosis based on history, physical examination findings, and clinical suspicion. Defer phlebotomy, IV line placement, and attempts to visualize the epiglottis or posterior pharynx until personnel capable of providing a definitive airway are present. Children should be allowed to maintain an airway protective position that they have likely assumed, classically sitting up in a sniffing position until medical personnel are ready for intubation. Patients in extremis can undergo bag-valve-mask ventilation only if necessary until a definitive airway can be placed. A lateral neck radiograph may be obtained in a clinically stable patient for whom the diagnosis is not clear. The film may show classic signs of epiglottitis including a swollen epiglottis, thickened aryepiglottic folds, and obliteration of the vallecula.

Airway management should plan not only for endotracheal intubation but also for the potential need for a surgical airway. Further evaluation and intubation most commonly occurs in the operating room with an otolaryngologist present. Direct laryngoscopy should be performed as soon as feasible under controlled circumstances looking for a cherry red, edematous, and swollen epiglottis. A surface culture may be obtained at this time if possible. Endotracheal tube (ETT) size will commonly need to be smaller than expected because of airway edema.

Once the airway is controlled, an IV line should be placed and blood culture results obtained. The CBC will most commonly show a leukocytosis. The blood culture will be positive in 80% to 90% of cases of epiglottitis due to *H. influenzae* type b. Antibiotics should be given as soon as IV access has been established. Empiric antibiotic choices are:

Ceftriaxone 50-100 mg/kg/day IV divided q12-24h (max 4 g/day)
OR
Cefotaxime 200 mg/kg/day IV divided q6h (max 12 g/day)
OR
Ampicillin-sulbactam (Unasyn) 200-300 mg ampicillin component/kg/day IV divided q6h (max 12 g ampicillin/day)

The patient should be admitted to an ICU. If transport to another facility is required, the patient should not be transported without a secure airway. Personnel skilled in management of the difficult airway should accompany the patient.

 ## BACTERIAL TRACHEITIS

Bacterial tracheitis is an uncommon infection in childhood, but when it occurs, it may be the result of a superinfection of croup or secondary to tracheal trauma or intubation. Bacterial infection of the trachea results in laryngotracheal inflammation, edema, purulent secretions, and possible pseudomembrane formation that may contribute to acute airway obstruction and/or significant respiratory distress. Common bacterial pathogens are *S. aureus* (most common), group A β-hemolytic streptococci, *S. pneumoniae*, *Streptococcus pyogenes*, *H. influenzae* type b, *Mycobacterium catarrhalis*, *Klebsiella* species, *Peptostreptococcus*, and *Bacteroides*.

Clinically the presentation is similar to that of a child with severe croup (see Chapter 30, Respiratory Distress). The diagnosis of tracheitis is often suspected after a lateral neck film reveals irregularity of the tracheal border.

Symptoms
- Fever
- Audible stridor
- Cough, may be "barky"
- Decreased oral intake

Signs
- Respiratory distress
- Stridor at rest
- Toxic appearance

Workup
- Blood culture.
- AP and lateral neck radiographs, which would show tracheal narrowing or irregularity of the tracheal border.
- Diagnosis confirmed with direct laryngoscopy.
- Culture and Gram stain of tracheal secretions.
- CBC may show leukocytosis.

Comments and Treatment Considerations
As with epiglottitis the first priority is to secure an adequate airway. Intubation is frequently necessary to stabilize the airway. Because of the swelling within the trachea, the ETT size is often smaller than usual and there is a frequent need for suctioning. A tracheostomy may be necessary if intubation is unsuccessful. Intravenous antibiotic therapy with adequate

staphylococcal coverage such as ampicillin-sulbactam (Unasyn) 200 mg of ampicillin component/kg/day IV divided q6h (max 8 g of ampicillin/day) or clindamycin 40 mg/kg/day IV divided q6-8h (max 4.8 g/day) should be given. Admission to an ICU is recommended.

PERITONSILLAR/RETROPHARYNGEAL ABSCESS/LUDWIG'S ANGINA

Peritonsillar and retropharyngeal abscesses may cause fever and neck pain (see Chapter 26, Mouth and Throat Pain).

KAWASAKI DISEASE

Fever lasting >5 days and cervical adenopathy can be a manifestation of Kawasaki disease. Given the serious sequelae of coronary aneurysms, it is imperative to consider this diagnosis (see Chapter 14, Fever).

CERVICAL LYMPHADENITIS

Cervical adenopathy is the most common cause of a neck mass in children. The most common cause of acute cervical adenopathy is a viral upper respiratory tract infection, which typically causes bilateral enlarged and minimally tender soft nodes. Bacterial cervical adenitis is most commonly caused by group A β-hemolytic streptococci or *S. aureus*, atypical mycobacteria, and *M. tuberculosis*; oral anaerobes must also be considered. Lymph nodes that are hard and fixed may require a biopsy to evaluate for malignancy.

Symptoms
- Neck pain
- Neck mass
- Fever

Signs

- Firm tender mass, most commonly unilateral and along anterior cervical chain
- Erythema
- Warmth
- Fluctuance

Workup

- US or CT scanning with contrast, to identify those nodes that are fluctuant and may require surgical drainage.
- PPD tuberculin test and CXR if atypical mycobacteria or tubercular infection is suspected.

Comments and Treatment Considerations

Bacterial adenitis in an ill-appearing child or a child who has failed outpatient oral antibiotic therapy should be treated with antibiotics as described in the previous section. These antimicrobials provide good coverage against both gram-positive cocci and oral anaerobic bacteria. Outpatient oral antibiotic choices may include amoxicillin-clavulanic acid (Augmentin) dosed at 25 to 45 mg amoxicillin component/kg/day PO divided tid (max 500 mg/dose) or clindamycin 30 mg/kg/day PO divided q6-8h (max 1.8 g/day). If atypical mycobacteria or *M. tuberculosis* infection is suspected, an excisional biopsy will be required for diagnosis. Atypical mycobacteria infection generally causes unilateral adenopathy just under the mandible that is slow growing. This typically occurs in younger children and is rarely associated with systemic symptoms. However, *M. tuberculosis* lymphadenitis typically occurs in children older than 5 years, involves the posterior cervical chain, and often has associated pulmonary or systemic involvement. Tuberculosis infections will require 6 to 9 months of antitubercular therapy and must be reported to public health authorities.

 INFECTIOUS MONONUCLEOSIS

Epstein-Barr virus (EBV), the causative agent of infectious mononucleosis, commonly causes cervical lymphadenopathy, particularly in the posterior chain. The classic presentation consists of fever, malaise, tonsillopharyngitis, and hepatosplenomegaly (see Chapter 39, Weakness/Fatigue).

 ## CAT-SCRATCH DISEASE

Cat-scratch disease is caused by *Bartonella henselae*. It is a subacute regional lymphadenitis that occurs after cutaneous inoculation. Most commonly, the vector is a cat (particularly kitten) scratch or bite, although cases have been reported after injury from dogs, monkeys, fish hooks, thorns, or no injury at all. Affected nodes are usually tender, warm, and enlarged for 4 to 6 weeks, with persistence up to 12 months. Fever occurs in 30% of patients. Parinaud oculoglandular syndrome occurs when the site of primary inoculation is the conjunctiva and conjunctivitis accompanies the primary lesion.

Treatment is supportive as most patients with cat-scratch disease have a benign course with spontaneous resolution. Needle aspiration may provide relief for patients with unusually large, tender suppurative nodes (excision should be avoided because of the risk of creating sinus fistulas). A few patients may require antibiotic treatment for systemic symptoms with trimethoprim (TMP)-sulfamethoxazole (Bactrim) 6 to 12 mg TMP/kg/day PO divided bid (max 320 mg TMP/day), ciprofloxacin for patients older than 18 years dosed at 20 to 30 mg/kg/day PO divided bid (max 1.5 g/day), or azithromycin 10 mg/kg/day PO × 1 day (max 500 mg) then 5 mg/kg/day PO q day × 4 days (max 250 mg/day).

 ## NECK TUMORS AND CONGENITAL MALFORMATION

Although neck masses in children are fairly common, tumors are quite rare. Congenital malformations of the head and neck include hemangioma, branchial cleft cyst, thyroglossal duct cyst, and cystic hygroma. Hemangiomas are vascular formations that may occur anywhere on the neck. Cystic hygroma is a lymphatic malformation that occurs in the lateral neck of infants, which may grow rapidly and cause airway compromise. Branchial cleft cysts (lateral) and thyroglossal duct cysts (midline) are embryologic remnants. Malignant masses are most commonly found as a single mass in the posterior triangle, or multiple or matted masses involving both anterior and posterior triangles.

Symptoms
- Painless swelling
- Rapidly progressive growth
- Constitutional symptoms such as fever, night sweats, and weight loss

Signs
- Nontender, nonmobile, hard or firm mass
- Size > 3 cm
- Hepatosplenomegaly, bruising, or cachexia should raise suspicion for malignancy

Workup
- A thorough examination of the head and neck is mandatory because many primary tumors originate in the nasopharynx or involve sites such as the orbit and tongue.
- CT to define mass.
- A biopsy is indicated for any mass suspected to be malignant.

Comments and Treatment Considerations
Treatment is based on etiology. Otolaryngology consultation is warranted in any case of congenital malformation because these lesions often can become infected if not surgically excised. Oncology consult should be obtained if there is a suspicion of malignancy.

 ## *TORTICOLLIS*

Torticollis in children may be congenital or acquired. Congenital torticollis affects infants within the first few days to weeks of life. It is due to swelling and contracture of the ster-nocleidomastoid muscle and most commonly occurs from fetal malposition or birth trauma.

Rotary atlantoaxial subluxation subsequent to trauma is frequently confused with inflammatory torticollis but can be differentiated based on the direction of head tilt. In rotary subluxation, the head is turned toward the affected side, in contrast to inflammatory torticollis in which muscle spasm causes the head to turn away from the affected sternocleidomastoid muscle.

Neurologic, ophthalmic, or vestibular dysfunction may produce head tilt or torticollis as a means of compensation for the imbalance. Dystonic reactions, presenting as torticollis or oculo-gyric crisis, can be seen in children treated with metoclopramide (Reglan), prochlorperazine (Compazine), or phenothiazines.

Symptoms
- Head deviation
- Difficulty moving neck
- Neck pain or spasm

Signs
- Limited range of motion of neck
- Palpable mass or contracture of sternocleidomastoid muscle
- Head deviation

Workup
- Careful neurologic examination.
- Cervical spine radiograph findings are usually negative for bony abnormality in the absence of trauma.
- Lateral neck radiograph may be considered in the evaluation of the febrile or toxic-appearing child for diagnosis of a retropharyngeal abscess (see Chapter 26, Mouth and Throat Pain).
- Consider cervical CT for persistent torticollis of unclear etiology.

Comments and Treatment Considerations
Acquired cervical muscle spasm in children is usually self-limited and resolves within 2 weeks. Treatment is primarily

supportive and includes heat, massage, analgesics, and muscle relaxants. Diazepam can be used in children for muscle relaxation and is generally dosed at 0.2 to 0.8 mg/kg/day PO divided q6-8h (usual adult dose 2 to 10 mg/dose). Alternatively, cyclobenzaprine may be useful in adolescents and adults and is generally dosed at 5 to 10 mg/dose PO tid for no longer than 2 weeks. A soft collar may provide additional comfort. Treatment of an acute dystonic reaction consists of intravenous diphenhydramine at a dose of 1 to 1.25 mg/kg (max 50 mg/dose) and may require repeated dosing. Any patient with an abnormal neurologic examination finding or bony abnormality on radiographs should remain C-spine immobilized and have appropriate consultation with neurosurgery or orthopedics. Patients with persistent torticollis not improving after 1 to 2 weeks should be referred to a pediatric orthopedist.

REFERENCES

Bernstein T, Brilli R, Jacobs B: Is bacterial tracheitis changing? A 14-month experience in a pediatric intensive care unit, *Clin Infect Dis* 27(3):458-462, 1998.

Brown RL, Azizkhan RG: Pediatric head and neck lesion, *Pediatr Clin North Am* 45(4):889-905, 1998.

Butler KM, Baker CJ: Cervical lymphadenitis. In Feigin RD, Cherry JD, editors: *Textbook of pediatric infectious diseases*, 4th ed, Philadelphia, 1998, WB Saunders.

Fleisher GR, Ludwig S, editors: *Textbook of pediatric emergency medicine*, 4th ed, Philadelphia, 2000, Lippincott Williams & Wilkins.

Kahn ML, Davidson R, Drummond DS: Acquired torticollis in children, *Orthop Rev* 20(8):667-674, 1991.

Marci SM: Cervical adenitis, *Pediatr Infect Dis* 4(3; suppl):S23, 1985.

Ross M, Dufel S: Torticollis, *eMed J* 2(5):1, 2001.

Stroud RH, Friedman NR: An update on inflammatory disorders of the pediatric airway: epiglottitis, croup and tracheitis, *Am J Otolaryngol* 22(4):268-275, 2001.

Wubbel L, McCracken GH Jr: Management of bacterial meningitis, *Pediatr Rev* 19(3):78-84, 1998.

Zitelli BJ: Evaluating the child with a neck mass, *Contemp Pediatr* 7:90-112, 1990.

CHAPTER 28

Pallor

LOIS K. LEE

Pallor is associated with various medical problems, not all of which have a hematologic etiology. It can be the result of a chronic problem or can develop acutely and may be associated with a life-threatening illness. If caused by anemia, pallor can be clinically appreciated when the hemoglobin concentration is between 8 and 9 g/dl.

 ## HYPOTENSION

Pallor may be seen in a patient with volume loss of any etiology and subsequent early shock or hypotension (see Chapter 20, Hypotension/Shock).

 ## SEPSIS

Pallor may be seen in a patient with sepsis of either bacterial or viral causes (see Chapter 14, Fever).

 ## HEMOLYSIS

Hemolytic anemia occurs when there is increased RBC destruction. This may be due to inherent RBC abnormalities, environmental factors, or a combination of the two. Signs, symptoms, and initial evaluation are independent of etiology.

Differential (Partial)

- RBC membrane defects (hereditary spherocytosis)
- RBC enzyme defects (pyruvate-kinase deficiency, G6PD deficiency)
- Hemoglobin defects (sickle cell disease)

    In the patient with sickle cell disease, anemic crises arise from three potential mechanisms: a transient decrease in the rate of RBC production usually caused by bone marrow suppression from a viral illness (particularly parvovirus); by splenic sequestration (associated with a rapidly enlarging spleen, particularly in children younger than 5 years); or increased RBC destruction, again often caused by viral illness (more common in patients who are sickle and G6PD deficient).
- Autoimmune mediated IgG, IgM, or autoimmune hemolytic anemia [AIHA]
- Environmental factors (certain drugs, foods, or infections)

Symptoms

- Pallor
- Jaundice
- Lethargy
- Abdominal pain
- Fever
- Hemoglobinuria
- Vomiting (acute hemolysis in G6PD)
- Diarrhea (acute hemolysis in G6PD)

Signs

- Hepatomegaly
- Splenomegaly

Workup

- CBC with differential and peripheral smear will usually reveal a normocytic normochromic anemia with reticulocytosis (unless aplastic crisis, i.e., sickle cell disease). The smear may show spherocytes, schistocytes, and/or nucleated RBCs.

- Direct Coombs' antiglobulin test results will be positive in AIHA.
- Osmotic fragility test for evaluation of RBC membrane disorders (may consider after consultation with hematologist).
- Hemoglobin electrophoresis if undiagnosed sickle cell anemia is suspected. Sickle cell disease is most common in African Americans but may occur in any ethnic group.
- Fluorescent RBC assay if G6PD deficiency is suspected and not previously diagnosed. G6PD deficiency is very common in African Americans and to a lesser degree in people of Mediterranean, Middle Eastern, or Chinese descent. Although it may be seen in any ethnic group, G6PD deficiency is uncommon in whites of non-Mediterranean descent.
- Reticulocyte count (lack of elevation in the setting of anemia indicates lack of appropriate increase in production) that may need to be repeated every few days to follow bone marrow function.

Comments and Treatment Considerations

Patients with severe hemolysis and anemia of any etiology may require emergent transfusion. In some cases, it may be helpful to consult a pediatric hematologist before providing initial therapy. For life-threatening symptoms a PRBC transfusion should be started with 10 to 20 ml/kg. Typed and cross-matched blood is preferable, although O-negative blood may be used. Unless there is acute massive blood loss or shock, transfusion should be given no faster than 2 to 3 ml/kg/hr over at least 4 hours. Volume of transfusion for non–life-threatening situations may be estimated by the following formula:

$$\text{Volume of PRBCs (ml)} = \text{EBV (ml)} \times \frac{\text{Desired Hct} \times \text{Actual Hct}}{\text{Hct of PRBCs}}$$

where EBV is the estimated blood volume, which varies by age but in an emergency can be approximated to 80 ml/kg. Hematocrit (Hct) of PRBCs is usually 55% to 70%.

Patients with sickle cell disease may benefit from exchange transfusion instead of simple transfusion based on the suspected etiology of the anemia and the patient's specific medical history. Patients with G6PD and hemolysis will additionally require removal of the inciting agent.

Patients with AIHA present a particular challenge for therapy. For stable patients, therapy should be instituted only after consultation with a hematologist. Those with AIHA and life-threatening anemia may need blood transfusion with the "least incompatible" blood while beginning steroids or intravenous immune globulin (IVIG). Corticosteroids or IVIG are effective for approximately 80% of patients with IgG-induced AIHA. Methylprednisolone (Solu-Medrol) dosed at 1 to 2 mg/kg/day IV divided q6-12h or prednisone dosed at 1 to 2 mg/kg/day PO divided q6-12h is commonly used. Higher doses have been administered for resistant cases. Alternatively or in conjunction with corticosteroids, IVIG dosed at 1 to 2 g/kg given over 1 to 2 days can also be used in patients with AIHA. IgM-mediated cold agglutinin disease–mediated AIHA is not usually responsive to corticosteroids or IVIG. Exchange transfusion and plasmapheresis may also be considered for some types of AIHA (particularly nonresponsive IgM-mediated cold agglutinin disease); however, further hemolysis may occur and the procedure needs to be done carefully under supervision of a blood bank specialist/hematologist.

 ANEMIA

Anemia is defined as the decrease in hemoglobin level in the blood. This can be due to decreased RBC or hemoglobin production, increased RBC destruction (see earlier section on hemolysis), RBC sequestration outside the circulating blood volume, or blood loss. This section focuses on decreased RBC or hemoglobin production. Signs, symptoms, and initial evaluation are independent of etiology.

Differential (Partial)

- Iron deficiency
- Acquired aplastic anemia
- Congenital anemias
- Leukemia (see earlier section)
- Transient erythroblastopenia of childhood (TEC)

- Sickle cell disease with splenic sequestration
- Sickle cell disease with aplastic anemia crisis (usually associated with parvovirus B19 infection)

Symptoms
- Pallor
- Fatigue
- Irritability/behavioral disturbances
- Dyspnea
- Orthopnea
- Abdominal pain (splenic sequestration in sickle cell disease)
- Vomiting (splenic sequestration in sickle cell disease)

Signs
- Tachycardia
- Cardiac murmur
- Finger and toenail changes (iron deficiency anemia) ++
- Occult gastrointestinal tract bleed (iron deficiency anemia) +++
- Splenomegaly (splenic sequestration in sickle cell disease) +++++
- Hypotension (splenic sequestration in sickle cell disease)

Workup
- CBC with differential and peripheral blood smear.
  Iron deficiency anemia will show a hypochromic microcytic anemia, low mean corpuscular volume (MCV), and increased RBC distribution width (RDW). TEC will show a normochromic, normocytic anemia.
- Reticulocyte count (low in iron deficiency, TEC, and aplastic anemia; elevated in splenic sequestration crisis).
- Serum iron, total iron-binding capacity, and serum ferritin if concerned about iron deficiency anemia.
- Hemoccult stool for gastrointestinal tract bleeding (iron deficiency anemia).
- Bone marrow aspiration may be done by a hematologist/oncologist to differentiate between acute leukemia and aplastic or other types of anemia.

Comments and Treatment Considerations

If the patient is symptomatic from anemia (or has a hemoglobin <8 g/dl), a PRBC transfusion should be given very slowly (see previous section). An etiology for the anemia then needs to be determined to direct further care. A pediatric hematologist should be consulted for almost all causes of anemia with unclear etiologies.

Iron deficiency anemia is treated with oral iron therapy. Enteral iron should be dosed as the elemental form at 3 to 6 mg/kg/day PO divided tid (max 6 mg elemental iron/kg/day or 240 mg elemental iron/day, whichever is less). Table 28-1 presents elemental content of the iron salts.

Treatment of TEC is usually conservative unless the patient has a significant or symptomatic anemia, which requires blood transfusion. Patients with sickle cell disease who have profound anemia caused by splenic sequestration or aplastic crisis may require support with blood transfusions until the marrow regenerates. Patients with sickle cell and aplastic anemia will often have a concomitant viral infection, most commonly parvovirus (see Chapter 29, Rash). Splenectomy may be indicated for severe sequestration crises. For anemia thought to be secondary to malignancy, see Chapter 6, Bleeding and Bruising.

Table 28-1   Element Content of Iron Salts

Iron Salt	Elemental Iron Content (% of Salt Form)	Approximate Equivalent Doses (mg of Iron Salt)
Ferrous fumarate	33	197
Ferrous gluconate	11.6	560
Ferrous sulfate	20	324
Ferrous sulfate, exsiccated	30	217

Adapted from Taketomo CK, et al: *Pediatric dosage handbook*, 8th ed, Hudson, Ohio, 2001, Lexicomp.

INTUSSUSCEPTION

Parents of children with intussusception will commonly describe an acutely pale child with intermittent episodes of crying or abdominal pain (see Chapter 1, Abdominal Pain).

 ## LEUKEMIA

Leukemia refers to the family of hematopoietic neoplasms where the accumulation of immature malignant white blood cells interrupts blood cell production, resulting in anemia that may clinically manifest itself as pallor (see Chapter 6, Bleeding and Bruising).

REFERENCES

Cohen A: Pallor. In Fleisher GR, Ludwig S, editors: *Pediatric emergency medicine*, Baltimore, 2000, Williams & Williams.

Ebb DH, Weinstein HJ: Diagnosis and treatment of childhood acute myelogenous leukemia, *Pediatr Clin North Am* 44(4):847–862, 1997.

Kelly KM, Lange B: Oncologic emergencies, *Pediatr Clin North Am* 44(4):809–830, 1997.

Oski F: Iron deficiency in infancy and childhood, *N Engl J Med* 329(3):190–193, 1993.

Oski F: The nonhematologic manifestations of iron deficiency, *Am J Dis Child* 133(3):315–322, 1979.

Poplack DG, Reaman G: Acute lymphoblastic leukemia in childhood, *Pediatr Clin North Am* 35(4):903–932, 1988.

Rackoff WR, Lange B: Oncologic emergencies. In Fleisher GR, Ludwig S, editors: *Pediatric emergency medicine*, Baltimore, 2000, Williams & Williams.

Sackey K: Hemolytic anemia: part 1, *Pediatr Rev* 20(5):52–58, 1999.

Sackey K: Hemolytic anemia: part 2, *Pediatr Rev* 20(6):204–208, 1999.

Schreiber AD: Autoimmune hemolytic anemia, *Pediatr Clin North Am* 27(2):253–267, 1980.

Segal GB: Anemia, *Pediatr Rev* 10(3):77–88, 1988.

Taketomo CK, et al, editors: *Pediatric dosage handbook*, 8th ed, Hudson, Ohio, 2001, Lexicomp.

Young G, Toretsky JA, Campbell AB, et al: Recognition of common childhood malignancies, *Am Fam Physician* 61(7):44–54, 2000.

CHAPTER 29

Rash

KAREN D. GRUSKIN

A rash is a common presenting complaint for a child or family seeking medical attention. The etiologies of pediatric rashes are diverse and the rash itself is often just one clue among a constellation of historical and physical findings. Many etiologies of rashes are not urgent; however, a number of potentially life-threatening diseases require immediate diagnosis, appropriate management, and therapy. Conversely, there are a number of common rashes that if diagnosed can alleviate fears of more serious disease. When initially evaluating a rash, the clinician often cannot make a diagnosis and further evaluation or consultation will be needed. See Table 29-1 for definitions of basic dermatology descriptors used in this chapter.

This chapter presents common patterns of rash and then discusses those etiologies most consistent with that pattern (Table 29-2). Potentially life-threatening disorders are discussed first in each subset. This chapter is not meant to be an exhaustive review but an aid in the diagnosis of potentially severe disorders with skin manifestations.

 MACULOPAPULAR DISORDERS

ROCKY MOUNTAIN SPOTTED FEVER

Rocky Mountain spotted fever (RMSF) is caused by infection with *Rickettsia rickettsii,* an obligate intracellular pathogen, and is transmitted to humans by the bite of a tick. Disease course can be rapidly progressive and fatal if untreated. Most of the symptomatology appears to be due to its vasculitic effects that can affect any organ system. The classic triad of fever, rash, and

Table 29-1	Basic Dermatology Descriptors
Macule	Flat circumscribed changes of the skin that vary in size or shape but are not raised or depressed.
Papule	Circumscribed raised lesions of any shape <1 cm in diameter.
Vesicle/bullae	Sharply circumscribed, raised fluid-containing lesions that are <0.5 cm or >0.5 cm.
Eczematous	An adjective to describe eczema-like changes of the skin including dryness and thickening.
Petechial	Minute, red, hemorrhagic spots caused by vascular injury; nonblanching.
Purpuric	Red-blue or blue-purple lesion caused by larger hemorrhage into the skin; nonblanching.
Wheals or urticaria	Distinctive type of skin elevation caused by local superficial edema. Color can range from pale to deep red and lesions are often effervescent and transient. Lesions may appear target, with central clearing in some disorders.

tick exposure is seen in only 67% of patients overall and in only 3% of patients during the first few days of illness. A high level of clinical suspicion with particular attention to potential exposure history is imperative so early diagnosis and treatment can occur to prevent morbidity and mortality.

Symptoms
- History of a tick bite ++++
- Seasonal presentation, more common in April through October
- Residency or travel to an endemic area, which despite its name, is most commonly the southern Atlantic, southeastern and south central states in the United States
- Rash usually appears by the second or third day (approximately 50%) but may be delayed to the sixth day of illness (Fig. 29-1)

Table 29-2   Disease Rash Patterns*

MACULOPAPULAR

Rocky Mountain Spotted Fever[†]

Erythema multiforme/Stevens-Johnson syndrome[†]

Bacterial causes
Scarlet fever
Disseminated gonorrhea
Secondary syphilis

Viral illnesses
Measles[†]
Coxsackie
Roseola infantum
Erythema infectiosum (fifth disease)
Epstein-Barr virus
Varicella (early or after immunization)

Other
Kawasaki syndrome[†]
Pityriasis rosea

URTICARIAL/ANGIOEDEMA

Type 1 hypersensitivity reactions

PURPURIC/PETECHIAL

Meningococcemia[†]

Rocky Mountain Spotted Fever[†]

Trauma—especially inflicted[†] *injury*

Disseminated intravascular coagulation/bleeding disorders[†]

Henoch-Schönlein purpura

ECZEMATOUS

Atopic dermatitis
Contact dermatitis
Nummular eczema
Scabies

VESICOBULLOUS

Toxic shock syndrome[†]
Staphylococcal scalded skin[†]/toxic epidermal
    necrolysis
Erythema multiforme
Allergic contact dermatitis
Rhus
Viral infections
    Herpes infection
    Varicella
    Coxsackie
    Nonspecific

ERYTHEMATOUS

Toxic shock syndrome[†]
Staphylococcal scalded skin[†]/toxic epidermal
    necrolysis
Necrotizing fasciitis[†]
Lyme disease (erythema migrans)
Id reactions: tinea, scabies, candida
Photoallergic reaction

---

*Note that many disease entities can exhibit more than one pattern and evolve from one pattern to the other. Location within this chapter is based on the most common presentation and is noted by the name being *italicized*.
[†]Potentially life-threatening conditions.

- The rash often begins at the wrists and ankles as a blanching macular rash that then spreads proximally becoming more maculopapular ++++
- In some cases the rash may become petechial and/or hemorrhagic +++ and often involves the palms/soles ++++
- The rash may be absent in 10% to 20% of patients, making diagnosis more difficult

Early Signs (Develop 2 to 14 Days after Exposure)

- Fever +++++
- Headache ++++ (often intense and persistent)
- Myalgia ++++
- Confusion ++
- Nausea/vomiting +++
- Abdominal pain ++

Late Signs (Especially if Untreated)

- Shock ++
- Arrhythmia ++
- Myocarditis ++
- Seizures ++
- Pulmonary involvement ++
- Renal insufficiency

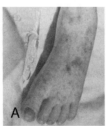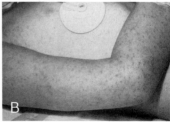

Fig. 29-1 Rocky Mountain spotted fever. **A,** The exanthem characteristic of this disease first appears distally on wrists, ankles, palms, and soles. **B,** In this child the rash has become generalized. Both petechial and blanching erythematous lesions are present. See Color Insert. (From Zitelli B, Davis H: *Atlas of pediatric physical diagnosis,* 4th ed, St. Louis, 2002, Mosby. Courtesy Ellen Wald, MD, Children's Hospital of Pittsburgh.)

- Meningitis ++
- Neurologic abnormalities +++
- Dissemination intravascular coagulation (DIC) ++
- Hepatic dysfunction ++

Workup

- Fourfold or greater rise in antibody titer by immunofluorescent antibody (IFA) ++++/+++++, complement fixation +++, latex agglutination ++++, or indirect hemagglutination assay ++++/+++++, or a single titer ≥64 by IFA assay or ≥16 by complement fixation.
- Immunofluorescence staining of skin or organ tissue ++++.
- CBC may show bandemia +++ and/or anemia ++.
- Thrombocytopenia +++.
- Electrolytes may show hyponatremia ++/+++.
- Liver function test (LFT) elevation +++ and hyperbilirubinemia ++.
- CSF (if obtained) may reveal minimal leukocytosis.

Note: Cultures are not routinely obtained because of the danger to laboratory personnel.

Comments and Treatment Considerations

Delay in diagnosis increases morbidity and mortality. Diagnosis can be confirmed by a fourfold or more increase in titers between acute- and convalescent-phase serum specimens but needs to be suspected based on clinical presentation. Therapy of choice for patients of any age is doxycycline as the benefits outweigh the risk of teeth staining. Doxycycline dosed at 4 mg/kg/day PO or IV divided q12h (max 200 mg/day) until patient is afebrile for at least 2 to 3 days. Despite therapy, some children may not have complete resolution of neurologic sequelae, leading to learning disabilities or decreased school performance. RMSF has a fatality rate of 5% with antimicrobial treatment and 12% to 40% without such treatment.

ERYTHEMA MULTIFORME/STEVENS-JOHNSON SYNDROME

Erythema multiforme (EM) is believed to result from an immune-mediated acute hypersensitivity reaction following exposure to a sensitizing antigen. Based on severity patients are classified as having EM minor or EM major (also called Stevens-Johnson syndrome). EM major is characterized by extensive skin and mucosal involvement associated with significant extravascular fluid loss. In particularly severe cases, EM major is associated with significant morbidity and in rare cases, mortality.

EM minor is characterized by cutaneous skin involvement alone or mucosal involvement that is limited to one surface (usually the mouth) and minimal systemic symptoms.

Symptoms

- Exposure to a common offending antigen such as:
  - Drugs: especially trimethoprim-sulfamethoxazole, cefaclor, and phenytoin
  - Foods: especially nuts and shellfish
  - Infections: including viral, bacterial, protozoal, or fungal infections; herpetic and *Mycoplasma pneumoniae* rank among the most common infectious causes

Signs

- Rash: The rash of EM is characterized by diffuse erythematous macules with central clearing often called a *target* or *iris lesion* (Fig. 29-2). Lesions may also include erythematous papules, macules, urticarial raised lesions, vesicles, or bullae.
- Major form: fever, chills, malaise, and ulceration of mucosal surfaces
- Conjunctivitis and keratitis may lead to permanent scarring and require ophthalmologic referral

Workup

- The diagnosis is predominately clinical.
- Laboratory values such as electrolytes, UA, and/or BUN or creatinine may be obtained to help manage systemic symptoms, especially regarding fluid losses in patients with large areas of denuded skin.

Comments and Treatment Considerations

Treatment is predominantly supportive with special attention to fluid management. Large areas of involved skin may ulcerate

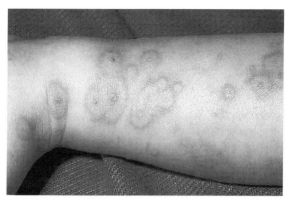

Fig. 29-2 Early fixed papules with a central dusky zone on the dorsum of the forearm of a child with erythema multi-forme caused by herpes simplex virus. See Color Insert. (From Weston W, Lane A, Morelli J: *Color textbook of pediatric dermatology,* 3rd ed, St. Louis, 2002.)

and slough with significant extravascular fluid losses. Mortality rates of 5% to 15% have been reported in severe cases.

Potentially inciting drugs or possible inciting agents should be discontinued immediately. Patients severely affected should be admitted to the hospital because they may require fluid support, pain medication, and observation for evidence of possible secondary infection. Systemic corticosteroids, such as methylprednisolone prescribed at 1 to 2 mg/kg/day, are of unproven benefit.

For less severe cases, pruritus can be treated with antihistamines. Diphenhydramine 1 mg/kg/dose (max 50 mg/dose) IV/PO q6-8h or hydroxyzine 2 mg/kg/day IV/PO divided q6-8h can be used. Oral applications of a 1:1 mixture of diphenhydramine and Maalox with or without viscous lidocaine 2% may provide pain relief from oral involvement. Use caution as lidocaine toxicity may occur if applied too frequently.

BACTERIAL DISORDERS
Scarlet Fever

The rash of scarlet fever (caused by group A streptococcal infection) is usually described as a fine, raised, generalized maculopapular rash with a coarse or sandpapery feel on palpation. It tends to spare the circumoral area and after 3 to 5 days may show fine to extensive peeling. Rheumatic fever is a complication that may develop in untreated patients (see Chapter 26, Mouth and Throat Pain).

Disseminated Gonorrhea

Disseminated gonorrhea may cause a range of cutaneous lesions, including small erythematous papules, petechiae, or vesicular pustules on a hemorrhagic base. These lesions usually develop on the trunk but may occur anywhere on the extremities. Suggested primary antibiotic regimens include ceftriaxone or cefotaxime. Parenteral antibiotics should be continued for 24 hours after symptom reduction, followed by a 7-day course of cefixime or ciprofloxacin.

Secondary Syphilis

Skin manifestations of secondary syphilis usually occur 6 to 8 weeks after the appearance of the primary lesion, which may have gone unnoticed. The exanthem extends rapidly and is usually pronounced, lasting for only hours or persisting for up to several months. The rash is characterized by a generalized cutaneous eruption, usually composed of brownish, dull-red macules or papules that range from a few millimeters to 1 cm in diameter. Lesions are generally discrete and symmetrically distributed, particularly over the trunk, where they follow the lines of cleavage. The palms and soles may be involved. Skin lesions of syphilis can be variable and easily confused with other entities, particularly pityriasis rosea. Intramuscular benzathine penicillin G is the treatment of choice. Dose and length of treatment depend on the duration of infection.

VIRAL ILLNESS
Measles

Measles is caused by an RNA-containing virus of the Paramyxovirus family. Infection rates have decreased significantly with increased vaccination rates since 1992, but measles infection can cause significant illness when it occurs.

Symptoms
- Most commonly seen in inadequately vaccinated persons
- Known exposure to an infected person

Signs
- Classic measles
  - Prodrome lasting from 1 to 6 days but most commonly 3 to 4 days of the following:
    - Temperature of 38.3° to 40.0° C
    - Chills
    - Malaise
    - Headache
    - Cough usually a persistent dry hacking cough
    - Coryza with mucopurulent discharge
    - Conjunctivitis
- Koplik's spots: A pathognomonic enanthem can be seen as whitish elevations on the buccal mucosa resembling grains of sand 12 to 24 hours before the rash develops
- Rash: Usually appears on days 3 and 4 of illness, beginning as a erythematous maculopapular eruption first on the scalp and hairline then spreading downwards to include the trunk and extremities; rash fades in the same order as appearance and the skin many have some fine desquamation

Modified Measles

As its name implies, modified measles has a more modified course with minimal to mild prodromal symptoms, but characteristic rash occurs in children who have received serum immune globulin after exposure. In addition, a mild rash may appear around the site of injection following MMR vaccination. Occasionally, a mild diffuse rash may develop 48 to 72 hours after vaccination.

Workup
- Diagnosis is often made on a clinical basis but can be confirmed by a positive serologic test result for measles immunoglobulin M (IgM) antibody. If test results are negative and the specimen was drawn from a patient with a rash <72 hours, it should be repeated. An increase in

measles immunoglobulin G (IgG) between paired acute and convalescent serum specimens can also be confirmatory.

Comments and Treatment Considerations

Immune globulin dosed at 0.25 ml/kg IM × 1 dose (max 15 ml/dose) can be given to prevent or modify measles in a susceptible person within 6 days of exposure. Immunocompromised children should receive immunoglobulin at the higher dose of 0.5 ml/kg IM × 1 dose (max 15 ml/dose). Once disease is present, care is primarily supportive. Ribavirin can be considered in severely affected and immunocompromised children. There is some evidence that oral vitamin A supplementation of 100,000 units/day if 6 months to 1 year and 200,000 units/day if >1 year for 2 days may decrease morbidity and mortality. Supplementation is recommended for hospitalized patients age 6 months to 2 years, as well as for older patients at risk of vitamin A deficiency. After the removal of vitamin A oral preparations from the U.S. market, the parenteral preparation has been given orally.

Complications include: otitis media, bronchopneumonia, laryngotracheobronchitis, diarrhea, acute encephalitis (occurs in 1 per 1000 cases and often results in permanent neurologic injury), and subacute sclerosing panencephalitis (a rare central nervous system [CNS] degenerative disease can develop years after the initial infection from persistent measles virus infection).

Death primarily caused by respiratory and neurologic complications occurs in 1 to 3 per 100 cases in younger and immunosuppressed patients.

Roseola Infantum

Roseola infantum has recently been attributed to human herpes virus type 6 (HHV-6) and is characterized by the onset of a maculopapular rash after a 3- to 4-day febrile illness. The rash is widely disseminated, appearing as small pinkish macules. The occurrence of the rash within 24 hours of defervescence, rather than the morphologic characteristics of the rash, leads to the correct diagnosis.

Erythema Infectiosum (Fifth Disease)

Erythema infectiosum, or fifth disease, is a benign disease that has been attributed to parvovirus B19, the same virus that can cause an acute aplastic crisis in patients with sickle cell anemia and transient erythroblastopenia of childhood in healthy children. It presents in a highly characteristic fashion, with a lacy macular rash on the flexor extremities of the arms and legs and a characteristic facial erythema, the so-called *slapped cheeks.* The acute phase of the rash lasts for a few days. The rash may recur with exposure to strong sunlight for several weeks. Because parvovirus can cause an aplastic crisis or fetal hydrops, patients with fifth disease should be isolated, especially from patients with hemoglobinopathies or pregnant women.

Epstein-Barr Virus (Mononucleosis)

Between 5% and 15% of patients with infectious mononucleosis (Epstein-Barr virus infection) have a maculopapular rash, and more than 50% (some investigators report nearly 100%) will develop a rash if they have received amoxicillin or ampicillin. The typical rash consists of erythematous macules or maculopapular lesions that are discrete. The exanthem is most prominent on the trunk and proximal extremities and usually lasts 2 to 7 days (see Chapter 39, Weakness/Fatigue).

INFESTATIONS
Scabies

Scabies is a commonly seen infestation of the *Sarcoptes scabiei* female mite.

Symptoms

- Total body itch, not limited to the location of the rash ++++

Signs

- The pathognomonic primary lesion is a linear, gray-brown, threadlike burrow a few millimeters in length with a central black dot (the mite). The more usual lesions are erythematous papules that may be excoriated and possibly secondarily infected because of intense pruritus. On occasion, generalized urticarial or "id" reactions develop. In older patients, usual sites of infestation are somewhat localized to interdigital webs, ankles, buttocks, genitals, lower abdomen, or anterior axillary lines; however, involvement in younger children may be more diffuse and occur in the additional areas of the palms, soles, scalp, and neck (Figs. 29-3 and 29-4).

Workup

- Diagnosis is usually based on clinical suspicion, although definitive confirmation can be made by identifying the adult mite on microscopic examination of a scraping of a suspicious burrow.

Comments and Treatment Considerations

The treatment of choice is the topical application of permethrin 5% cream that may be repeated in 1 week if live mites reappear. Pruritus often persists for several weeks, even after the mites have been eliminated and can be treated with antihistamines and/or topical steroid creams. Close contacts should be treated as well. The mites cannot survive away from human hosts or at high temperatures. All clothing, bedding, and stuffed animals should be laundered in water at least 50° C (120° F) or stored for several days in plastic bags.

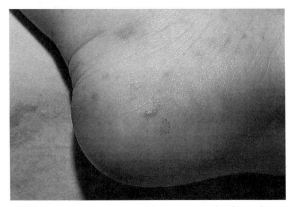

Fig. 29-3 Scabies. Papules and burrows on the foot of an infant. See Color Insert. (From Weston W, Lane A, Morelli J: *Color textbook of pediatric dermatology,* 3rd ed, St. Louis, 2002.)

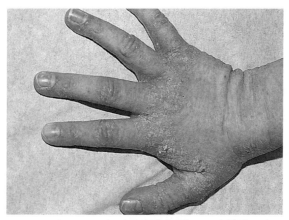

Fig. 29-4 Scabies. Involvement of the dorsa of the hands and interdigital webs in a child. See Color Insert. (From Weston W, Lane A, Morelli J: *Color textbook of pediatric dermatology,* 4th ed, St. Louis, 2002, Mosby.)

OTHER
Kawasaki Disease
The most commonly associated rash with Kawasaki disease is a generalized exanthem with raised erythematous plaques; however, the rash may also present with an erythematous maculopapular, morbilliform, scarlatiniform, or erythema marginatum–like pattern. In order to prevent serious sequelae, the diagnosis of Kawasaki disease should be considered in any ill-appearing child with a fever of >5 days duration and a rash (see Chapter 14, Fever).

Pityriasis Rosea
Pityriasis rosea is a benign self-limited disorder of presumed viral etiology. It tends to affect older children and adolescents. The rash begins with an oval-shaped "herald" patch in 80% of cases that is followed about 2 weeks later by a more generalized rash consisting of erythematous papulosquamous ovals that follow the skin lines of the trunk in a "Christmas tree" pattern of distribution.

The rash may be pruritic and antihistamines may give symptomatic relief. Exposure to ultraviolet light or sunshine tends to hasten resolution, which may take 2 to 4 weeks.

✳ URTICARIA

Urticaria, or hives, is a common cutaneous vascular reaction caused by the release of histamine and other vasoactive and chemotactic substances by the body in response to an offending antigen. If deeper structures of the respiratory, cardiovascular, and gastrointestinal system are affected, then life-threatening symptoms including angioedema (Fig. 29-5), stridor, shortness of breath, wheezing, laryngospasm, hypotension, vomiting, diarrhea, and/or abdominal pain can develop.

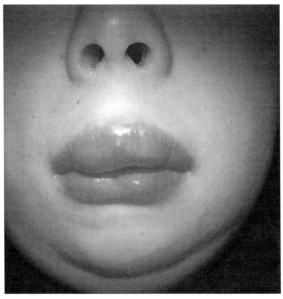

Fig. 29-5 Angioedema of the lips after ingestion of aspirin. (From Shah B, Laude T: *Atlas of pediatric clinical diagnosis*, Philadelphia, 2000, WB Saunders.)

Urticarial reactions are usually considered to be an IgE-mediated or type I hypersensitivity reaction. The skin develops erythematous papules or wheals from edema in the upper dermis with a surrounding flare of erythema caused by vasodilation (Fig. 29-6). Individual lesions can be transient with frequent resolution and reappearance (evanescent).

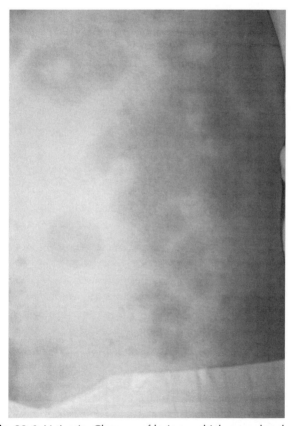

Fig. 29-6 Urticaria. Close-up of lesions, which are pale edematous plaques with irregular margins and a surrounding erythematous flare. See Color Insert. (From Shah B, Laude T: *Atlas of pediatric clinical diagnosis,* Philadelphia, 2000, WB Saunders.)

Etiologies vary and are often not elicited at first presentation. Among common offending agents are the following:

Food: peanuts, eggs, chocolate, shellfish, milk, strawberries, dyes, and preservatives

Drugs: penicillin derivatives, sulfa drugs, opiates, anticonvulsants, contrast dye, aspirin, NSAIDs

Infectious: hepatitis, streptococci, viral illnesses, and parasitic infestation

There are also hereditary forms and urticaria that is associated with malignancy or immunologic disorders such as juvenile rheumatoid arthritis (JRA).

Symptoms
- History of known allergy
- History of hereditary angioedema
- Strong family history of atopy
- History of reactive airways disease

Signs
- Urticaria (Fig. 29-6)
- Possible systemic involvement as noted earlier

Workup
Laboratory and radiographic studies would be dictated by any systemic symptoms. No workup is necessary in acute urticarial disease. Patients manifesting urticaria for >6 weeks (considered chronic urticaria) should undergo testing for associated infectious, immunologic, or genetic disease.

Comments and Treatment Considerations
Attention to the ABCs is always the first priority. Serious allergic reactions may be treated with epinephrine (1:1000) 0.01 ml/kg/dose (max of 0.5 ml/dose) IM q15-20 min until stable. Diluted epinephrine (1:10,000) 0.01-0.1 ml/kg/dose may be used IV once access is established in a patient with shock. Antihistamines such as diphenhydramine 1 mg/kg/dose (max 50 mg/dose) IV/IM/PO q6-8h or hydroxyzine 2 mg/kg/day IV/IM/PO divided q6-8h can be used as well. In severe or persistent cases (including all that require epinephrine), systemic

corticosteroids and H_2 antagonists (ranitidine, famotidine) are also recommended. Epinephrine auto-injectors should be prescribed for any patient who has had an anaphylactic reaction. Auto-injectors are available as EpiPen Jr 0.15 mg for children younger than 8 years (<30 kg) and EpiPen 0.3 mg for patients 8 years or older (≥30 kg).

All patients receiving a prescription for an Epi-Pen should be taught how to use an autoinjector before leaving the ED.

PURPURIC/PETECHIAL

MENINGOCOCCEMIA

Meningococcemia is caused by any of 13 serotypes of *Neisseria meningitides*, although types A, B, C, and increasingly Y account for >90% of clinical disease. The bacteria is spread person to person via contact with nose or throat secretions of infected individuals or asymptomatic carriers. There is an increased risk among persons with deficiencies in terminal complement, asplenia, and those with diseases or therapies causing immunosuppression. Early clinical diagnosis and rapid administration of antibiotics are required as this disease can be rapidly progressive and lead to death within hours.

Signs
- Early signs may be nonspecific
- Age younger than 5 years with a peak of 3 to 5 months and epidemic type of outbreaks (although <5% of cases) in older adolescent populations
- Fever
- Chills
- Malaise

Symptoms
- Rash of some sort is ultimately apparent in two thirds of cases and may be urticarial, maculopapular, petechial, or in its most severe form classic "purpura fulminans" (Figs. 29-7 and 29-8)
- Fever

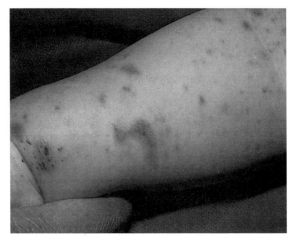

Fig. 29-7 Meningococcemia. Petechiae are more apparent in this close-up of an infant. Gram stain of petechial scrapings may reveal organisms. See Color Insert. (From Zitelli B, Davis H: *Atlas of pediatric physical diagnosis,* 4th ed, St. Louis, 2002, Mosby.)

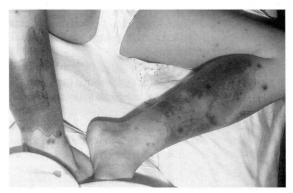

Fig. 29-8 Meningococcemia. Purpura may progress to form areas of frank cutaneous necrosis, especially in patients with disseminated intravascular coagulation. See Color Insert. (From Zitelli B, Davis H: *Atlas of pediatric physical diagnosis,* 4th ed, St. Louis, 2002, Mosby. Courtesy Kenneth Schmidt, MD.)

Workup

- CSF cell counts, glucose and protein concentration to diagnosis potential meningitis.
- Gram stain of CSF, blood, or joint fluid looking for gram-negative diplococci.
- Bacterial antigen-detection tests such as latex agglutination; polymerase chain reaction (PCR) testing available in some areas.
- Cultures of blood and CSF.
- Consider baseline electrolytes and BUN/SCr.
- DIC panel. Fibrinogen level >250 is associated with a favorable prognosis.
- CBC with platelet count.

Comments and Treatment Considerations

Early treatment with IV antibiotics is essential. All patients should be admitted for intravenous antibiotics and observation of systemic symptoms of septic shock (see Chapter 20, Hypotension/Shock). Antibiotic therapy usually consists of high-dose penicillin G, cefotaxime, ceftriaxone, or chloramphenicol (in cases of penicillin allergy). Studies suggest that corticosteroids (given concurrently or just before the first dose of antibiotics) in the form of dexamethasone at a dose of 0.15 mg/kg/dose (max of 10 mg) should be considered in the patient with septic shock or meningitis.

Chemoprophylaxis with rifampin, ceftriaxone, or ciprofloxacin is recommended for close contacts and exposed health care workers. Close contacts are defined as household members, childcare associates, people sleeping in proximity, and anyone directly exposed to oral secretions through kissing or sharing drinks/utensils, or cigarettes within the last 7 days. Prophylaxis is recommended for health care workers exposed to oral secretions during intubation or nasogastric suctioning without appropriate precautions.

TRAUMA

Inflicted injuries can mimic a purpuric etiology. Suspicion is the key to diagnosis (see Chapter 2, Abuse/Rape).

DISSEMINATED INTRAVASCULAR COAGULATION OR BLEEDING DISORDERS

Disseminated intravascular coagulation (DIC) or a platelet disorder can cause a petechial, and if severe, a purpuric rash. The patient in DIC will usually be systemically ill, whereas the patient with a bleeding disorder will have a positive history or laboratory study results (see Chapter 6, Bleeding and Bruising).

HENOCH-SCHÖNLEIN PURPURA

Henoch-Schönlein purpura is an immunologically mediated inflammatory disorder of unknown etiology that causes a purpuric rash usually most evident on the buttocks and lower legs, which is classically described as palpable purpura in the dependent regions (see Chapter 6, Bruising and Bleeding).

 VESICOBULLOUS

CONTACT DERMATITIS

Severe cases of contact dermatitis produced either by local exposure to a primary irritating substance (primary irritant dermatitis) or by an acquired allergic response to a sensitizing substance (allergic contact dermatitis) can lead to extensive skin manifestations.

PRIMARY IRRITANT DERMATITIS
Symptoms

- Exposure to an irritant such as harsh soaps, bleaches, detergents, solvents, oils, bubble baths, talcum particles, urine, feces, or intestinal secretions

Signs

- Erythematous, eczematous, or vesicobullous rash in area of contact

Comments and Treatment Considerations

Treatment consists of a barrier to an ongoing irritant such as a diaper ointment to protect the skin of a baby from urine or feces. For more severe cases a low- to medium-potency topical corticosteroid cream may be used.

ALLERGIC CONTACT DERMATITIS/RHUS

Rhus dermatitis caused by poison ivy or oak is the most common and classic form of allergic contact dermatitis, although exposure to any antigen (especially metals, shoes, preservatives, or fragrances) may cause dermatitis. Rhus dermatitis is caused by the allergen oleoresin in the leaves of the plant.

Symptoms
• Known or possible exposure to allergen

Signs
• The rash is characterized by intense pruritus, redness, papules, vesicles, and bullae. A linear distribution, the Koebner reaction, with an irregular spotty distribution is highly characteristic (Fig. 29-9). The rash usually develops

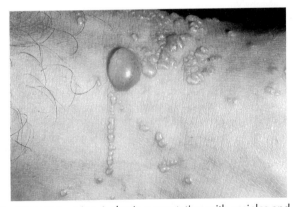

Fig. 29-9 Poison ivy. A classic presentation with vesicles and blisters. A line of vesicles (linear lesions) caused by dragging the resin over the surface of the skin with the scratching finger is a highly characteristic sign of plant contact dermatitis. See Color Insert. (From Habif T: *Clinical dermatology,* 3rd ed, St. Louis, 1996, Mosby.)

within 1 to 3 days of exposure and can occur anywhere that the skin has been in contact with the resin. The resin may be spread diffusely by direct contact or from vaporized resin from leaf burning.

Comments and Treatment Considerations

Obviously the best treatment is prevention by avoiding contact with known antigens. In the case of rhus dermatitis one should immediately wash in soapy water any body surfaces, clothing, and shoes that may still contain residue because the resin can continue to cause sensitization. Family pets contaminated with the plant residue may also need to be bathed, because they can be a source of repeated exposure. The rash itself or fluid from the vesicles is not contagious. Mild cases can be treated with topical cold compresses and oral antihistamines for pruritus. In more severe cases administration of topical steroids or even systemic corticosteroids such as prednisone dosed at 1 mg/kg/day for 5 days may be useful. Tapering of corticosteroids may be necessary if a resurgence of the rash occurs.

VIRAL INFECTIONS
Herpes Simplex Virus

Primary herpes simplex virus (HSV) infections may be widespread and severe in immunocompromised patients and in patients with severe eczema (eczema herpeticum). In severe attacks, crops of vesicles appear, which may coalesce over 7 to 9 days, causing widespread disruption of skin integrity and resulting in fluid, protein, and electrolyte losses. Systemic symptoms of high fever and malaise may be prominent. Diagnosis may be made by antigen-detection methods such as enzyme-linked immunosorbent assay or immunofluorescent techniques applied to the scraping from the base of a vesicular lesion. In addition to supportive care for fluid loss, oral or intravenous acyclovir should be considered for all severe cases. Intravenous acyclovir is effective treatment for immunocompromised patients or in severe cases.

Varicella

Primary infection with the virus causes chickenpox, whereas reactivation of latent infection causes the oftentimes painful herpes zoster (shingles). Varicella or zoster may be particularly severe in an immunocompromised host (see Chapter 21, Immunocompromised Patients: Special Considerations). Primary varicella infections have decreased with the introduction of the varicella vaccine licensed in 1995.

Symptoms
- Known exposure within 10 to 21 days (usually 14 to 16 days), with an infected contact
- Peak incidence during late winter or early spring
- Prodrome of fever, headache, and malaise

Signs
- The highly pruritic rash characteristically begins as small macules on the nape of the neck, scalp, and face and then spreads downwards to the trunk and extremities. The macules then evolve into small vesicles of clear liquid often described as a "teardrop" before becoming crusted. New crops of lesions develop over 3 to 5 days, which progress through these same stages of evolution. The distal extremities tend to be spared, but mucosal membranes are often involved (Fig. 29-10).

Workup
- Diagnosis can usually be made clinically on the basis of the rash with lesions in all phases of evolution: macules, "teardrop" vesicles, and crusted lesions. Diagnosis may be difficult early in the course or in atypical cases. When necessary confirmatory tests can be done, which include culture, direct fluorescent antigen (DFA) testing, indirect fluorescent antibody testing, complement fixation, and PCR. The Tzanck smear is no longer recommended given the newer, better diagnostic studies. DFA has the advantages of a rapid turnaround, good sensitivity, and ability to differentiate varicella from HSV.

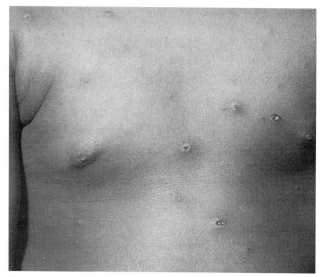

Fig. 29-10 Varicella/chickenpox. The typical feature of lesions in all stages of evolution is seen on the trunk of this child. Note the presence of papules, vesicles, and umbilicated and scabbed lesions, all within a small area. (From Zitelli B, Davis H: *Atlas of pediatric physical diagnosis,* 4th ed, St. Louis, 2002, Mosby.)

Comments and Treatment Considerations

Chickenpox and shingles may be treated with intravenous or oral acyclovir, valacyclovir, famciclovir, or foscarnet in patients at risk of more severe disease. Therapy is not recommended for healthy young children but should be considered in patients older than 12 years, persons with chronic cutaneous or pulmonary disorders, persons receiving long-term salicylate therapy, and patients on inhaled, oral, or systemic corticosteroid therapy. The treatment dose and frequency of acyclovir therapy depend on the immunologic competency of the patient. Some experts also recommend the use of oral acyclovir for secondary household cases in which the disease tends to be is more severe.

Therapy must be initiated as soon as possible after onset of rash and preferably within 24 to 48 hours because most viral replication has stopped after 72 hours. Varicella-zoster immune globulin (VZIG) prophylaxis at a dose of 125 units/10 kg (max 625 units/dose) IM × one dose may be considered for susceptible patients at high risk of severe disease if it can be given within 96 hours of exposure. Do not give >2.5 ml of VZIG in one site but rather administer in multiple sites.

Complications of varicella include bacterial superinfection of skin lesions, pneumonia or pneumonitis, thrombocytopenia, arthritis, hepatitis, cerebellar ataxia, encephalitis, meningitis, and/or glomerular nephritis. Serious invasive group A streptococcal disease has been reported as a common etiology of complications. Pulmonary complications are more common in older patients. Severe and fatal varicella infection has been reported in otherwise healthy children who have been receiving corticosteroid therapy and in immunocompromised hosts.

Patients are most contagious 1 to 2 days before the onset of rash to shortly after rash development. Contagiousness continues until all lesions are crusted. When in doubt, consult a pediatric infectious disease expert for additional guidance as many cases are atypical or have special considerations in an immunocompromised host (see Chapter 21, Immunocompromised Host, Approach To).

Coxsackie

The disease caused by coxsackie A16 virus is a characteristic exanthem in association with constitutional symptoms. The rash usually occurs in a child who has sore throat, malaise, anorexia, and often fever. The enanthem usually occurs 1 to 2 days after the onset of fever and shortly before the cutaneous lesions. The oral lesions are vesicular, 4 to 8 mm, and usually occur on the tongue, buccal mucosa, and posterior pharynx. The skin lesions are most common on the hands and feet, although the buttocks, legs, and arms also may be involved, hence, its nickname hand, foot, and mouth disease. Macules appear first and progress to papules and then to vesicles. The cutaneous lesions usually last <1 week.

Nonspecific Viral Exanthems

A nonspecific vesicobullous rash can be seen with many viral infections and is usually of no clinical concern. It is critical to make sure the lesions blanch and do not represent petechiae that would require further evaluation.

Id Reactions/Autosensitization

Id reactions, or autosensitization, is a term used to describe an immune sensitization of the body to circulating antibody or activated lymphocytes. This response may be due to exposure to any number of antigens but most commonly to scabies, tinea, and candidal infections. The rash often develops after initiation of medical therapy and is a diffuse papulovesicular eruption that can cover both extremities and the trunk. Severe cases may be treated with systemic corticosteroids.

 ERYTHEMATOUS

TOXIC SHOCK SYNDROME

Toxic shock syndrome is a clinical syndrome caused by exotoxin-producing strains of *Staphylococcus aureus* or *Streptococcus pyogenes* (group A strep) in persons without protective anti-bodies. In both types the clinician will find that the skin exhibits a diffuse macular erythematous rash in a clinically toxic or ill-appearing child. Clinical diagnosis is based on a set of criteria for each type (see the following section).

Signs and Symptoms

Staphylococcal toxic shock syndrome clinical criteria

A *definitive case* is defined as meeting 6/6 clinical findings or 5/6, with death occurring before the symptom of desquamation develops. A *probable case* is defined as meeting 5/6 clinical findings.

- Fever ≥38.9° C
- Diffuse macular erythroderma
- Desquamation beginning usually at 1 to 2 weeks after onset commonly involving palms and soles

- Hypotension: ≤90 mm Hg for adults, ≤5% of lower limit of normal in a pediatric patient, orthostatic drop in diastolic blood pressure ≥15 mm Hg, or orthostatic dizziness or syncope
- Multisystem involvement of three of the follow systems:
  - Gastrointestinal: vomiting or diarrhea at onset of illness
  - Muscular: severe myalgia and creatine phosphokinase (CPK) two times the upper limit of normal for age
  - Renal: BUN or SCr two times normal or UA with >5 WBC/hpf with no evidence of UTI
  - Hepatic: total bilirubin, AST, or ALT two times normal
  - Hematologic: platelet count $<100 \times 10^3$ upper limit
  - CNS: alteration without fever or hypotension present
- Negative results on the following if obtained:
  - Cultures of blood, throat, or CSF except for *S. aureus*
  - Serologic tests for RMSF, leptospirosis, or measles

Streptococcal toxic shock syndrome clinical criteria
A definite case is defined by meeting criteria IA, IIA, and IIB. A *probable case* is defined by meeting IB, IIA, and IIB.
  I. Isolation of group A β-hemolytic streptococci from
    A. A normally sterile site such as blood, CSF, peritoneal fluid, or tissue biopsy
    B. A nonsterile site such as throat, sputum, or vagina
  II. Clinical signs of severity
    A. Hypotension <90 mm Hg for adults or <5% of lower limit for age
    B. Two or more of the following:
      1. Renal impairment: SCr >2 mg/dl or two times upper limit of normal for age
      2. Coagulopathy: platelets $<100 \times 10^3$ or DIC
      3. Hepatic involvement: total bilirubin, AST, or ALT two times normal
      4. Adult respiratory syndrome
      5. A generalized erythematous macular rash that may desquamate
      6. Soft-tissue necrosis including necrotizing fasciitis, myositis, or gangrene

Given the clinical similarities and the inability to distinguish between them initially, work-up and initial management is the same for both types. If positive cultures are obtained, then therapy can be tailored more selectively.

Workup

- Initial diagnosis is clinical.
- General labs for a patient in a toxic condition screening for multi-system involvement would include CBC, platelets, electrolytes, BUN, SCr, LFTs, PT, PTT, fibrinogen, UA.
- Blood cultures will be positive in <5% of staphylococcal cases and >50% of streptococcal cases.
- ASLO titers may be useful later if cultures are negative to indicate recent streptococcal infection.
- Cultures from sites of local infections such as bone, skin, or tissue.

Comments and Treatment Considerations

All patients should be admitted to the hospital and consultation with a pediatric infectious disease specialist is strongly recommended. Severe cases will require rapid and aggressive fluid replacement and anticipatory management of multisystem organ failure. Parenteral antimicrobial therapy should consist of two agents able to have a bactericidal effect against both staphylococcal and streptococcal infection (i.e., a β-lactamase–resistant anti-staphylococcal agent such as nafcillin or oxacillin) and the ability to halt enzyme, toxin, or cytokine production (i.e., a protein synthesis inhibitor such as clindamycin). Dosing is as follows:

Nafcillin 100-200 mg/kg day IV divided by q4-6h (max 12 g/day)

OR

Oxacillin 100-200 mg/kg/day IV divided q4-6h (max 12 g/day)

AND

Clindamycin 40 mg/kg/day IV divided q6h (max 4.8 g/day)

Intravenous immune globulin dosed at 150 mg/kg/day for 5 days may be considered for refractory or severe cases.

STAPHYLOCOCCAL SCALDED SKIN SYNDROME/TOXIC EPIDERMAL NECROLYSIS

Staphylococcal scalded skin syndrome (SSSS) is caused by an epidermolytic toxin produced by certain strains of staphylococci. The disorder occurs primarily in children who are thought to lack antibodies against the organism. Clinically the disorder is indistinguishable from toxic epidermal necrolysis (TEN) of other etiologies (such as drug induced).

Signs
- Age younger than 2 years +++, younger than 6 years ++++
- Malaise
- Fever
- Irritability

Symptoms
- Rash appears initially like a "sunburn." Neck, intertriginous areas, and periorbital and perioral areas are initially involved with spread to the trunk and extremities. In severe forms, vesicles can coalesce into bullae and entire sheets of skin can be denuded leaving an oozing surface similar to a burn. Patients will have a positive Nikolsky sign, in which rubbing of the skin can lead to blistering (Fig. 29-11).
- Tenderness of the skin when touched.

Workup
- Electrolytes to assess hydration status and potential electrolyte imbalance.
- CBC and UA are generally not helpful.
- Blood cultures are usually negative.
- If needed, histologic examination of skin biopsy specimen to differentiate SSSS from drug-induced TEN and the two disorders cause skin shearing at different microscopic levels.

Comments and Treatment Considerations
All patients should be admitted to the hospital and consultation with a pediatric infectious disease specialist is strongly recom-

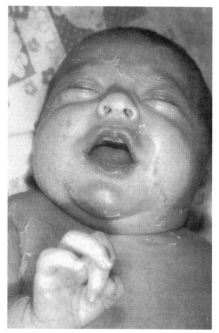

Fig. 29-11 Staphylococcal scalded skin syndrome. Epidermolysis in a 3-week-old infant. (From Davis M, Votey, S, Greenough PG: *Signs and symptoms in emergency medicine,* St. Louis, 1999, Mosby.)

mended. Intravenous fluids may be needed to maintain hydration and electrolyte balance if significant areas of skin are involved. Intravenous antistaphylococcal antibiotics (listed previously in the Toxic Shock Syndrome Section) should be considered to treat any underlying bacterial infection. Consider "burn-type" management of involved skin surfaces with bacitracin, Silvadene, or Xeroform dressings. Observe closely for signs of secondary infection. Avoid corticosteroids because they have not been shown to be effective and may exacerbate dermatitis.

NECROTIZING FASCIITIS

Necrotizing fasciitis is a progressive, rapidly spreading inflammatory infection located in the deep fascia, with secondary necrosis of the subcutaneous tissues. Though first described more than a century ago, necrotizing fasciitis has been recently "re-recognized," as a result of lay-press reports about "flesh-eating bacteria." The process can be difficult to recognize in its early stages but can progress rapidly and typically requires aggressive therapy to prevent significant morbidity or mortality.

Group A β-hemolytic streptococci (GABHS) ("flesh-eating bacteria") is the most commonly identified bacteria causing necrotizing fasciitis in the pediatric population. Other bacterial pathogens include *Staphylococcus aureus, Bacteroides, Clostridium, Peptostreptococcus,* Enterobacteriaceae, coliforms, *Proteus, Pseudomonas,* and *Klebsiella.* For children, prior varicella infections (chickenpox) have been frequently implicated. In adults, trauma, injections, and surgical procedures are frequently found to precede the event.

Symptoms

- Pain, often severe and initially with few physical findings +++++
- Swelling
- Paresthesia
- Itching

Signs

- Erythema that spreads rapidly, typically without a clear demarcation; may be absent in early disease
- Swelling
- Tenderness
- Overall toxic appearance
- Necrotic skin (signifies significant progression)

Workup

- CT or MRI will better differentiate the sites of involvement by demonstrating necrosis, asymmetric fascial thickening, or the presence of gas within the tissue planes ++++.
- Blood and wound cultures, including anaerobic culture.

- Gram stain of any discharge from wound site.
- CBC.
- Plain films may reveal the presence of gas in subcutaneous tissue planes.

Comments and Treatment Considerations

Necrotizing fasciitis can progress extremely rapidly. It is imperative to consult surgery as soon as there is a concern because debridement of the necrotic tissue (often done serially) is the key to therapy. In pediatrics, broad-spectrum antibiotic coverage for group A β-hemolytic streptococci, *S. aureus,* anaerobes, and gram-negative organisms should be initiated as soon as possible. Once the organism (or organisms) can be identified, coverage may be narrowed. Intravenous penicillin G 400,000 units/kg/day IV divided q4h is recommended in addition to an antistaphylococcal penicillin and an aminoglycoside for gram-negative coverage. Several experts advocate the addition of clindamycin as adjuvant empiric therapy based on improved survival in studies of animal models with GABHS necrotizing fasciitis. Clindamycin should not be used as the sole agent secondary to increased resistance and bacteriostatic properties. Clindamycin dosing is 40 mg/kg/day IV divided q6h (max 4.8 g/day). Although data are limited, hyperbaric oxygen therapy increases local oxygen concentrations, which may be bacteriocidal, as well as aiding wound healing.

LYME DISEASE

Lyme disease results from infection and immune response to the spirochete *Borrelia burgdorferi.* The disease is transmitted by infected tick vectors (*Ixodes* genus). The clinical findings can be divided into three stages, each with its own distinctive features: early localized, early disseminated, and late. Furthermore, treatment of early localized disease almost always prevents later sequelae. As a result, clinicians must have a strong index of suspicion for Lyme disease, particularly in endemic areas, which include the eastern seaboard from Maryland to Massachusetts, upper Midwest including Wisconsin and Minnesota, and the West including California, Nevada, Utah, and Oregon.

Early Localized

The most common manifestation of early localized disease is the rash, erythema migrans (Fig. 29-12). The incubation period from tick bite to the appearance of the rash can range from 3 to 31 days and typically appears between day 7 and 14. Subtle systemic symptoms may accompany the rash.

Symptoms

After rash alone:
- Fever
- Malaise
- Headache
- Neck stiffness
- Myalgia
- Arthralgia

Signs

- Erythema migrans: an erythematous macule or papule forms at the site of the tick bite, which gradually enlarges to form a large, annular, plaquelike lesion; the border is usually

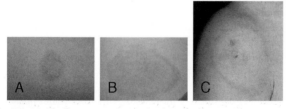

Fig. 29-12 Erythema migrans. **A,** This 2- to 3-cm lesion is just starting to clear centrally. **B,** This larger plaquelike lesion had a bluish center the day before, which has faded to pink. **C,** Central clearing is nearly complete, and within the erythematous border the puncta of two tick bites are evident. See Color Insert. (From Zitelli B, Davis H: *Atlas of pediatric physical diagnosis,* 4th ed, St. Louis, 2002, Mosby. **A** and **B,** Courtesy Sylvia Suarez, MD, Centerville, VA. **C** Courtesy Ellen Wald, MD, Children's Hospital of Pittsburgh.)

erythematous and flat and middle may show clearing but may also be necrotic or vesicular (Fig. 29-12)
- Malar rash
- Conjunctivitis
- Pharyngitis

Early Disseminated

Early disseminated disease follows early localized disease by days to weeks. The most common manifestation of early disseminated disease is multiple erythema migrans.

Symptoms
- Arthralgia
- Myalgia
- Fever
- Headache
- Fatigue
- Neck ache

Signs
- Multiple erythema migrans
- Cranial nerve palsies (particularly cranial nerve VII)
- Aseptic meningitis
- Carditis (characterized by various degrees of heart block, exceedingly uncommon in children)
- Other neurologic complaints such as ataxia, chorea, and/or radiculopathies

Late Disease

Late disease can present months to years after initial presentation. Late disease is characterized most commonly by recurrent arthritis (see Chapter 24, Joint Pain and Swelling). CNS manifestations include subacute encephalopathy, chronic fatigue, and polyradiculopathy.

Workup

The evaluation for Lyme disease is the same for all stages. Diagnosis is made clinically during the early stages of Lyme disease if erythema migrans is present.

- Routine laboratory testing is usually nonspecific and not helpful. Diagnosis can be confirmed by enzyme immunoassay with confirmation by Western immunoblot testing. PCR may replace this two-stage approach once its clinical usefulness is proven.
- Serologic testing can be difficult to interpret. IgM-specific antibody typically peaks 3 to 6 weeks after onset of infection; IgG-specific antibody increases slowly and is generally highest weeks to months after infection but may persist for years despite cure of the disease.
- LP for Lyme testing if any neurologic symptoms are present.

Comments and Treatment Considerations

Treatment of early disease almost always prevents development of later stages of Lyme disease. First-line treatment options are listed below. Penicillin-allergic patients may be treated with cefuroxime (if reaction to penicillin is rash only) or erythromycin. Clinical response to therapy is often slow, and signs and symptoms may persist for weeks even in successfully treated patients. Erythema migrans lesions often resolve within several days of initiating treatment.

Early Localized Disease

Older than 8 years	Doxycycline, 100 mg PO bid for 14 to 21 days
All ages	Amoxicillin, 25 to 50 mg/kg/day divided bid for 14 to 21 days (max 500 mg/dose)

Early Disseminated and Late Disease

Multiple erythema migrans	21 days of oral regimen as above
Isolated facial palsy	21 to 28 days of oral regimen as above
Arthritis	28 days of oral regimen
Persistent or recurrent arthritis	Ceftriaxone 75 to 100 mg/kg IV/IM qd for 14 to 21 days (max 2 g/dose and 4 g/day)
Carditis, meningitis, or encephalitis	Penicillin G, aqueous 300,000 units/kg/day IV divided q4h for 14 to 21 days (max 24 million units/day)

PHOTOALLERGIC REACTIONS

Photoallergic reactions may occur after the use of systemic or topical medications. These reactions usually manifest as a erythematous rash in sun-exposed areas as a result of absorption of ultraviolet radiant energy. Common drugs causing these reactions include sunscreens containing paraaminobenzoic acid, phenothiazines, sulfonamides, tetracyclines, anticonvulsants, and thiazide diuretics.

ECZEMATOUS

The term *eczema* is used to describe a constellation of signs and symptoms that result in the skin manifestations of erythema, edema, exudation, clustered papulovesicles, scaling, crusting, and when long-standing, lichenification. Atopic dermatitis is the form most commonly seen in children.

ATOPIC DERMATITIS/ECZEMA

Atopic dermatitis is the term commonly used for the skin manifestations that are related to allergic-type responses in susceptible individuals.

Symptoms

- Parents and/or siblings with eczema
- History of asthma or hay fever +++
- Dry skin +++
- Pruritus
- Worsening of symptoms in winter

Signs

- Eczematous rash with common age-based locations:
  - Infants: face (particularly cheeks) and scalp
  - Young children: extensor surfaces of arms and legs
  - Older children/adults: antecubital and popliteal fossa, face, and neck

Workup

Diagnosis is usually based on clinical signs and symptoms. Difficult or unclear cases may be referred to a dermatologist.

Comments and Treatment Considerations

Treatment is symptomatic and aimed at reducing dryness and pruritus. A mainstay of therapy is to decrease frequency of bathing because the cleaning process seems to remove lipoprotein complexes on the skin, which hold in moisture. Topical lubricants should be used frequently. Dove or Neutrogena soap is recommended for bathing. Within 3 minutes of exiting the tub, a lotion such as Vaseline, Aquaphor, or Eucerin cream should be generously applied. Mild cases may respond well to Aveeno cream. Topical corticosteroids or tacrolimus ointment (Protopic) can be used for flares and should be prescribed at the lowest effective dose possible. Systemic corticosteroids should be avoided in pediatric patients unless absolutely necessary and these patients should be managed in consultation with a dermatologist.

The most common complications are secondary infection with staphylococcal or streptococcal organisms. If signs of secondary infection exist, topical and/or systemic antibiotics should be prescribed. It is not uncommon for a flare to improve after treatment with an antibiotic alone. HSV infections can be particularly severe in atopic individuals (see the section Herpes Simplex Virus, earlier in this chapter).

NUMMULAR ECZEMA

Nummular eczema is used to describe coin-shaped plaques that are erythematous with crusts and/or tiny papules or vesicles. Lesions are most common on extremities and may occur in children with dry skin and irritation, as well as those that are truly atopic. Lesions may be confused with impetigo or granuloma annulare. Therapy is the same as that for atopic dermatitis (see earlier section).

REFERENCES

American Academy of Pediatrics: Lyme disease. In Pickering LK, editor: *2000 red book: report of the Committee on Infectious Diseases,* 25th ed, Elk Grove Village, Ill, 2000, American Academy of Pediatrics.

Brady WJ, DeBehnke D, Crosby DL: Dermatological emergencies, *Am J Emerg Med* 12(2):217, 1994.

Cartwright KA: Early management of meningococcal disease, *Infect Dis Clin North Am* 13(3):661, 1999.

Centers for Disease Control and Prevention: Case definitions for infectious conditions under Public health surveillance, *MMWR Morb Mortal Wkly Rep* 46(RR-10), 1997.

Diaz PS: The epidemiology and control of invasive meningococcal disease, *Pediatr Infect Dis J* 18:631, 1999.

Durongpisktkul K, Gururaj VJ, Park JM, Martin CF: The prevention of coronary artery aneurysm in Kawasaki disease: a meta-analysis on the efficacy of aspirin and immunoglobulin treatment, *Pediatrics* 96(6):1057, 1995.

Esterly N: Viral exanthems: diagnosis and management, *Semin Dermatol* 3(2):140, 1984.

Gilbert DN, Moellering RC, Sande MA: *The Sanford guide to antimicrobial therapy,* 31st ed, Hyde Park, 2001, Antimicrobial Therapy Inc.

Gruskin KG: Maculopapular rash. In: Fleisher GR, Ludwig S, editors: *Textbook of pediatric emergency medicine,* 4th ed, Philadelphia, 2000, Lippincott Williams & Wilkins.

Helmick CG, Bernard KW, D'Angelo LJ: Rocky mountain spotted fever: clinical, laboratory, and epidemiological features of 262 cases, *J Infect Dis* 150(4):480, 1984.

Hurwitz S: *Clinical pediatric dermatology. A textbook of skin disorders of childhood and adolescence,* 2nd ed, Philadelphia, 1993, WB Saunders.

Jan DG, Diederik VB, for the European Dexamethasone in Adulthood Bacterial Meningitis Study Investigators: Dexamethasone in adults with bacterial meningitis, *N Engl J Med* 347(20):1549, 2002.

National Vaccine Advisory Committee: The measles epidemic: the problems, barriers, and recommendations, *JAMA,* 266(11):1547, 1991.

Nelson WE, editor: *Nelson textbook of pediatrics,* 15th ed, Philadelphia, 1996, WB Saunders.

Pickering LK, editor: *2000 red book: report of the Committee on Infectious Diseases,* 25th ed, Elk Grove Village, Ill, 2000, American Academy of Pediatrics.

Resnick RD: New aspects of exanthematous diseases of childhood, *Dermatol Clin* 15(2):257, 1997.

Scheld WM, Tunkel AR: Corticosteroids for everyone with meningitis? *N Engl J Med* 247(20):1613, 2002.

Shapiro ED: Tick-borne diseases, *Adv Pediatr Infect Dis* 13:187, 1998.

Shulman ST, Inocencio JD, Hirsch R: Kawasaki disease, *Pediatr Clin North Am* 42(5):1205, 1995.

Silber JL: Rocky mountain spotted fever, *Clin Dermatol* 14:245, 1996.

Spach DH, Liles WC, Campbell GL, et al: Tick-borne diseases in the united states, *N Engl J Med* 329(13):936, 1993.

Stechenberg BW: Lyme disease. In: Feigin RD, Cherry JD, editors: *Textbook of pediatric infectious diseases,* 4th ed, Philadelphia, 1998, WB Saunders.

Taketomo CK, Hodding JH, Kraus DM: *Pediatric dosage handbook,* 8th ed, Hudson, Ohio, 2001, Lexicomp.

Todd J, Fishaut M, Kapral F, Welch T: Toxic-shock syndrome associated with phage-group-I staphylococci, *Lancet* 1978.

Walker DH: Tick-transmitted infectious diseases in the united states, *Ann Rev Dept Public Health* 19:237, 1998.

Weber DJ, Walker DH: Rocky mountain spotted fever, *Infect Dis Clin North Am* 5(1):19, 1991.

Working Group on Severe Streptococcal Infections: Defining the group A streptococcal toxic shock syndrome: rationale and consensus definition, *JAMA* 269(3):390, 1993.

CHAPTER 30

Respiratory Distress

DEBRA L. WEINER AND RICHARD GARY BACHUR

Respiratory distress is one of the most common chief complaints in children. Rapid evaluation, anticipation, and aggressive management are essential to optimize outcome. If not recognized and properly managed, almost any form of respiratory distress can lead to respiratory failure. Respiratory failure is the underlying cause of 95% of cardiac arrest in children. The etiology of respiratory distress may be within the respiratory system or within organ systems that affect respiration. Establishing a diagnosis depends on localizing the cause of respiratory distress and is key to providing definitive treatment.

Pediatric normal respiratory rates vary with age (Table 30-1).

Early indicators of respiratory compromise include restlessness, anxiety, combativeness, tachypnea, nasal flaring, retractions, grunting, tachycardia, pallor, and decreased perfusion. Late indicators that signal severe hypoxia possibly, with hypercarbia, include somnolence, lethargy, coma, seizure, bradypnea, apnea, bradycardia, dysrhythmia, and cyanosis. Upper airway respiratory sounds include snoring, gurgle, dysphonia/aphonia, barky cough, and stridor. Lower airway sounds include expiratory wheeze, rales, and rhonchi.

Patients in respiratory distress must be constantly monitored and reassessed. Transcutaneous oxygen saturation monitoring is a useful bedside test, provided one is aware that pulse oximetry is not reliable in patients with poor perfusion; with abnormal hemoglobin, such as in sickle cell anemia; and with carbon monoxide poisoning. Additionally, ventilation may be significantly impaired (e.g., asthma) while oxygen saturation is maintained. It is important to recognize which diagnoses should be made clinically, when diagnostic tests are appropriate, and which tests should be performed. Maneuvers to establish an airway and

Table 30-1 Normal Pediatric Respiratory Rates	
Age	Respiratory Rate (breaths/min)
Neonate	35-50
Infant/toddler	30-40
Early school age	20-30
Older child/adolescent	12-20

relieve impediments to ventilation must be initiated without delay to improve respiratory status and prevent further compromise.

LIFE-THREATENING ETIOLOGIES OF RESPIRATORY DISTRESS

For patients in extremis, respiratory distress is often secondary to trauma resulting in airway injury, pneumothorax, hemothorax, pericardial tamponade, flail chest, CNS injury (see Chapter 3, Altered Mental Status), and/or massive hemorrhage (see Chapter 20, Hypotension/Shock). Atraumatic etiologies include foreign body aspiration and epiglottitis. A high index of suspicion and careful attention to airway, breathing, and circulation are essential to manage patients with these life-threatening conditions. Those that are most immediately life threatening are laryngotracheal foreign body, tension pneumothorax, pericardial tamponade, and epiglottitis.

LARYNGOTRACHEAL FOREIGN BODY: PATIENT UNABLE TO PHONATE

If the patient is unable to phonate, there is a true airway emergency. Foreign body aspiration (FBA) is a significant cause of accidental death in infants and toddlers, with the greatest risk to children from birth to age 5 years, peaking at age 1 to 2 years. FBA is most commonly caused by aspiration of food such as popcorn, grapes, peanuts, hot dog, hard candy, or a smooth object with low mass/volume ratio. One must have a high index of suspicion for FBA in the young child with sudden onset of respiratory distress, even if there is no evident history. See p. 424 for management of patients able to phonate.

Symptoms
- Choking ++++
- Aphonia +++++
- Dysphagia +++
- Stridor ++
- Loss of consciousness +

Signs
- Anxiety early, decreased level of consciousness late +++++
- Tachycardia early +++
- Hypoxia +++, pallor +++, cyanosis ++
- Aphonia, cough, or attempted cough ++++
- Stridor ++
- Facial erythema ++++
- Petechiae of the face and trunk (above nipple line) secondary to choking ++
- Retractions +++
- Bradypnea, dysrhythmia, or apnea are late ominous findings

Workup
- In a patient with respiratory compromise, no workup is needed, but immediate maneuvers to remove foreign body are required.
- If patient is stable, confirmatory diagnosis with x-ray, fluoroscopy, laryngoscopy, or bronchoscopy.

Comments and Treatment Considerations
Support the ABCs, attempting immediate foreign body removal according to the American Heart Association's guidelines as outlined below. If a foreign body is suspected and the patient is unable to phonate, the appropriate method of treatment is back blows and chest thrusts if younger than 1 year old and the Heimlich maneuver if older than 1 year. If the foreign body is visible in oral pharynx, remove using fingers, McGill's forceps, or

Kelly's clamp. Blind finger sweep of the mouth is contraindicated. In a patient who is not breathing and has no history of FBA/foreign body ingestion, attempt bag-valve-mask ventilation. If unable to deliver breaths, proceed to intubation and direct visualization. If unable to establish an airway, needle or surgical cricothyroidotomy is indicated (see Chapter 36, Trauma). Surgical removal, laryngoscopy, or bronchoscopy should be attempted if the foreign body is not retrievable. Hospital admission is required if the patient demonstrates altered level of consciousness before foreign body removal, airway instability, and/or respiratory compromise that persists after foreign body removal.

TENSION PNEUMOTHORAX (PNEUMOTHORAX/HEMOTHORAX)

Pneumothorax occurs when air enters the potential space between the lung and the chest wall. A tension pneumothorax occurs when pressure builds in this space as a result of continued leakage of air so the lung, heart, and potentially the trachea are shifted to the contralateral side. Tension pneumothorax may lead to shock by impairing venous return. Tension pneumothorax requires immediate identification and emergent management.

Tension pneumothorax can occur secondary to penetrating or blunt trauma, including mechanical ventilation and cardiopulmonary resuscitation. Tension pneumothorax may be associated with hemothorax, flail chest, cardiac contusion, or cardiac tamponade. Clinical presentation may mimic cardiac tamponade. Subcutaneous emphysema of the chest, neck, and abdomen may be present with pneumothorax.

Hemothorax is defined as bleeding into the pleural space, usually as a result of penetrating trauma, and is often associated with other injuries.

Symptoms

- Respiratory distress (severe with large pneumothorax)
- Anxiety
- Chest pain
- History of trauma

Signs

- Tachypnea, hypoxia, pallor, cyanosis
- Tachycardia early, bradycardia late
- Breath sounds may be decreased or absent over the area of pneumothorax (clinical diagnostic pitfall in children is that breath sounds are easily transmitted and may seem to be present on the side of the pneumothorax; to minimize risk of hearing only transmitted breath sounds, position stethoscope on the midaxillary line during auscultation)
- Altered mental status
- Resistance to bag-valve-mask ventilation
- Ipsilateral hyperexpansion
- Ipsilateral hyperresonance
- Electromechanical dissociation, cardiac arrest
- In tension pneumothorax:
  - Hypotension, narrow pulse pressure
  - Pulsus paradoxus drop in blood pressure >10 mm Hg during inspiration
  - Tracheal deviation to contralateral side (not always seen in young children)
  - Jugular venous distention secondary to compromised venous return—may be absent with hypovolemia

Workup

Tension pneumothorax must be clinically suspected and/or diagnosed. Immediate treatment should not be delayed by obtaining a radiograph. X-ray will reveal hyperlucency on the affected side (pleural space filled with air alone outside of the collapsed lung) and mediastinal shift (Fig. 30-1). CXR is appropriate after chest tube insertion to evaluate for residual air leak, fluid accumulation, associated thoracic trauma, chest tube position, and to follow clinical course. CXR should be obtained in a stable patient in whom a pneumothorax or hemothorax is suspected. Further workup is as indicated for associated trauma.

Comments and Treatment Considerations

For all cases of suspected respiratory compromise resulting from pneumothorax ABCs must be managed with immediate

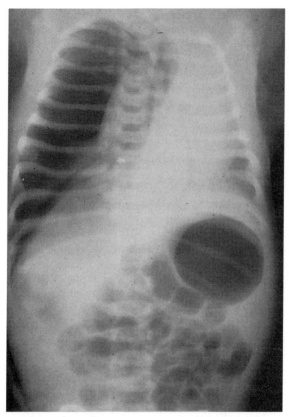

Fig. 30-1 This chest film shows typical radiologic signs of tension pneumothorax: mediastinal shift, flattening of the diaphragm, and widening of the intercostal spaces. (From Zitelli B, Davis H: *Atlas of pediatric physical diagnosis,* 4th ed, St. Louis, 2002, Mosby.)

needle thoracostomy using a large-bore needle inserted into the second intercostal space in the midclavicular line. This maneuver converts a tension pneumothorax to a simple pneumothorax. If there is no improvement after thoracostomy, perform a thoracentesis on the contralateral side. Definitive treatment requires the placement of a chest tube after initial needle decompression. In less emergent circumstances, chest tube placement may proceed without prior needle thoracostomy.

Hemothorax, unless small, usually requires chest tube drainage for diagnostic and therapeutic purposes. If the hemothorax is large or expanding, the patient may become hypotensive, requiring volume resuscitation, blood transfusion, or surgical intervention. A small spontaneous pneumothorax may be treated with 100% oxygen and close monitoring depending on the mechanism and level of concern for expansion.

Consider antibiotics and tetanus prophylaxis if open wounds are present. Empiric antibiotics should include adequate staphylococcal and streptococcal coverage. Cefazolin dosed at 75 to 100 mg/kg/day IV divided q8h (max 2000 mg/dose) is commonly chosen. See tetanus prophylaxis recommendations in Chapter 5, Bites. Management of associated trauma is necessary and these patients often require head, chest, C-spine, and/or abdominal imaging. These patients require admission and consultation with a pediatric surgeon for further management.

PERICARDIAL TAMPONADE

A high index of suspicion and immediate decompression are necessary to save the life of a patient with pericardial tamponade. When blood, serous fluid, or air fills the pericardial sac, venous return to the heart is compromised.

Acute-onset pericardial tamponade is usually secondary to trauma, particularly penetrating cardiac injury, which is rare in children. More common causes of pericardial tamponade include pericarditis, oncologic disease (especially mediastinal lymphoma), or a complication of cardiac surgery. Clinical presentation may mimic tension pneumothorax. Even a small amount of pericardial fluid that acutely enters the pericardial space can lead to hemodynamic compromise, although a slow accumulation may allow large pericardial effusions that are not hemodynamically significant to develop.

Symptoms
- Severe respiratory distress, dyspnea, increased work of breathing
- Anxiety
- Chest pain
- History of trauma, infectious disease, inflammatory process, or recent cardiac surgery

Signs
- Tachypnea, hypoxia, pallor, cyanosis
- Tachycardia early, bradycardia late
- Hypotension, narrow pulse pressure, pulsus paradoxus >10 mm Hg
- Altered mental status
- Beck's triad: muffled heart sounds, jugular venous distention, and hypotension (only one third of patients will have all three)
- Weak apical pulse
- Friction rub with small amount of fluid, may be absent with larger amounts
- Poor peripheral perfusion
- Pulseless electrical activity, cardiac arrest

Workup
Pericardial tamponade is a diagnosis made when significant cardiorespiratory compromise is present. Do not delay treatment for diagnostic testing. However, if the patient is stable, perform the following:
- Echocardiography showing fluid in the pericardial space provides definitive diagnosis and may be useful to follow patients. Other tests are of limited value.
- Electrocardiogram (ECG) may show tachycardia; low QRS voltage, especially in the precordial leads, nonspecific ST-segment and T-wave changes.
- Portable CXR is useful to rule out other etiologies. An enlarged cardiac silhouette is seen in tamponade.

- Laboratory studies, as clinically indicated, to include pericardial fluid cell count, gram stain, cultures, immunofluorescent assays if concern of possible infection, and morphology if concern of malignancy.
- Further workup is as indicated for associated trauma, infection, or malignant processes.

Comments and Treatment Considerations

Support the ABCs and perform emergent pericardiocentesis. Echocardiogram guidance may be valuable if it is immediately available and if the patient is stable. Aspiration of just a few milliliters of fluid may temporarily decompress tamponade. Consider repeating an unsuccessful pericardiocentesis if the index of suspicion remains high. If clotted blood is suspected, open pericardiocentesis may need to be performed. Open thoracotomy may be considered if other measures fail. This can be lifesaving, particularly in children with penetrating trauma to the chest in which a pericardial tamponade is the cause of hemodynamic instability.

Empiric antibiotics are recommended if a bacterial etiology is suspected; tetanus prophylaxis is recommended for open wounds (see Chapter 5, Bites). Associated trauma or malignant processes will require additional evaluation. Patients should be admitted to the hospital with appropriate consultations.

FLAIL CHEST

Flail chest develops when multiple rib fractures allow for an abnormally mobile portion of the chest wall (see Chapter 36, Trauma).

CENTRAL NERVOUS SYSTEM INJURY

Any significant head injury can cause bradypnea or apnea (see Chapter 3, Altered Mental Status).

MASSIVE HEMORRHAGE

Any significant decreases in circulating blood volume can cause respiratory distress (see Chapter 20, Hypotension/Shock, and Chapter 36, Trauma).

EPIGLOTTITIS

Epiglottitis is the most acute life-threatening etiology of stridor. Supraglottic obstruction caused by inflammation, edema of the epiglottis, aryepiglottic folds, and/or false vocal cords is a classic finding (see Chapter 27, Neck Pain/Masses).

 STRIDOR

Acute stridor results from upper airway edema or inflammatory narrowing of the larger airways. Acute etiologies of stridor include infection, trauma, and anatomic obstruction. Chronic etiologies, which will not be further discussed here, include laryngomalacia, hemangioma, subglottic stenosis, laryngeal web, and vascular sling. Vocal cord dysfunction can be an episodic or a chronic cause of stridor.

INFECTIOUS ETIOLOGIES
Epiglottitis

See the earlier section on Life-Threatening Etiologies of Respiratory Distress and Chapter 27, Neck Pain/Masses.

Croup (Laryngotracheobronchitis)

Croup is the most common etiology of acute stridor. Subglottic obstruction occurs as a result of inflammation and edema. Croup is usually viral in etiology, with the most common pathogens parainfluenza type 1 and 3. Other causative etiologies include parainfluenza type 2, influenza, adenovirus, and occasionally respiratory syncytial virus (RSV), rhinovirus, coxsackie, enterovirus, measles, and *Mycoplasma pneumoniae*. Approximately 3% who seek medical care require hospitalization, and 0.5% to 2.0% of those hospitalized require intubation. Prolonged, severe, or recurrent croup may warrant airway evaluation for underlying structural or functional airway narrowing contributing to stridor.

A subset of patients have "spasmodic" croup. These children present with recurrent episodes of acute-onset croup that is thought to be allergic in etiology. Treatment is the same as for its infectious counterpart.

Symptoms

- Age most commonly 6 months to 3 years for viral and school age for spasmodic or allergy-mediated croup
- Male/female ratio 2:1
- Occurs year round, but more prevalent late spring to fall for viral croup; anytime for spasmodic croup
- Onset of infectious croup is usually insidious with a few days of upper respiratory tract infection prodrome, followed by the onset of a barky or seal-like cough ++++
- Spasmodic or allergic croup is usually heralded by the abrupt onset of a barky cough ++++
- Worse at night
- Low grade fever <39° C +++
- Hoarse voice ++
- Increased work of breathing ++
- Improved with warm humidified air (from shower) or cool night air +++

Signs

- Nontoxic appearing ++++
- Anxious ++
- Tachypnea ++, pallor +, cyanosis +
- Tachycardia ++
- Oxygen saturation is usually normal ++++; low oxygen saturation suggests severe obstruction or lower airway disease
- Hoarseness ++
- Barky cough +++++
- Inspiratory stridor +++, occasionally with expiratory stridor + (reflects obstruction at level of intrathoracic trachea or major bronchi)
- Nasal flaring ++, retractions of accessory muscles of respiration ++
- Decreased air entry ++
- Respiratory failure +

Workup

- Usually a clinical diagnosis, with a barky cough alone adequate for diagnosis.

- Do not agitate child if concerned about inducing further airway compromise.
- Pulse oximetry.
- Consider x-ray of airway to rule out other etiologies if diagnosis of croup is uncertain. Anteroposterior x-ray will show subglottic tracheal narrowing, referred to as a "steeple sign," on inspiratory film but may appear as a false positive on expiratory film (Fig. 30-2).
- CBC and blood culture are not indicated unless considering alternative diagnoses such as retropharyngeal abscess, tracheitis, or bacterial superinfection.
- ABG analysis is seldom necessary and may result in increased patient anxiety, worsening the obstruction.

Comments and Treatment Considerations

Croup is usually benign and self-limited, is occasionally severe, and is rarely fatal. Peak severity of viral croup usually occurs on the second night, with resolution in nearly 80% of patients after the third night, 95% after the fifth night, with rare cases lasting >10 days. Spasmodic croup resolves more quickly. Measures of severity are stridor at rest; use of accessory muscles; and decreased aeration, oxygenation, and level of consciousness. Intubation may be required in severe cases and may require the use of a smaller endotracheal tube size than would normally be selected for the child's age.

Usual treatment consists of humidified air (preferably cool), supplemental oxygen if hypoxic, racemic epinephrine, and corticosteroids. Racemic epinephrine may be given as Vaponephrine 2.25% solution dosed at 0.25 to 0.5 ml via inhalation, diluted in 2 to 3 ml of 0.9% NaCl. L-Epinephrine (1:1000) can be used in place of racemic epinephrine, with 10 mg of racemic epinephrine equal to 5 mg of L-epinephrine; therefore use 2.5 to 5 ml of L-epinephrine. For stridor at rest, may repeat q1-2h PRN, and as frequently as q20 minutes if required. Although rare, systemic toxicity can occur with large doses. Symptoms usually improve dramatically within 30 minutes of administration. The patient must be observed for 2 to 3 hours after the racemic epinephrine dose to ensure symptoms do not re-emerge after the peak drug effect has passed.

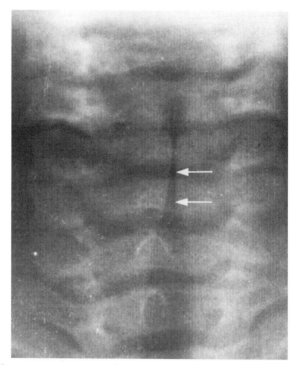

Fig. 30-2 Croup. Frontal view shows typical funnel-shaped subglottic narrowing (steeple sign). (From Cummings C et al: *Otolaryngology–head and neck surgery*, 3rd ed, St. Louis, 1998, Mosby-Year Book.)

Dexamethasone (Decadron) 0.6 mg/kg IM/PO × 1 (max 10 mg/dose) results in improvement, even with mild croup within 1 to 5 hours of administration, and decreases rebound visits. Although efficacy remains unknown, additional doses of dexamethasone may be considered (0.6 mg/kg PO × one dose 24 hours after the first dose or 0.25 mg/kg/dose PO q6-24h for one to four doses), especially if the patient presents on the first night of illness or with severe symptoms. Prednisolone (Prelone, Orapred) dosed at 2 mg/kg load PO × one dose followed by 1 mg/kg/dose PO qd to bid for 4 days is often used by pediatricians in place of dexamethasone because of availability and improved tolerance, but data regarding efficacy are limited. Recent data suggest that humidified oxygen is valueless.

Mildly symptomatic patients may be discharged home without any therapy with instructions for caregiver to provide humidified air by vaporizer, steaming up a bathroom, or taking the child out into the cooler night air. If stridor at rest was responsive to racemic epinephrine without recurrence 2 to 3 hours after the dose and the patient received corticosteroids, then the patient may be discharged to home. Consider hospitalization for patients demonstrating a higher severity of illness, history of severe croup, underlying anatomic abnormalities, and day or early evening presentation. If there is stridor at rest despite racemic epinephrine within 2 to 3 hours and/or respiratory compromise, admit the patient to the hospital.

Consider consultation with an otolaryngologist for direct laryngoscopy and/or bronchoscopy if atypical course or multiple recurrences to rule out anatomic abnormalities.

Retropharyngeal Abscess

Abscesses of the retropharyngeal area may result in respiratory distress (see Chapter 26, Mouth and Throat Pain).

Bacterial Tracheitis

Tracheitis is a bacterial infection of the trachea resulting in laryngotracheal inflammation, edema, purulent secretions, and possible pseudomembrane of the trachea—all of which may contribute to acute airway obstruction or significant respiratory distress (see Chapter 27, Neck Pain/Masses).

 ## *TRAUMA*

Any trauma of the upper airway can result in stridor. Emergent control of the airway when symptoms of respiratory distress and airway trauma are present is required because delay may lead to worse airway obstruction and inability to secure an airway. The usual supportive resuscitation maneuvers should be instituted with early consultation of an otolaryngologist (see Chapter 36, Trauma).

ANATOMIC CAUSES

Foreign Body Aspiration: Tracheal or Esophagus (Patient Able to Phonate)

Foreign bodies of the esophagus include food, small objects, and most commonly coins. Most ingested foreign bodies enter the esophagus. Forty percent of patients are asymptomatic at presentation. The diagnosis is based on history of reported or suspected ingestion. Lack of history does not rule out foreign body. Symptoms may be due to soft-tissue injury, with the foreign body no longer present in the upper airway or esophagus. Presentation is often delayed until the patient develops symptoms secondary to movement of the foreign body, secondary infection, and/or erosion of soft tissue compressed by the foreign body. Anyone in significant respiratory distress should be managed for a potential tracheal foreign body as described in the section on life-threatening etiologies (p. 411).

Symptoms
- Most common age 1 to 5 years
- Choking or gagging episode ++
- Fever ++ suggests infection
- Localized pain or discomfort of throat or at site of foreign body +++
- Dysphonia +, dysphasia +++, drooling +
- Shortness of breath +
- Cough +
- Stridor + (inspiratory if extrathoracic trachea, expiratory or biphasic if intrathoracic)

Signs
- Anxious +
- Tachypnea +, pallor+
- Tachycardia +
- Oropharyngeal trauma +
- Retractions of accessory muscles of respiration +

Workup

- If patient is stable, x-rays of the lateral neck and the anteroposterior chest should be obtained. Coins in the esophagus are seen on the edge on lateral views and as a full circle on anteroposterior views. Consider abdominal x-ray for objects for which there is a concern for potential of gastrointestinal (GI) tract perforation (batteries) or those that may fail to pass. An abdominal view is not necessary for coins because nearly all pass within a week once they are beyond the gastroesophageal (GE) junction.
- Metal detectors in experienced hands can replace x-ray for coins but are not 100% sensitive, especially in obese children or if multiple coins have been ingested.

Comments and treatment considerations

All foreign bodies in the trachea and those that are potentially caustic or are persistently above the GE junction in the esophagus should be removed. Button batteries lodged in the esophagus must be removed urgently to prevent erosion of esophagus. Delaying removal of noncaustic objects to provide an opportunity for the foreign body to pass spontaneously remains controversial.

 ## WHEEZE

Wheezing is the result of lower airway inflammation and obstruction. The differential diagnosis most commonly includes lower airway foreign body, asthma, and bronchiolitis. Wheezing associated with allergic reactions is discussed in Chapter 29, Rash. Some children with pneumonia, pulmonary edema, pulmonary embolism, and aspiration pneumonia will wheeze (see later sections in this chapter on intrathoracic and pulmonary causes of respiratory distress). Less common causes, which are not discussed here, include vocal cord dysfunction, cystic fibrosis, immotile cilia syndrome, bronchopulmonary dysplasia, bronchiectasis, congestive heart failure (CHF), anaphylaxis, and anatomic abnormalities (laryngeal web, tracheoesophageal fistula, vascular ring, mediastinal or pulmonary mass, or extrapulmonary mass).

LOWER AIRWAY FOREIGN BODY

Consider lower airway foreign body in any child, particularly those younger than 5 years, with a history of choking episode, unilateral wheeze (particularly if right middle lobe), first time wheeze, and persistent or recurrent pneumonia. Often no history suggestive of foreign body ingestion can be elicited and diagnosis is delayed until respiratory infection develops, usually several days to >1 week after aspiration. Foreign body is more common in the right lung than the left, especially the right middle lobe. Objects most commonly aspirated are those with higher surface/mass ratio (e.g., balloons) and those that are round or cylindrical with smooth surfaces (e.g., grapes, marbles). If dental trauma has occurred, consider the possibility of a tooth aspiration. Foreign bodies in the esophagus compressing the lower airway may result in symptoms similar to those from lower airway foreign body.

Signs
- Choking episode ++
- Cough +++
- Labored or painful respirations +
- Fever if infection secondary to retained foreign body ++

Symptoms
- Tachypnea ++
- Fever ++
- Asymmetric breath sounds such as a focal decrease in breath sounds or unilateral rales and/or wheeze ++

Workup
- Guided by level of suspicion based on history and physical examination findings.
- CXR may reveal radiopaque foreign body, infiltrate, and less commonly, lung abscess or focal bronchiectasis. Inspiratory and forced expiratory films may suggest foreign body by showing an area of unilateral hyperinflation

(Fig. 30-3). Decubitus films may show airtrapping in a patient unable to cooperate for forced expiration radiographs.
- Fluoroscopy may show abnormal airway movement, focal airtrapping, mediastinal shift away from foreign body during inspiration, and/or paradoxic diaphragm movement suggestive of foreign body. Fluoroscopy is particularly useful in a child too young to cooperate for inspiratory/expiratory films.
- CT is more sensitive than CXR and fluoroscopy but is not usually required.

Comments and Treatment Considerations

Do not administer bronchodilators or perform chest physiotherapy unless absolutely necessary because either may result in dislodging the foreign body. Rigid bronchoscopy is the definitive therapy for foreign body removal. Consider bronchoscopy if there is a high level of suspicion despite negative radi-

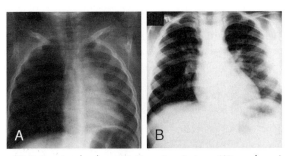

Fig. 30-3 Foreign body aspiration: inspiratory **(A)**, and expiratory **(B)** radiographs. A, This inspiratory film taken during fluoroscopy suggests hyperinflation of the right lower and middle lobes. This becomes much more evident on exhalation, when the hyperinflation persists and the mediastinum shifts to the opposite side. (From Zitelli B, Davis H: *Atlas of pediatric physical diagnosis*, 4th ed, St. Louis, 2002, Mosby. Courtesy Robert Gochman, MD, Schneider Children's Hospital, Long Island Jewish Medical Center, Long Island, NY.)

ographic study findings. Antibiotics should be prescribed if there is evidence of pneumonia or pulmonary abscess.

ASTHMA

Asthma is the most common chronic childhood disease, affecting at least 5% to 15% of children, with a higher incidence in urban areas. There is a known genetic predisposition. Most children with asthma wheeze, although a subset of children have what is called *cough-variant asthma,* whose primary manifestation is cough rather than wheeze.

Precipitating environmental factors most commonly include upper respiratory tract infection, cigarette or fireplace smoke, aerosolized chemical irritants, environmental allergens (dust mites, cockroaches, animal dander, pollen, mold), change in weather, exercise, stress, aspiration of gastric contents, and medications (β-blockers, aspirin, NSAIDs). Asthma is often associated with eczema, underlying pulmonary disease or cardiopulmonary abnormalities, and family history of asthma or atopy. Diagnosis is based on response to bronchodilators. During the first 2 years of life, viral bronchiolitis is a common etiology of wheeze. Thirty percent of children who wheeze with bronchiolitis are eventually diagnosed with asthma.

Risk factors for death from asthma include adolescent age, history of life-threatening episode requiring intensive care unit admission with or without requirement for intubation, more than two hospital admissions or more than three ED visits in the previous year, inadequate medical care/noncompliance, abuse of asthma medications, and lack of access to care.

Symptoms

- Wheeze ++++
- Cough that may be chronic or recurrent; cough-variant asthma is unusual in infants and is more common in adolescents; however, cough is often part of a precipitating viral illness
- Chest tightness ++++ or chest pain ++
- Increased work of breathing, dyspnea, and/or shortness of breath ++++

Signs

- If severe:
  - Restlessness, agitation +++, fatigue, decreased level of consciousness or somnolence, confusion ++
  - Tripod position ++
  - Diaphoresis +
  - Cyanosis +
- Nasal flaring ++
- Retractions of accessory muscles +++
- Tachypnea ++++
- Tachycardia ++++
- Thoracoabdominal dissociation (respiratory alternans)—paradoxic breathing whereby chest collapses on inspiration and abdomen protrudes +++
- Wheeze (expiratory ++++, with inspiration +); may be absent if severe obstruction +
- Cough instead of wheeze ++
- Prolonged expiratory phase (normal 1:1) +++
- Rales and/or rhonchi, especially if in association with respiratory tract infection +++
- Asymmetric breath sounds, diminished aeration +++
- Fever +++ caused by associated illness
- Dyspnea or difficulty speaking in full sentences ++

Workup

- Cardiorespiratory monitoring, especially if moderate or severe.
- Pulse oximetry; initial oxygen saturation <91% indicates a severe asthma exacerbation and predicts need for hospitalization independent of response to initial management. Oxygen saturation may be preserved until ventilation is seriously compromised. Saturation may decrease for 10 to 20 minutes after inhaled nebulization treatments because of transient ventilation/perfusion mismatch.
- Peak expiratory flow rate (PEFR) to evaluate severity and response to treatment. Measurements <70% of expected or personal best indicate moderate disease, and those <50% indicate severe disease. It is difficult for young children

(younger than 5 years) to use a peak flow meter and yield accurate results.

- CXR as clinically indicated to rule out infiltrate or air leak (i.e., pneumothorax or pneumomediastinum). If first wheezing episode, consider CXR to rule out other causes of wheezing, particularly foreign body ingestion or anatomic abnormality. Findings consistent with asthma include hyperinflation, peribronchial thickening, and patchy atelectasis.

- ABG analysis may occasionally be useful if severe distress. Pco_2 initially low because of hyperventilation, normal Pco_2 suggests tiring, and elevated Pco_2 suggests respiratory failure or impending failure. If available, continuous end-tidal CO_2 monitoring is proving a useful tool for following ventilation status.

- CBC is not indicated for workup of asthma. If clinically indicated to evaluate for other processes, try to obtain before administering β-agonist therapy or corticosteroids, which may elevate WBC.

- Serum theophylline level (therapeutic 10 to 20 mcg/ml) if patient is taking theophylline.

Comments and Treatment Considerations

In severe cases support the ABCs as needed, including oxygen for saturations <95%; then begin $β_2$-agonists and give an intravenous loading dose of corticosteroids (see the following paragraph for dosing). Additional agents discussed in the following paragraph include ipratropium, magnesium sulfate, terbutaline, and ketamine.

For most patients $β_2$-agonists and corticosteroids are the mainstay of therapy. The primary $β_2$-agonist used is albuterol, which can be given via nebulization (0.5% solution) 0.03 ml/kg to max 1 ml/dose or via inhaler (90 mcg/puff) 2-4 puffs every 20 minutes by spacer/mask. Repeated doses, usually three to six within a 6-hour period, are routinely given at 20-minute intervals until the patient improves or a decision is reached to admit the patient to the hospital. Nebulization therapy given within 4 hours of arrival to the ED should be included in the total count. Patients who improve with treatment should be observed for a minimum of 30 to 60 minutes before discharge home. If severe distress is evident, continuous nebulized albuterol dosed at 0.5 mg/kg/hr may be initiated (max 15 mg/hr). Continuous nebulization or repeated doses of albuterol is safe and may be lifesaving. Efficacy of albuterol nebulization versus inhalation via MDI plus spacer is similar for patients age older than 2 years, but few data exist for use in those younger than 2 years. Racemic epinephrine is as effective as nebulized albuterol but has a higher rate of side effects.

Epinephrine (1:1,000) 0.01 ml/kg/dose (max 0.5 ml/dose) given IM may be used emergently if respiratory failure is imminent and may be repeated q5-10 minutes until improvement is noted.

Intubation should be avoided whenever possible because of the risk of barotrauma and air leak. If intubation becomes necessary, ketamine 1 to 2 mg/kg IV is the recommended drug of choice as an induction agent. As a potent bronchodilator, ketamine is the best sedative/analgesic agent for rapid sequence intubation of children in status asthmaticus (please note that a history of asthma is a relative contraindication for the use of ketamine for procedural sedation due to the risk of laryngospasm and increased secretions.)

Magnesium sulfate infusion may be beneficial in moderate to severe exacerbations and is dosed at 40 mg/kg (max 2000 mg) and run over 20 minutes. ECG monitoring should be ongoing throughout the infusion. Apnea and heart block can result if magnesium is infused too rapidly.

Terbutaline, an injectable β_2-agonist, can be given as a load of 2 to 10 mcg/kg SC or IV over 10 minutes, followed by an infusion of 0.4 mcg/kg/min, titrated by 0.2 mcg/kg/min increments to a maximum of 3 to 10 mcg/kg/min. As with all β-agonists, terbutaline can cause cardiac toxicity and patients should be monitored by serial ECGs and CPK troponin levels. The total β-agonist dose should be kept at <20 mg/hr if possible, although there are reports of higher tolerable total doses in the literature. Tachycardia is most often the dose-limiting factor.

Levalbuterol (Xopenex) is a stereospecific isomer of albuterol and may be used in place of albuterol. Initial studies suggested fewer side effects when compared to albuterol, although subsequent studies have failed to find clinically important differences for most patients. Empiric dosing is suggested at 0.31 mg for children age 6 to 12 years and 0.63 mg for children older than 12 years. Controversy surrounds the use of levalbuterol routinely in place of albuterol because of concerning efficacy data and substantially higher cost.

Side effects of β-agonists include restlessness, tachycardia, palpitations, hypertension, headache, and nausea. Consider spacing or withholding β-agonist therapy for young patients with a heart rate of >200 beats per minute and for adolescent with a heart rate of >150 beats per minute; however, never withhold β-agonists if severe respiratory distress is caused by bronchospasm. Caution should be used when administering β-agonists to patients with preexisting cardiovascular disease, hypertension, history of arrhythmia, seizure disorder, hyperthyroidism, and diabetes. Severe drug-drug interactions can occur if β-agonists are used concurrently with monoamine oxidase inhibitors, tricyclic antidepressants, and β-blocking agents.

Ipratropium bromide (Atrovent) is an anticholinergic agent that may provide additional bronchodilation, especially in moderate to severe exacerbations. Ipratropium 0.02% solution is commonly dosed at 0.25 mg/dose for patients younger than 2 years and at 0.5 mg/dose for those 2 years or older and may be mixed in the nebulizer with albuterol. Give one to three doses initially and then q6-8h prn. Initial studies showed a decrease in the rate of hospitalization and shorter hospitalization stays with use of ipratropium, but several subsequent studies have failed to substantiate these findings.

Corticosteroids should be prescribed for all patients with moderate or severe exacerbations, or if symptoms are not resolved after initial β-agonist therapy. Corticosteroids are contraindicated if there is a history of recent varicella exposure in a nonimmune patient or recent varicella vaccination within the past 4 to 6 weeks. Prednisolone or prednisone are frequently used and dosed at 2 mg/kg PO load (max 80 mg/dose) followed by 1 mg/kg/dose PO divided qd-bid (max 80 mg/dose, 120 mg/day). If the exacerbation is severe or the patient is unable to tolerate oral corticosteroids, methylprednisolone (Solu-Medrol) 2 mg/kg IV × one dose initially then 1 mg/kg/dose IV q6h may be used, converting to oral dosing when able to tolerate. Enteral and parenteral corticosteroids are equally effective, but oral corticosteroids are commonly refused and/or vomited by many children because of poor palatability. Newer formulations of prednisolone have become available with improved taste. Corticosteroids should be continued for a minimum of 5 days. Use of corticosteroids for >7 days or as frequent short courses requires a tapered wean.

Theophylline is rarely used as maintenance therapy and is no longer recommended routinely.

Disposition should be guided by duration of symptoms, response to therapy over initial 2 to 4 hours, and parental knowledge in assessing and managing symptoms. Patients should be admitted if in moderate to severe respiratory distress or if they have underlying medical or social issues. If considering discharging a patient to home, a good rule of thumb is to add at least one medication (e.g., a 5-day course of an oral corticosteroid) or to increase dose or use of medication that he or she was using before the exacerbation. Close follow-up is recommended.

BRONCHIOLITIS

Bronchiolitis begins as an upper respiratory tract illness and in 40% of children younger than 1 year, progresses over 1 to 2 days to lower airway inflammation, edema, bronchoconstriction, and mucous plugging. Bronchiolitis accounts for approximately 500 deaths/year and 100,000 hospitalizations/year for children in their first year of life. Mortality is 0.5% to 2.0% of those hospitalized and 3% to 5% if underlying cardiopulmonary disease is present.

Patients at greatest risk of severe disease are premature infants born at ≤36 weeks of gestation, age younger than 6 months if premature or younger than 6 weeks if full term, underlying cardiopulmonary condition, or immunodeficiency. Other patients at risk for more severe disease include those with airway anomalies, neuromuscular disease, Down syndrome, and history of recurrent aspiration.

The most common pathogen is RSV (20% to 40%). Other causes are parainfluenza (10% to 30%), influenza (10% to

20%), adenovirus (5% to 15%), and metapneumovirus (2% to 10%). The illness can be seen at anytime during the year, but epidemics are more common in the winter months from October to March, with a peak in January and February. By age 2 years, >90% of children have measurable antibodies to RSV. Preventive RSV immune globulin preparations that decrease the incidence and severity of RSV infection are now routinely available for at-risk children who meet specific criteria.

Symptoms

- Age younger than 2 years, peak 2 to 8 months
- Nasal congestion, copious nasal secretions ++++
- Increased respiratory effort +++
- Decreased oral intake ++
- Fever, usually <39° C +++
- Cough ++++
- Apnea may be presenting manifestation, particularly in patients younger than 6 weeks if full term and younger than 6 months if preterm +
- Dehydration as a result of fever, tachypnea, or decreased oral intake, especially patients younger than 4 months

Signs

- Nontoxic ++++, anxious ++
- Tachycardia +++
- Tachypnea +++, apnea/bradypnea +, cyanosis +
- Fever, usually <39° C
- Nasal flaring ++, retractions +++
- Grunt +
- Wheeze ++++
- Rales/rhonchi ++++
- Palpable liver and spleen secondary to pulmonary hyperinflation

Workup

- CXR is usually obtained to rule out other etiologies of respiratory illness. In cases of bronchiolitis, CXR will show hyperinflation, air trapping, peribronchial cuffing, patchy atelectasis/infiltrates, and flattened diaphragms (Fig. 30-4).

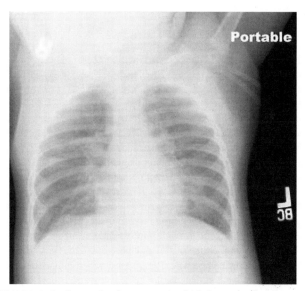

Fig. 30-4 Radiograph of a 3-month-old infant who has lower respiratory syncytial virus disease showing characteristic hyperinflation and area of consolidation in the right middle lobe.

- Nasal swab for RSV immunofluorescent antibody testing or enzyme-linked immunosorbent assay can confirm diagnosis. Testing is necessary only if the result will affect management decisions (i.e., determine admission for very young infants) or patient cohorting for infection control purposes ++++.

Comments and Treatment Considerations

ABCs, oxygen, and supportive care as needed. Infants may require intubation for apnea or severe respiratory distress. Fullterm infants <6 weeks of age and premature infants <6 months of age are at increased risk of apnea and admission for observation even without respiratory distress is recommended. Nasal suction relieves some distress, particularly while attempting to feed. Duration of illness is usually 7 to 10 days, although residual cough and wheeze may last longer.

Although bronchodilators are generally not effective for bronchiolitis, a trial of albuterol or racemic epinephrine may be warranted if wheezing is present. Albuterol (0.5% solution) nebulizer 0.03 ml/kg in 2 ml of NS or racemic epinephrine (2.25% solution) 0.35 mg/kg, max 0.5 ml, nebulized in 2 ml of NS q2-4h may be tried and continued if the treatment decreases respiratory rate and/or wheezing. Patients who demonstrate improvement are thought to be those with a predisposition to reactive airways disease. Be aware that some patients may worsen with nebulization therapy because of initial ventilation/perfusion mismatch.

Systemic corticosteroid use is controversial and thus is not routinely recommended. They may be helpful in patients with reactive airways disease or with a genetic predisposition to reactive airways disease. Antibiotics are recommended only for associated bacterial infections such as otitis media or in the case of questionable bacterial pneumonia (25% of patients with bronchiolitis have atelectasis vs. infiltrate on x-ray). Ribavirin is no longer recommended.

If the patient is younger than 3 months and fever is present, consider infant fever evaluation (see Chapter 14, Fever). Serious bacterial infection is unusual in patients with bronchiolitis and evaluation in patients older than 2 months should be based on clinical judgment.

If the patient is stable enough to be discharged home, consider albuterol nebulizer or inhaler with spacer device q4-8h if responsive to a trial of bronchodilator therapy and arrange follow-up within 24 hours especially if the patient is younger than 1 year. Hospitalization is warranted for moderate to severe respiratory distress; tachypnea with a respiratory rate of >60 breaths per minute, concern for apnea particularly if younger than 6 weeks, respiratory fatigue/failure, hypoxia, hypercarbia, inability to maintain hydration, history of prematurity, or underlying cardiopulmonary disease or immunodeficiency.

Complications of bronchiolitis include pneumothorax, pneumomediastinum, bronchiolitis obliterans, respiratory failure, acute respiratory distress syndrome, the syndrome of inappropriate antidiuretic hormone secretion, chronic lung disease, cardiomyopathy, arrhythmia, bacterial infection, central apnea, and death. Bacterial superinfection/coinfection is unusual: bacteremia occurs in <1%, urinary tract infection <3%, and meningitis <1%. Reinfection is common within the first 2 years of life. Thirty percent of patients who develop bronchiolitis are later diagnosed with asthma.

 ## OTHER PULMONARY CAUSES OF RESPIRATORY DISTRESS

PNEUMONIA

Pneumonia, broadly defined as parenchymal inflammation of the lung, is usually of an infectious origin. Pneumonia is a relatively common infection that afflicts approximately 2% of children annually. Viral and bacterial etiologies (Table 30-2) are roughly equal.

Uncommon causes of pneumonia include: *Staphylococcus aureus, Klebsiella,* and *Neisseria meningitidis.* In unimmunized

Table 30-2	Etiologies of Bacterial Origins Vary by Age
First week of life	Group B *Streptococcus* and enteric gram-negative organisms predominate
2 wk to 2 mo	*Chlamydia pneumoniae* in addition to the neonatal pathogens should be considered
Beyond the neonatal period	*S. pneumoniae* predominates at every age, but its frequency in the post–pneumococcal vaccine era should decrease; mycoplasma should be considered in children older than 3 years. *C. pneumoniae* may be seen in the adolescent

patients, *H. influenzae* type B should be considered. Children with neoplasms, human immunodeficiency virus, and other immunodeficiencies are at risk of infection with unusual pathogens such as *Pneumocystis carinii*. Noninfectious causes of pneumonia such as aspiration and inhalation are discussed separately.

Symptoms
- Fever (bacteria +++, atypical bacteria +, viral +)
- Cough (may be absent early) +++
- Rhinorrhea (viral ++)
- Chest pain
- Dyspnea
- Labored respirations
- Wheeze (viral +)

Signs
- Tachypnea ++
- Retractions (absent with small pneumonia)
- Focal decreased breath sounds + (with associated effusion ++)
- Rales (focal with bacterial, focal or diffuse with atypical, diffuse with viral)
- Grunting (infants) +
- Nasal flaring (infants) +
- Cyanosis (severe) +

Workup
Guided by degree of distress or uncertainty of diagnosis.
- No diagnostic tests are needed if minimal distress, typical history, and examination findings consistent with pneumonia.
- Pulse oximetry.
- Moderate distress or any infant younger than 1 year:
  - CXR to confirm diagnosis and guide therapy. A focal consolidation associated with high fever is most consistent with bacterial pneumonia; multiple infiltrates are more consistent with viral and atypical bacterial pneumonia; effusions may occur with bacterial and atypical bacterial infections and are rare with viral etiologies; cavitary pneumonias imply specific pathogens.

- CBC and blood culture in patients with high fever, age younger than 6 months, or large pneumonia. Elevated WBC count is common with bacterial pneumonia and a normal WBC count is likely with viral and atypical bacteria. Elevated eosinophils may be seen with chlamydial infections.
- ABG analysis for severe distress or concern of respiratory failure.
- Nasopharyngeal aspirate in infants for virus (generally not useful except in immunocompromised children or for inpatient cohorting of patients, i.e., RSV).
- Consider mycoplasma titers and cold agglutinins (if age appropriate), though generally not useful.

- Thoracentesis for moderate to large effusions for diagnosis and alleviation of respiratory distress.

Comments and Treatment Considerations

Ensure adequacy of airway, provide supplemental O_2, and support ABCs. For those with moderate or severe distress cardiorespiratory monitoring and intravenous access should be established. Hospital admission should be considered in patients who exhibit signs of the following:

- Toxic appearance
- Hypoxia (O_2 saturation <93%)
- Tachypnea with a respiratory rate of >60 breaths per minute infant, >40 preschool age, or >30 school age
- Increased work of breathing: grunting, flaring, or deep retractions
- Age younger than 3 months with any suspicion of pneumonia
- Age younger than 1 year with presumed bacterial pneumonia
- Inability to maintain hydration or take oral antibiotics
- Failure to respond to outpatient antibiotics
- Risk of respiratory failure based on chronic medical condition

Antibiotics should be prescribed when bacterial pneumonia is presumed. Specific agents are based on age (Table 30-3).

If a macrolide antibiotic is indicated in an infant <6 weeks of age, azithromycin should be considered instead of erythromycin in light of reports of erythromycin's association with the development of pyloric stenosis. Ceftriaxone is generally

Table 30-3 Empiric Antibiotic Dosing Recommendations for Pneumonia Treatment

Age-group	Antibiotic
Neonatal (<3 wk)	Ampicillin 200-300 mg/kg/day IV divided q8-12h + gentamicin 4 mg/kg/day IV q24h OR Ampicillin 200-300 mg/kg/day IV divided q8-12h (interval dependent on age) + cefotaxime 200 mg/kg/day IV divided q6-12h (interval dependent on age)
3 wk to 3 mo	*Outpatient (assumes Chlamydia pneumoniae):* Macrolide (choose one): Azithromycin 10 mg/kg IV/PO × 1 day, then 5 mg/kg/day IV/PO q24h × 4 days Clarithromycin 15 mg/kg/day PO divided q12h Erythromycin base 30-40 mg/kg/day IV/PO divided q6h *Inpatient:* Macrolide (as above) + ceftriaxone 50-100 mg/kg/day IV divided q12-24h* OR Macrolide (as above) + cefuroxime 75-150 mg/kg/day IV divided q8h
4 mo to 4 yr	*Outpatient:* Amoxicillin 80-100 mg/kg/day PO divided q8h

Continued

Table 30-3 Empiric Antibiotic Dosing Recommendations for Pneumonia Treatment—Cont'd

Age-group	Antibiotic
	Inpatient:
	Ampicillin 200 mg/kg/day IV divided q6h
	OR
	Ceftriaxone 50-100 mg/kg/day IV divided q12-24h*
	OR
	Cefuroxime 75-150 mg/kg/day IV divided q8h
5-15 yr	*Outpatient:*[†]
	Macrolide (as above)
	OR
	Doxycycline (if patient older than 8 yr) 4 mg/kg/day PO divided q12h (max 200 mg/day)
	Inpatient:
	Macrolide (as above) + ampicillin 200 mg/kg/day IV divided q6h (max 8 g/day)
	OR
	Macrolide + ceftriaxone 50-100 mg/kg/day IV divided q12-24h (max 2 g/dose, 4 g/day)*
	OR
	Macrolide + cefuroxime 75-150 mg/kg/day IV divided q8h (max 6 g/day)

*Cefotaxime 200 mg/kg/day IV divided q6h (max 12 g/day) may be used in place of ceftriaxone.
[†]Consider adding amoxicillin 80-100 mg/kg/day PO divided q8h for focal consolidation.

avoided until 14 days of life secondary to bilirubin displacement from albumin-binding sites. This is particularly important in patients who are jaundiced before institution of therapy.

Viral pneumonia is most common in the 4-month to 4-year-old age-group and requires no antimicrobial therapy. Consider adding macrolide to amoxicillin as first-line therapy for children 2 to 5 years old, especially if atypical organisms are suspected. Amoxicillin or ceftriaxone may be added to outpatient treatment for the 5- to 15-year-old age-group if severe consolidated infiltrates.

ASPIRATION PNEUMONIA

Aspiration pneumonia should be suspected in any child who has a history of acute onset of distress after vomiting or gagging, as well as in patients at high risk of aspiration. Elevated risk is based on a combination of oropharyngeal dysfunction (such as children with cerebral palsy, developmental delay, or muscle weakness) and GE reflux. Respiratory distress usually develops within 2 hours after aspiration. Aspiration pneumonia may be due to any of the following: bacterial flora from the mouth, chemical insult from gastric secretions, or particulate matter from the stomach or mouth.

Symptoms
- History of vomiting/choking/gagging +
- Sudden onset of distress ++
- Cough +++
- Fever +
- Lack of upper respiratory tract symptoms +
- Respiratory distress ++

Signs
- Tachypnea ++, retractions +, grunting +
- Tachycardia +
- Pallor ++; cyanosis in severe cases
- Rales ++
- Wheeze +
- Rhonchi +

Workup

- CXR reveals lobar infiltrates. Radiographs may be falsely reassuring immediately after aspiration.
- Consider CBC and blood culture in very young or ill-appearing children with fever.
- ABG analysis for severe distress.

Comments and Treatment Considerations

Treatment is mainly supportive. Support the ABCs and provide supplemental oxygen as needed. Antibiotic therapy is controversial, although many experts recommend treating when there is a strong suspicion of aspiration pneumonia. Empiric antibiotics may include either aqueous penicillin G dosed at 250,000 to 400,000 units/kg/day IV divided q6-12h (interval based on age; max 24 million units/day) or clindamycin 30 to 40 mg/kg/day IV divided q6-8h (max 4.8 g/day). Complicated aspiration pneumonia may require broader spectrum antibiotics such as ampicillin-sulbactam dosed at 200 mg of ampicillin/kg/day IV divided q6h (max 8 g of ampicillin component/day) or the addition of an aminoglycoside such as gentamicin dosed at 4 to 7.5 mg/kg/day IV divided q8-24h (dose and interval dependent on age). Most children with significant disease, especially with underlying conditions, will require hospital admission for at least 24 hours to observe the initial course of disease and to monitor for respiratory distress or failure.

PULMONARY EMBOLISM

Pulmonary embolism is rare in healthy children. Classic symptoms include sudden onset of dyspnea, pleuritic chest pain, cough, and hemoptysis. Dyspnea, distress, and hypoxia are often out of proportion to auscultatory or radiographic findings (see Chapter 8, Chest Pain).

PULMONARY EDEMA

Pulmonary edema refers to fluid accumulation in alveolar spaces and bronchioles caused by increased hydrostatic pressure, decreased oncotic pressure, or increased permeability of the alveolar membranes. Onset of pulmonary edema may be rapid. Causes include CHF (due to myocarditis, cardiomyopathy, congenital heart lesions with increased flow to left ventricle or left-sided outlet obstruction, and severe anemia), nephrosis, liver disease, burns, sepsis, renal failure, upper airway obstruction, altitude sickness, and poisonings (such as barbiturates, alcohol, narcotics, hydrocarbons, and smoke inhalation).

Symptoms
- Shortness of breath +++
- Cough ++
- Chest pain
- Exertional dyspnea +++, nocturnal dyspnea +, orthostatic dyspnea +
- Peripheral edema (variable)

Signs
- Tachypnea +++, rales ++, grunting +
- Tachycardia +++
- Copious clear to blood tinged sputum +
- Pallor +, cyanosis (late)
- Poor perfusion (especially with cardiac etiology)
- Peripheral edema (CHF, renal failure, hypoalbuminemia) +
- Gallop rhythm, hepatomegaly, jugular venous distention (cardiac etiologies)

Workup
- CXR may show multiple abnormalities: Kerley's A and B lines may represent interstitial fluid accumulation, may see pleural effusion etiology, and enlarged cardiac size with primary cardiac or hypervolemic states. Coexisting pulmonary conditions may make it difficult to judge the amount of edema. Early pulmonary edema may be difficult to detect.
- ABG analysis may assist in some cases.
- ECG if cardiac etiology suspected.
- Current body weight comparison to recent previous weight is helpful in young infants with underlying pulmonary or cardiac disease.

- General screening labs for electrolyte imbalance, renal disease, protein wasting etiology, or infection include electrolytes, UA, BUN, SCr, albumin, total protein, triglycerides, cholesterol, and CBC.
- Carboxyhemoglobin level if suspicion of smoke inhalation exists.

Comments and Treatment Considerations

Management is initially supportive and then guided by etiology of edema. Support ABCs. Initial therapy may include morphine sulfate dosed at 0.05 to 0.1 mg/kg/dose IV/SC q3-4h prn to reduce anxiety and dyspnea with careful attention to possible respiratory depression; diuretics such as furosemide 1 to 2 mg/kg/dose IV/PO q6h prn for hypervolemia and CHF; vasopressors to improve contractility in cases with decreased myocardial function (see Chapter 20, Hypotension/Shock); afterload reducers to counter cardiac poor contractility; renal failure may require dialysis; and albumin infusion (slow) with a diuretic such as furosemide can be used for hypoalbuminemic states.

Consider intubation before respiratory failure occurs, as additional benefits include reducing fluid filtration into alveoli, decreasing pulmonary vascular volume, and raising intrathoracic pressure. Early intubation is also recommended for smoke inhalation associated with thermal injury of the airway and for maximizing oxygenation in CO poisoning (see Chapter 7, Burns). Patients with pulmonary edema will require hospital admission, usually to an intensive care unit. Consultation with an intensivist is recommended.

Consider central venous pressure monitoring with a Swan-Ganz catheter to assess left atrial pressures. Consider blood transfusion for CHF associated with severe anemia, usually given slowly with diuretics. Appropriate early consultation should be sought with the appropriate subspecialist based on etiology.

PERTUSSIS

Whooping cough is caused by infection with *Bordetella pertussis*. The incidence of pertussis increases cyclically, with reported peaks every 3 to 4 years. Although adolescents and young adults account for the majority of cases, pertussis is the most severe and potentially life threatening for infants who are not fully immunized against the disease. Clinical syndrome varies by age and prior immunization. Three distinct stages have been defined but may not always be seen: the catarrhal stage (1 to 2 weeks) involves typical symptoms of a nonspecific upper respiratory tract infection; the paroxysmal stage (2 to 4 weeks) with severe cough and associated "whoop" with inspiration; and the convalescent phase as cough improves.

Symptoms
- Mild cough, coryza, conjunctivitis, and low-grade fever (catarrhal stage)
- Severe cough +++, paroxysms of coughing ++, posttussive emesis + (paroxysmal stage)
- Poor feeding (infants)
- Confusion, somnolence, and irritability are rare manifestations of associated encephalitis or intracranial hemorrhage

Signs
- Catarrhal stage:
  - Cough
  - Rhinorrhea
  - Conjunctivitis
- Paroxysmal stage:
  - Coughing paroxysms +++ (may be inducible by gagging with tongue blade)
  - Whoop + (whoop often absent in infants, adolescents)
  - Cyanosis with cough +
  - Apnea + (infants)
  - Respiratory arrest from mucous plug (infants)
  - Subconjunctival hemorrhage
  - Dehydration (infants)
- Seizures, altered mental status (encephalitis or intracranial hemorrhage are rare)
- Prolonged cough (may be the only manifestation in immunized individuals, especially adolescents and young adults)

Workup

- Fluorescent antibody staining of nasal pharyngeal swab or aspirate is diagnostic, although results are not immediately available in most laboratories.
- CXR allows differentiation from pneumonia and findings are usually normal but may have a characteristic "shaggy" right heart border.
- CBC can reveal an absolute lymphocytosis (inconsistent in infants younger than 6 months).

Comments and Treatment Considerations

Pertussis should be suspected in any child, especially infants, with paroxysms of coughing.

All children younger than 6 months with suspected or proven pertussis should be admitted for monitoring because they are at risk of apnea, choking, and dehydration (see Chapter 4, Apnea). Older children showing signs of respiratory compromise (cyanosis with coughing) or who may have secondary bacterial pneumonia should be admitted. High fever is unusual with pertussis and if present should suggest possible secondary bacterial pneumonia. Treatment for pertussis is thought to be therapeutic if started during the catarrhal, and if started after the cough is established, to have minimal therapeutic effect but limits the spread of organisms to others. Treatment consists of a macrolide, the drug of choice being erythromycin base 40 mg/kg/day (max 2000 mg base/day) PO divided q6h × 14 days. Both azithromycin 10 mg/kg/day PO q24h (max 500 mg/day) × 5 to 7 days and clarithromycin 15 mg/kg/day (max 1000 mg/day) PO divided q12h × 7 to 14 days have been used successfully. Of note, the increasing reports of pyloric stenosis in young infants exposed to erythromycin may render azithromycin or clarithromycin preferable in this population. Chemoprophylaxis is ideally instituted as early as possible after exposure and is of little benefit if >3 weeks has elapsed since exposure. All household and close contacts should receive prophylaxis; the antibiotics and doses are the same as for treatment.

PLEURITIS

Pleuritis, or pleurisy, represents inflammation of the pleura usually associated with pneumonia or other underlying diseases.

Associated underlying diseases include subdiaphragmatic infections, pancreatitis, collagen vascular disease, neoplasms with associated pleural metastasis or lymphatic obstruction, CHF, hypoproteinemic states, and trauma. When associated with large amounts of pleural fluid, respiratory distress ensues. The fluid may be any combination of transudate, exudate, or blood. *Dry pleurisy* refers to chest pain associated with dry cough in a patient with an upper respiratory tract infection and minimal or no effusion.

Symptoms
- Pleuritic chest pain +++
- Fever +
- Cough + (if associated pneumonia +++)
- Shortness of breath +
- History of trauma or collagen vascular disease

Signs
- Tachypnea ++, retractions, grunting
- Fever (depends on etiology) +
- Splinting due to pain +
- Decreased breath sounds +
- Dullness to percussion +; egophony; decreased tactile and vocal fremitus
- Associated rales caused by adjacent pneumonia +
- Pleural rub +
- Abdominal pain (only subdiaphragmatic causes)
- Chest wall pain to palpation

Workup
- CXR to determine presence of effusion. Decubitus films can help determine whether effusion is present and free flowing.
- Further evaluation should be guided by the primary underlying disorder.
- Thoracentesis is indicated when fluid accumulation is contributing to respiratory distress or for diagnostic purposes. If performed, fluid should be sent for appropriate cultures and Gram stain, cell count, pH, lactate dehydrogenase, protein, and glucose levels. Cytology should

be done for suspected malignancy. Generally, a pH level >7.3 represents sterile fluid. A pH level <7.3 limits the differential to empyema or collagen vascular disease. WBC count is not a good predictor of etiology or need for chest tube drainage. Exudative effusions, as well as those with a pH level <7.3, usually require tube thoracostomy.

Ultrasound guidance may be necessary for small effusions. Surgical consultation or CT may be necessary for drainage of loculated effusions.

- Consider
  - Sputum Gram stain and culture
  - Purified protein derivative test
  - Mycoplasma titers
  - Antinuclear antibody

Comments and Treatment Considerations

Support the ABCs and provide supplemental oxygen as needed. Care for "dry" pleurisy is supportive only, usually with NSAIDs such as ibuprofen dosed at 10 mg/kg/dose (max 800 mg/dose) PO q6-8h prn. Small effusions associated with significant pain may be treated with NSAIDs and if needed narcotic analgesics. Respiratory status should be closely monitored if any narcotics are used for pain control. Surgical consultation with or without chest CT is recommended for patients with large loculated effusions or if unable to distinguish between parenchymal disease and effusion. Closed tube thoracostomy is recommended for large effusions requiring further drainage. Antibiotics should be prescribed for associated bacterial pneumonia (see earlier section on pneumonia for empiric agents and dosing).

Most patients should be admitted to the hospital, with the exception of those without underlying disease, those with minimal symptoms, and those with small or no effusion.

�֍ NEUROLOGIC CAUSES OF RESPIRATORY DISTRESS

Patients with CNS issues (e.g., bleeding, ischemia, or inflammation) may present with difficulty maintaining upper airway patency or with abnormal breathing patterns (see Chapter 3, Altered Mental Status). Patients with spinal cord injury or disease may present with respiratory difficulty secondary to weak intercostal muscles (see Chapter 36, Trauma, and Chapter 39, Weakness/Fatigue). Peripheral nerve disease and muscle disorders may also lead to respiratory difficulty (see Chapter 39, Weakness/Fatigue).

✳ METABOLIC/TOXICOLOGIC CAUSES OF RESPIRATORY DISTRESS

Respiratory distress in the absence of pulmonary or intrathoracic disease can be due to metabolic disturbances, stimulation of the respiratory center, or primary neurologic disease. Ingestion of toxic substances may lead to distress by any of these three mechanisms. Most common metabolic causes include anion-gap acidosis and hyperammonemia. Common causes of anion-gap acidosis include lactate (sepsis, dehydration), diabetic ketoacidosis (DKA) (see Chapter 1, Abdominal Pain), poisonings/ingestions (see Chapter 35, Toxic Ingestion, Approach To), and inborn errors of metabolism. Common poisonings leading to metabolic acidosis include methanol, ethylene glycol, isopropyl alcohol, acetone, isoniazid, aspirin, cyanide, and carbon monoxide.

Mechanisms by which drugs and toxins leading to respiratory failure fall into two major categories: (1) depression of central drive such as is seen with barbiturates, opiates, alcohols, and clonidine or (2) paralysis of respiratory muscles such as is seen with organophosphates, selected venoms, botulinum toxin, tetanus, strychnine, and neuromuscular blockers (see Chapter 5, Bites; Chapter 35, Toxic Ingestion, Approach To; and Chapter 39, Weakness/Fatigue).

Symptoms
- Dyspnea +
- Absence of cough, upper respiratory tract symptoms
- Polyuria, polydipsia (DKA)
- Altered consciousness (toxicologic ++, DKA +, hyperammonemia +)

Signs

- Hyperpnea (metabolic acidosis, hyperammonemia) with no ausculatory findings ++
- Hypoventilation (toxicologic)
- Tachycardia and hypoperfusion +
- Confusion, somnolence, or coma (DKA, metabolic defects, ingestions, poisonings) ++
- Arrhythmias and seizures (poisonings and ingestions)

Workup

- Workup is guided by suspected etiology.
- Radiologic studies for CNS etiologies (CT of head for mass, bleed, edema; spinal magnetic resonance imaging for transverse myelitis, cord lesions).
- Cerebrospinal fluid analysis for CNS inflammation, meningitis, subarachnoid hemorrhage, or Guillain-Barré syndrome.
- CXR to differentiate from primary pulmonary etiologies.
- Electrolytes to assess for metabolic acidosis with associated metabolic derangements.
- Glucose to assess for hypoglycemia or hyperglycemia.
- ABG analysis to assess for degree of respiratory failure or evidence of a compensatory metabolic alkalosis in a primary metabolic acidosis.
- Carboxyhemoglobin if CO poisoning considered.
- Toxicologic studies.
- Ammonia for inborn errors of metabolism or liver disease, particularly if altered level of consciousness.
- Lactate, pyruvate, serum amino acids, and urine organic acids if suspect inborn error of metabolism.

Comments and Treatment Considerations

Support the ABCs. Assess and monitor for signs of respiratory failure. Patients with respiratory compensation for metabolic acidosis should have normal oxygen saturation, whereas those with hypoventilation will be hypoxic and have lowered oxygen saturation. Endotracheal intubation should be performed in any patient exhibiting respiratory difficulty caused by weakness or if signs of respiratory failure are present. When intubating the trachea of a patient who is hyperventilating as a result of metabolic acidosis as a compensatory mechanism, be careful to continue hyperventilation after intubation.

See Chapter 35, Toxic Ingestion, Approach To, for management. Bicarbonate can be given for correction of severe metabolic acidosis with adequate ventilation and for enhanced elimination of certain toxins (e.g., salicylates).

REFERENCES

American Academy of Pediatrics: Reassessment of the indications for ribavirin therapy in respiratory syncytial virus infections. American Academy of Pediatrics Committee on Infectious Diseases, *Pediatrics* 97:137-140, 1996.

Aoyama T, Sunakawa K, Iwata S, et al: Efficacy of short-term treatment of pertussis with clarithromycin and azithromycin, *J Pediatr* 129(5):761-764, 1996.

Ausejo M, Saenz Am Pham B, et al: The effectiveness of glucocorticoids in treating croup: meta-analysis, *BMJ* 319:595, 1999.

Bracken MB, Shepard MJ, Collins WF, et al: A randomized, controlled trial of methylprednisolone or naloxone in the treatment of acute spinal-cord injury. Results of the Second National Acute Spinal Cord Injury Study, *N Engl J Med* 322(20):1405-1411, 1990.

Centers for Disease Control and Prevention: Pertussis—United States, 1997–2000, *MMWR Morb Mortal Wkly Rep* 51(4):73-76, 2002.

Ciarallo L: Higher-dose intravenous magnesium therapy for children with moderate to severe acute asthma, *Arch Pediatr Adolesc Med* 154:979-983, 2000.

Cooper WO, Griffin MR, Arbogast P, et al: Very early exposure to erythromycin and infantile hypertrophic pyloric stenosis, *Arch Pediatr Adolesc Med* 156:647-650, 2002.

Craven D: Ipratropium bromide plus nebulized albuterol for the treatment of hospitalized children with acute asthma, *J Pediatr* 138:51-58, 2001.

Flores G, Horwitz RI: Efficacy of beta2-agonists in bronchiolitis: a reappraisal and meta-analysis, *Pediatrics* 100:233-239, 1997.

Glaser N, et al: Risk factors for cerebral edema in children with diabetic ketoacidosis. The Pediatric Emergency Medicine Collaborative Research Committee of the American Academy of Pediatrics, *N Engl J Med* 344(4):264-269, 2001.

Garrison MM, Christakis DA, Harvey E, et al: Systemic corticosteroids in infant bronchiolitis: a meta-analysis, *Pediatrics* 105:e44, 2000.

Jacobson SJ, et al: A randomized controlled trial of penicillin vs. clindamycin for the treatment of aspiration pneumonia in children, *Arch Pediatr Adolesc Med* 151:701-704, 1997.

Johnson DW, Jacobson S, Edney PC, et al: A comparison of nebulized budesonide, intramuscular dexamethasone, and placebo for moderately severe croup, *N Engl J Med* 339:498-503, 1998.

Kellner JD, Ohlsson A, Gadomski AM, Wang EE: Efficacy of bronchodilator therapy in bronchiolitis. A meta-analysis, *Arch Pediatr Adolesc Med* 150:1166-1172, 1996.

Kunkel NC, Baker MD: Use of racemic epinephrine, dexamethasone, and mist in the outpatient management of croup, *Pediatr Emerg Care* 12:156-159, 1996.

Kuppermann N, Bank DE, Walton EA, et al: Risks for bacteremia and urinary tract infections in young febrile children with bronchiolitis, *Arch Pediatr Adolesc Med* 151:1207-1214, 1997.

L'Hommedieu CS: The use of ketamine for emergency intubation of patients with status asthmaticus, *Ann Emerg Med* 16(5):568-571, 1987.

Mandelberg A, Tsehori S, Houri S, et al: Is nebulized aerosol treatment necessary in the pediatric emergency department? *Chest* 117:1309-1313, 2000.

Martinon-Torres F, Rodriguez-Nunez A, Martinon-Sanchez JM: Heliox therapy in infants with acute bronchiolitis, *Pediatrics* 109:68-73, 2002.

McIntosh K: Community-acquired pneumonia in children, *N Engl J Med* 346(6):429-437, 2002.

Meissner C: Uncertainty in the management of viral lower respiratory tract disease, *Pediatrics* 109:1000-1003, 2001.

Plint AC: The efficiency of nebulized racemic epinephrine in children with acute asthma: a randomized, double blind trial, *Acad Emerg Med* 7:1097-1103, 2000.

Qureshi F, Zaritsky A, Poirier MP: Comparative efficacy of dexamethasone versus oral prednisone in acute pediatric asthma, *J Pediatr* 139:20-26, 2001.

Scarfone RJ, Loiselle JM, Wiley JF, et al: Nebulized dexamethasone versus oral prednisone in the emergency treatment of asthmatic children, *Ann Emerg Med* 26:480-486, 1995.

Scarfone RJ: A randomized trial of magnesium in the emergency department treatment of children with asthma, *Ann Emerg Med* 36:572-578, 2000.

Schroeder LL, Knapp JF: Recognition and emergency management of infectious causes of upper airway obstruction in children, *Semin Resp Infect* 10:21-30, 1995.

Schuh S, Johnson DW, Callahan S, et al: Efficacy of frequent nebulized ipratropium bromide added to frequent high-dose albuterol therapy in severe childhood asthma, *J Pediatrics* 1264:639-645, 1995.

Schuh S: A comparison of inhaled fluticasone and oral prednisone for children with severe acute asthma, *N Engl J Med* 343:689-694, 2000.

Senior BA, Radkowsi D, MacArthur C, et al: Changing patterns in pediatric supraglottitis: a multi-institutional review, 1980–1992, *Laryngoscope* 104:1314-1322, 1994.

Stephanopoulos DE, Monge R, Schell KH, et al: Continuous intravenous terbutaline for pediatric status asthmaticus, *Crit Care Med* 26:1744-1748, 1998.

Streetman DD, Bhatt-Mehta V, Johnson CE: Management of acute, severe asthma in children, *Ann Pharmacother* 36:1249-1260, 2002.

Taketomo CK, Hodding JK, Kraus DM, editors: *Pediatric dosage handbook*, 8th ed, Hudson, Ohio, 2001, Lexicomp.

Westley CR, Cotton EK, Brooks JG: Nebulized racemic epinephrine by IPPB for the treatment of croup: a double blind study, *Am J Dis Child* 132:484-487, 1978.

Zorc JJ, Pucic MV, Ogborn CJ, et al: Ipratropium bromide added to asthma treatment in pediatric emergency departments, *Pediatrics* 103(4):748-752, 1999.

CHAPTER 31

Scrotal Pain or Swelling

CATHERINE E. PERRON

Acute scrotal pain or swelling in a child should be considered a potential surgical emergency. Although some causes of scrotal pain or swelling may be benign and require little more than observation, testicular torsion may lead to rapid loss of the testis if there is delay in diagnosis or treatment. Painful scrotal swellings include torsion of the testis, incarcerated inguinal hernia, trauma, torsion of a testicular appendage, and epididymitis. Painless causes of scrotal swelling include hydrocele, varicoceles, testicular tumors, infection and as a manifestation of a systemic reaction. For organizational purposes, painful and then painless scrotal swelling–associated entities are discussed in this chapter.

 ## TORSION OF THE TESTIS

Testicular torsion is the most significant condition causing acute scrotal pain and represents a true surgical emergency (Fig. 31-1). For the child with testicular torsion, time to the operating room for success in salvaging a testicle is measured in hours because irreversible testicular damage develops 4 to 6 hours after complete strangulation. After 12 hours of complete strangulation the testicle is usually unsalvageable; however, because it is impossible to determine exactly when and if complete or partial torsion occurred, testicular salvage should be considered even after 12 hours. When the diagnosis is clinically apparent, consultation with a urologist and transfer to the operating room should occur immediately.

Torsion results from an inadequate fixation of the testis to the intrascrotal subcutaneous tissue, resulting in a "bell-clapper

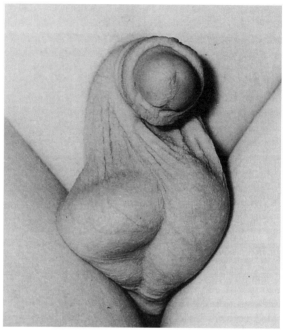

Fig. 31-1 Testicular torsion. Note the high-riding testicle with an abnormal transverse axis. (From Marconi D: *Emerg Med Clin North Am* 19(3): 547-568.)

deformity." The freely hanging testis may twist, producing torsion of the spermatic cord and infarction of the testis (Fig. 31-2). Testicular torsion is more common in the newborn period and during the early stages of puberty. Acute onset of severe testicular, groin, or lower abdominal pain may indicate torsion. A recent history of trauma may be offered but may be incidental and should not confuse the examiner about what is unrelated to trauma and truly represents spontaneous torsion.

Symptoms

- Sudden, severe scrotal pain ++++
- Nausea, anorexia, or vomiting +++

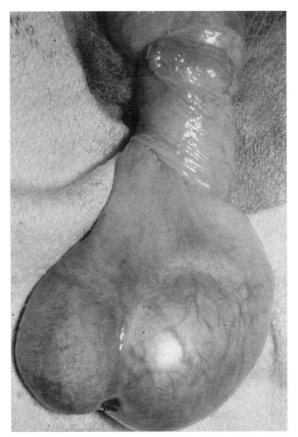

Fig. 31-2 Twisting of the spermatic cord in testicular torison. (From Marconi D: *Emerg Med Clin North Am* 19(3): 547-568.)

- Prior episodes of similar pain that resolved spontaneously +++
- Can be associated with increased physical activity or minor trauma ++
- Pain onset while sleeping or early morning ++

Signs

- Absent cremasteric reflex (may be present in incomplete or intermittent torsion) ++++
- Swollen, diffusely tender testicle ++++
- Elevated or abnormal lie (horizontal or transverse) of testicle in the scrotum +++
- Overlying scrotal erythema (later finding often similar to epididymitis)

Workup

- Radiologic imaging using color Doppler flow ultrasonography and scintigraphy may be helpful adjuncts but should never delay transfer to the operating room when the diagnosis of torsion is clear. In testicular torsion, color Doppler ultrasonography demonstrates decreased or absent testicular flow except in cases of spontaneous detorsion or intermittent torsion (in which case the flow may be normal).
- Nuclear scintigraphy may show a "cold spot," indicating impeded flow to the ischemic testicle. This study requires time and should not delay a clinically suggestive case of testicular torsion from proceeding to surgical exploration.

Comments and Treatment Considerations

Any patient, particularly the peripubertal child, with history or physical examination findings suggesting testicular torsion should have an immediate urologic or general surgical consultation for scrotal exploration, detorsion, and fixation of the affected and contralateral testis. Imaging studies should be reserved to support cases in which other diagnoses are more strongly suggested and should never delay surgical evaluation when testicular torsion is suggested.

❋ INCARCERATED INGUINAL HERNIA

An inguinal hernia (Fig. 31-3) can present with acute swelling and if incarcerated, acute pain and swelling. *Incarcerated* refers to a hernia that is not reducible, whereas *strangulated* refers to acute ischemia resulting from incarceration. Abdominal contents such as a loop of bowel or mesentery protruding

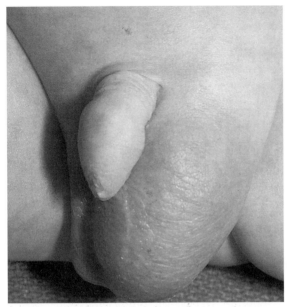

Fig. 31-3 A complete inguinal hernia extends into the scrotum, obscuring the testis. (From Zitelli B, Davis H: *Atlas of pediatric physical diagnosis,* 4th ed, St. Louis, 2002, Mosby.)

through a patent processus vaginalis is usually the cause of the hernia.

Symptoms
- Acute onset pain and swelling ++
- Prior intermittent inguinal fullness or known hernia ++++
- Nausea and vomiting ++
- Nonspecific fussiness or irritability in the small infant sometimes associated with poor feeding or pulling up of legs ++

Signs
- Fullness in inguinal area with normal palpable testicle +++
- Apparent tenderness and fullness when incarcerated ++++

Workup

Ultrasound may help differentiate other local causes of swelling such as adenitis or adenopathy when the diagnosis of hernia is not clear. Ultrasound may also ensure testicular integrity because torsion can also occur in an undescended testicle.

Comments and Treatment Considerations

Surgical repair is ultimately indicated, but an attempt at reduction is immediately necessary. Conscious sedation for reduction may be required. If the clinician is unable to reduce the incarcerated hernia, immediate surgical reduction is required. If the incarcerated hernia is reduced, elective surgical repair may be scheduled after a minimum of 2 to 3 days, allowing acute swelling to dissipate.

 TRAUMA

In children, scrotal trauma is usually due to a direct blow to the scrotum or a straddle injury, which forcefully compresses the testicle against the pubic bone. Penetrating injuries are less common, and the small size and greater mobility of the prepubertal testis make testicular injuries rare in this group. Scrotal trauma can result in minimal scrotal swelling or major trauma such as rupture of the testis presenting as a tense blood-filled tender scrotum. Unless the testis can be definitively determined to be normal and without tenderness, urgent surgical evaluation is required. Scrotal ultrasound can be useful in determining the location of fluid collections and the integrity of the testis. When testicular rupture is considered, surgical exploration is indicated because a ruptured testis has the best salvage rate when surgically repaired. The clinician must also consider that testicular torsion may present with a spurious history of trauma.

HEMATOCELES

Hematoceles, or blood within the tunica vaginalis, can represent severe testicular injury.

Signs
- Ecchymosis of the scrotal wall in the setting of trauma

Symptoms
- Scrotal pain, swelling, or discoloration
- Does not transilluminate in contrast to hydrocele

Workup
- Ultrasound will identify the more echogenic appearance of blood within the tunica when compared to a hydrocele.

Comments and Treatment Considerations
Testicular rupture requires scrotal exploration. Large hematoceles (without rupture of the testis) may heal more readily after drainage.

INTRATESTICULAR HEMATOMAS OR LACERATIONS OF THE TUNICA ALBUGINEA
Symptoms
- Localized testicular pain and swelling

Workup
- Sonography can determine the location of blood.

Comments and Treatment Considerations
If the tunica albuginea is determined to be intact, no surgical exploration is required; however, any question of possible laceration requires drainage of the hematoma and repair of the testicular laceration.

TRAUMATIC EPIDIDYMITIS
Traumatic epididymitis resulting from blunt trauma to the scrotum represents local inflammation and can develop within a few days of injury.

Symptoms
- Short-lived acute pain associated with trauma is followed by a pain-free period, after which pain returns

Signs

- Scrotal erythema, edema, and tenderness of the epididymis are found on examination

Workup

Urinalysis findings are negative because this does not represent an infectious process. Ultrasound demonstrates increased flow or hyperemia to the area and excludes any more severe injury.

Comments and Treatment Considerations

Treatment is supportive, including nonsteroidal antiinflammatory agents, supportive undergarments, and rest.

SCROTAL LACERATIONS

Scrotal lacerations require determination that the spermatic cord and testis are not injured.

Workup

- Ultrasound can delineate associated fluid collections and status of underlying testis.

Comments and Treatment Considerations

Examination by a urologist with the assistance of an inguinal block or general anesthesia may be required and sought if the integrity of the underlying structures is of concern. For simple lacerations, hemostasis and closure of the laceration with chromic gut is sufficient. If tolerated, ice packs may be helpful in minimizing swelling.

 ## TORSION OF A TESTICULAR APPENDAGE

Several vestigial embryologic remnants commonly attached to the testis or epididymis may twist around their bases, producing infarction and associated scrotal pain and swelling. Appendage torsion is most common in prepubertal children, with peak incidence from 7 to 12 years of age. Scrotal pain is the usual presenting feature and may be less acute or more insidious in onset than testicular torsion.

Symptoms
- Testicular pain, often less severe than with testicular torsion, has a crescendo pattern over the course of several days
- Nausea and vomiting are uncommon

Signs
Examination early in the course may reveal pathognomonic signs:
- Palpable, tender nodule in the superior portion of the testicle +++
- Discrete area of blue discoloration in the same area, called "blue dot sign" (specific when seen, but noted in as few as 4% of cases) ++++
- Torsed appendage visible with transillumination of the scrotum +++
- Testicle can be appreciated not to be enlarged +++

As the inflammatory process progresses, later examinations may reveal the following:
- Edema and erythema of entire scrotum
- Diffuse swelling and tenderness make differentiation from testicular torsion more difficult

Workup
- Color Doppler ultrasonography and scintigraphy demonstrate normal or increased flow to the affected testicle, representing inflammation.

Comments and Treatment Considerations
If the location of pain and tenderness can be reliably and reproducibly isolated to the superior pole of the testicle with the remainder of the testis nontender, the diagnosis of torsion of a testicular appendage is likely. Radiologic imaging studies may be helpful in supporting this diagnosis by documenting normal or increased flow to the involved testicle. If the clinician is confident in the diagnosis, no surgical exploration is needed. Analgesics or antiinflammatory agents, scrotal support (in severe cases run a thick piece of tape from the left thigh under the scrotum to the right thigh, making sure the sticky side is not against the scrotum), and rest usually result in resolution of the

symptoms in approximately 10 to 14 days. Follow-up in 48 hours is recommended. Rarely, severe pain refractory to analgesics and scrotal support may require surgical excision of the appendage.

 ## *EPIDIDYMITIS*

Epididymitis is the most common cause of acute scrotal pain and/or swelling beyond puberty. Overall, epididymitis accounts for more than one fourth of cases of acute scrotal pain in all age-groups. Epididymitis indicates inflammation of the epididymis and can be infectious, traumatic, or reactive. In adolescents, suspect sexually transmitted pathogens such as chlamydia and gonorrhea. In prepubertal boys, structural or functional genitourinary abnormalities are often present and result in retention of urinary coliform bacteria, causing epididymitis.

Symptoms
- Gradual onset of pain ++
- Dysuria ++++
- Fever +
- Urethral discharge ++++
- History of genitourinary abnormalities and/or surgery +++
- Recent sexual activity without barrier protection ++

Signs
- Early: localized swelling and tenderness of the epididymis +++
- Late: generalized tenderness, edema, and erythema of scrotum
- Urethral discharge ++++
- Fever >101° F +

Workup
- Urinalysis may show pyuria: >10 WBC/hpf in adolescents, >3 WBCs/hpf in a child.
- Urethral cultures for gonorrhea and chlamydia should be sent.

- Color Doppler ultrasonography shows normal or increased flow and decreased echotexture of epididymis, representing inflammation of the epididymis.
- Scintigraphy also shows normal or increased flow to the affected epididymis.

Comments and Treatment Considerations

Treatment is based on age. Sexually active males should be treated empirically for chlamydia and gonorrhea.

For epididymitis most likely caused by gonococcal or chlamydial infection:

Ceftriaxone 250 mg IM in a single dose
PLUS
Doxycycline 100 mg PO bid for 10 days

OR

Ofloxacin 300 mg PO bid for 10 days (for adolescent patients allergic to cephalosporins and/or tetracycline)

Prepubertal males should be treated for urinary pathogens (see Chapter 18, Hematuria, section on UTI).

Rest, scrotal support (in severe cases run a thick piece of tape from the left thigh under the scrotum to the right thigh making sure the sticky side is not against the scrotum), and analgesics or antiinflammatory agents. Follow-up is generally advised in 48 to 72 hours. Prepubertal children need urologic referral and imaging to evaluate for possible genitourinary abnormalities.

 ## *HYDROCELE*

An accumulation of fluid within the tunica vaginalis that surrounds the testis can be found in association with underlying testicular abnormalities, as occurs in torsion of the testis, torsion of an appendage, epididymitis, trauma, or tumor. If the testicle and overlying scrotal soft tissues are normal, this fluid collection represents an isolated hydrocele and is of developmental origin.

SIMPLE HYDROCELE

A simple hydrocele represents retained fluid after the processus vaginalis closes developmentally.

Symptoms
- Scrotal swelling that does not change in size over time; does not "wax and wane"

Signs
- Scrotal swelling that transilluminates
- Testicle size is normal

Comments and Treatment Considerations
Fluid usually resorbs in the first 12 to 18 months of life and requires only observation.

COMMUNICATING HYDROCELE
When the processus vaginalis remains patent, as it does in a communicating hydrocele, it can enlarge and permit the development of a hernia.

Symptoms
- Scrotal swelling with a history of change in size, particularly with crying or exertion
- Swelling transilluminates

Signs
- Scrotal swelling
- Testicle usually palpated to be normal
- Thickening of the spermatic cord structures as they are felt against the pubic tubercle is referred to as the "silk glove sign" ++

Comments and Treatment Considerations
Surgical exploration and high ligation of the processus vaginalis after decompression of the hydrocele is the appropriate treatment. Urologic referral is necessary but with documentation of normal testicle and a lack of tenderness, referral is not emergent.

VARICOCELES
Varicoceles, usually painless scrotal swelling caused by a collection of abnormally enlarged spermatic cord veins, is most

often found on routine examination of boys aged 10 to 15 years. Most varicoceles occur on the left side because of the sharp angle at which the spermatic vein drains into the renal vein in comparison to the right spermatic vein, which drains into the inferior vena cava. Occasionally a varicocele may present with mild swelling and discomfort.

Signs

- Full hemiscrotum without overlying skin changes ++
- Testis and epididymis are palpated as normal +++
- "Bag of worms" appreciated above the testicle represents a mass of varicose veins +++
- Varicocele more prominent when standing versus supine examination

Workup

Doppler ultrasound demonstrates normal flow to the testis and the collection of tortuous veins.

Comments and Treatment Considerations

Some large varicoceles may require internal spermatic vein ligation and can have an impact on testicular size and fertility. Most varicoceles are asymptomatic and benign.

 ## TESTICULAR TUMORS

Testicular or paratesticular tumors are rare in children. They usually present as painless, unilateral, firm to hard scrotal swellings. Leukemic infiltration of a testis can present bilaterally. Associated hydroceles may be found. In children younger than 2 years, the tumor is usually a yolk sac carcinoma or teratoma. After puberty, germinal cell tumors are seen.

Workup

Ultrasound is the primary tool for initial evaluation of a solid testicular mass.

Comments and Treatment Considerations

Surgical exploration through a groin incision allows control of the spermatic cord vessels and radical orchiectomy if malignancy is confirmed.

 OTHER PAINLESS SCROTAL SWELLING

Worth mention are several other causes of painless scrotal swelling including scrotal swelling associated with allergic reactions, insect bites, cellulitis, contact dermatitis, or a manifestation of an underlying illness causing generalized edematous states (see Chapter 11, Edema). Henoch-Schönlein purpura and Kawasaki disease are vasculitides known to produce scrotal pain and mild swelling, but they are usually identified by their other clinical findings.

REFERENCES

Baker LA, Sigman D, Matthews RI, et al: An analysis of clinical outcomes using color Doppler testicular ultrasound for testicular torsion, *Pediatrics* 105(3 Pt 1):604-607, 2000.

Burgher SW: Acute scrotal pain, *Emerg Med Clin North Am* 16(4):781-809, Nov 1998.

Jefferson RH, Perez LM, Joseph DB: Critical analysis of the clinical presentation of acute scrotum: a 9-year experience at a single institution, *J Urol* 158:1198-1200, 1997.

Kadish HA, Bolte RC: A retrospective review of pediatric patients with epididymitis, testicular torsion, and torsion of testicular appendages, *Pediatrics* 102(1):73-76, 1998.

Lewis AG, Bukowski TP, Jarvis PD, et al: Evaluation of acute scrotum in the emergency department, *J Pediatr Surg* 30(2):277-281, 1995.

Paltiel HJ, Connolly LP, Atala A, et al: Acute scrotal symptoms in boys with an indeterminate clinical presentation: comparison of color Doppler sonography and scintigraphy, *Radiology* 207:223-231, 1998.

CHAPTER 32

Seizures

VINCENT W. CHIANG

Seizures are the most common neurologic disorder in childhood and among the more common events that lead to an ED visit. Studies have shown that 4% to 6% of all children will have at least one seizure in the first 16 years of life. These can range from a brief self-limited nonrecurring episode to a prolonged life-threatening event.

The underlying abnormality in all seizures is hypersynchronous neuronal discharges. Cerebral manifestations include increased blood flow, increased oxygen and glucose consumption, and increased carbon dioxide and lactic acid production. Prolonged seizures (>20 minutes) can result in permanent neuronal injury. If appropriate oxygenation and ventilation are maintained, the increase in cerebral blood flow is usually sufficient to meet the initial increased metabolic requirements of the brain. Brief seizures rarely produce lasting effects.

STATUS EPILEPTICUS

Prolonged (>20 minutes) seizure activity, or status epilepticus, is a true medical emergency. Therapy should be initiated at presentation for any patient with seizure activity lasting >5-10 minutes. In one series, 88 of 239 patients who had convulsive status epilepticus for >1 hour had permanent neurologic sequelae. Treatment is directed at supporting respiratory and cardiac function (i.e., ABCs), halting the seizure activity, and treating any underlying cause of the seizure activity.

Systemic alterations that can occur with seizures result from a massive sympathetic discharge, leading to tachycardia, hypertension, and hyperglycemia. Failure of adequate ventilation, particularly in those patients in whom consciousness is impaired, can lead to hypoxia, hypercarbia, and respiratory acidosis. Patients with impaired consciousness may be unable to protect their airway and are at risk of aspiration. Prolonged skeletal muscle activity can lead to lactic acidosis, rhabdomyolysis, hyperkalemia, hyperthermia, and hypoglycemia.

Comments and Treatment Considerations

Initial treatment includes management of ABCs and measurement of oxygen saturation and glucose level. Hypoglycemia should be treated with a glucose containing IV fluid such as D25W 2-4 ml/kg IV. Benzodiazepines are the initial drug of choice for the treatment of seizures. Lorazepam (Ativan) dosed at 0.05 to 0.1 mg/kg IV (max 4 mg/dose) and diazepam (Valium) 0.1 to 0.2 mg/kg IV (max 10 mg/dose) are the most commonly used agents and may be repeated every 5 minutes if the initial dose does not stop the seizure activity. Airway management supplies should be readily available because multiple doses may cause respiratory depression, requiring intubation. If intravenous access cannot be obtained, undiluted diazepam injection may be given rectally (PR). The rectal dose of diazepam is 0.5 mg/kg (max 20 mg/dose) and may be repeated at a dose 0.25 mg/kg (max 10 mg/dose) in 10 minutes if needed.

Phenytoin (Dilantin) dosed at 10 to 20 mg/kg/dose IV and fosphenytoin (Cerebyx) dosed at 10 to 20 mg phenytoin equivalents (PE)/kg/dose IV are generally considered second-line agents. Infusion of phenytoin must not be faster than 1 mg/kg/min, at a maximum of 50 mg/min to prevent significant hypotension and bradycardia, which may result from rapid infusion. Fosphenytoin is a water-soluble prodrug of phenytoin and may be infused at a rate of 3 mg PE/kg/min, at a maximum infusion rate of 150 mg PE/min. Fosphenytoin may also be given IM if IV access cannot be obtained. Phenytoin should never be given IM.

Third-line agents include phenobarbital and valproic acid. Phenobarbital is commonly dosed at 10 to 20 mg/kg IV, administered no faster than 1 mg/kg/min, at a maximum of 30 mg/min for children and 60 mg/min for adults >60 kg. Phenobarbital may be repeated in 10 to 15 minutes, with the cumulative maximum dose not to exceed 30 mg/kg. Note that when benzodi-azepines and barbiturates are used together, there is a signifi-cant risk of respiratory depression requiring bag-mask ventilation or endotracheal intubation. Intravenous valproic acid may be useful in patients with allergies to either phenytoin or phenobarbital. Valproic acid is usually dosed at a 20 mg/kg load IV and administered at a rate no faster than 5 mg/kg/min. Valproic acid should not be used in children younger than 2 years secondary to a greater risk of hepatotoxicity.

If these therapies fail, patients may require continuous infusions of short-acting barbiturates (e.g., pentobarbital) or general anes-thesia (e.g., halothane and isoflurane) to abort the seizures. The level of anesthesia should be sufficient to maintain either a flat line or a burst-suppression pattern on the electroencephalogram (EEG). These patients will require intubation, admission to an intensive care unit, and continuous EEG monitoring. These patients may also require vasopressor support secondary to barbi-turate-induced hypotension.

After stabilization or cessation of seizure activity, con-sultation with a neurologist (if not already obtained) and further evaluation including EEG and head imaging are recommended.

CENTRAL NERVOUS SYSTEM INFECTIONS

Seizures associated with fever may be benign (see section on febrile seizures, later in this chapter) or the hallmark of an underlying CNS infection. In various studies 7% to 23% of patients with meningitis and 22% to 60% of patients with encephalitis developed seizures. Worldwide, calcifications sec-ondary to neurocysticercosis *(Taenia solium)* infection are one of the leading infectious causes of seizures.

Symptoms
- Altered level of consciousness
- Irritability
- Headache
- Vomiting
- Disorientation/confusion
- Somnolence

Signs

- Fever ++++
- Bulging fontanel ++
- Irritability ++
- Vomiting ++
- Lethargy ++
- Nuchal rigidity +++
- Kernig's sign ++
- Brudzinski's sign ++
- Abnormal mental status
- Coma

Workup

Consideration of the potential for an infectious cause of the seizure is critical. In patients without evidence of increased ICP and whose history and examination findings are not consistent with a simple febrile seizure (see the section Febrile, later in this chapter), an LP should be performed with CSF studies sent for cell count, chemistry (protein and glucose concentrations), gram stain, culture, and/or polymerase chain reaction (PCR). Imaging studies (CT or MRI) should be obtained in patients with focal seizure activity, in those with potentially elevated ICP, or if abscess/focal infection is suspected. Administration of antibiotics should not be significantly delayed for diagnostic studies and empiric treatment should be given promptly when CNS infection is being considered as the cause of seizure (see Chapter 3, Altered Mental Status, and Chapter 14, Fever).

HEAD TRAUMA

Although most head injuries are benign, seizures can result from traumatic depolarization of the cortex (immediately); from focal injury such as contusion, hemorrhage, ischemia, or edema (most within 24 hours but may occur up to a week after the trauma); or from scarring caused by vascular compromise, distortion, or mechanical irritation of the brain (>1 week after injury). A head CT scan should be obtained in all patients with posttraumatic seizures developing after the immediate traumatic event and considered in all patients with brief immediate seizures. Some recent studies suggest that immediate posttraumatic seizures have no prognostic implications for intracranial abnormalities. Nonaccidental trauma should be considered and an examination for other injuries undertaken if the findings are not consistent with the described mechanism of injury (see Chapter 3, Altered Mental Status, and Chapter 2, Abuse/Rape).

NEONATAL SEIZURES

The clinical manifestations of neonatal seizures are frequently quite subtle and can be overlooked. Because of the immaturity of the developing brain, infants (particularly those who are premature) may present with seizures that are not clearly clonic, tonic, or myoclonic.

Symptoms
- History of difficult birth
- Prematurity
- Increased tone

Signs
- Ocular phenomena (deviation of eyes with or without jerking of eyes or staring)
- Oral-buccal movements (chewing, lip smacking)
- Facial wincing
- Posturing
- Jerks
- Apnea
- Tachypnea
- Tachycardia
- Bradycardia

Workup
- EEG.
- Head CT or head ultrasound (to rule out hypoxic-ischemic encephalopathy or intracranial hemorrhage).
- Electrolytes (sodium, glucose, calcium, magnesium in particular).

- LP for CSF cell count, glucose and protein concentration, and culture.
- Serum amino and urine organic acids.

Comments and Treatment Considerations

The infant with evidence of repeated seizure activity must be treated promptly. First, as with older children and adults, adequacy of ventilation, oxygenation, and perfusion must be maintained.

If there is evidence of hypoglycemia, D10W at 2 ml/kg IV should be given and glucose-containing maintenance fluids begun. If hypoglycemia is not present, a benzodiazepine can be given followed by phenobarbital. Phenobarbital dosed at 20 mg/kg IV is the recommended first-line anticonvulsant agent for neonates. This can be given over 10 to 15 minutes with careful monitoring of respiratory effort. Phenobarbital can be repeated at 5 mg/kg/dose boluses up to a total cumulative dose of 40 mg/kg but watch for respiratory depression and need for airway management. Fosphenytoin or lorazepam can be given if the seizures persist (see dosing earlier in this chapter).

If there is evidence of hypocalcemia, calcium gluconate dosed at 4 ml/kg IV of a 5% solution can be given. Calcium should be infused via a central or large peripheral line; scalp and small hand and foot veins should be avoided. For hypomagnesemia, magnesium sulfate dosed at 0.2 to 0.4 mEq/kg (25 to 50 mg/kg) IV diluted to <200 mg/ml and infused over at least 10-20 minutes can be given. Be prepared to manage the airway because respiratory depression can be a side effect of a large, rapid magnesium load.

If seizures persist, pyridoxine deficiency should be considered as a rare cause of neonatal seizures and can be corrected with an empiric dose of pyridoxine 100 mg as a slow IV infusion.

Consult neurology for further management issues.

 ## CARDIAC ABNORMALITIES

Cardiac dysrhythmias may present as atypical seizures (see Chapter 34, Tachycardia)

METABOLIC ABNORMALITIES

Electrolyte and metabolic abnormalities may also cause seizures, particularly hyponatremia, hypoglycemia, hypocalcemia, and hypomagnesemia. In general, the routine screening for electrolyte abnormalities in a patient with seizures is a very low yield procedure. Unfortunately, seizures caused by electrolyte derangements are often refractory to anticonvulsant therapy and patients will continue with seizure activity until the underlying abnormality is corrected. Serum electrolytes should be measured in all patients with seizures and significant vomiting or diarrhea; those with underlying renal, hepatic, neoplastic or endocrinologic disease; those who are taking medications that may lead to electrolyte disturbances; or those who have seizures that are refractory to typical anticonvulsant management. Other patients may be evaluated on a case-by-case basis. Intravenous glucose, calcium, magnesium, or hypertonic (3%) sodium chloride should be used to treat the appropriate abnormal condition. In the case of hyponatremia, once the seizure activity has been stopped, the rate of sodium correction must be immediately reduced to avoid possible central pontine myelinolysis.

CENTRAL NERVOUS SYSTEM TUMOR

Any tumor of the CNS can cause seizures (see Chapter 3, Altered Mental Status).

INGESTION

Many ingestions or overdoses can cause seizures. Toxicologic screening may be helpful in the seizing patient because certain ingestions are managed with specific antidotes or treatments, remembering that not all substances are identifiable on toxicology screens. Typically the clinical scenarios are the young child with a possible unintentional ingestion or the adolescent seeking to "get high" or to commit suicide. In general, the toxicologic screen should be ordered to identify suspected agents known to cause seizures or those agents suggested by a clinical toxidrome.

Ingestions/toxins associated with seizures include the following:
- Camphor
- Carbon monoxide
- Cocaine
- Heavy metals (lead)
- Hypoglycemic agents
- Isoniazid
- Lithium
- Methylxanthines (theophylline or caffeine)
- Pesticides (organophosphates)
- Phencyclidine
- Sympathomimetics
- Tricyclic antidepressants
- Topical anesthetics

Consultation with a poison center specialist is recommended (see Chapter 35, Toxic Ingestion, Approach To).

 ## FEBRILE SEIZURES

Febrile seizures are the most common convulsive disorder in young children, occurring in 2% to 5% of the population. A consensus statement by the National Institutes of Health defines febrile seizures as a seizure occurring in anyone between 3 months and 5 years of age that is associated with a fever but without evidence of intracranial infection or other defined cause.

Febrile seizures can be of any type but most commonly are generalized tonic-clonic seizures. They are usually self-limited and last for only a few seconds to minutes. Febrile seizures are classified either as *simple* febrile seizures (which last <15 minutes and are generalized) or as *complex* febrile seizures (which are prolonged or focal and recur within 24 hours). Simple febrile seizures (85%) are much more common. There is also a familial tendency toward febrile seizures, but the exact inheritance pattern is uncertain.

Symptoms
- Fever

Signs
- Fever
- Nonfocal neurologic examination findings after seizure

Workup
LP for cell count, gram stain, glucose and protein concentration, and culture is recommended in children younger than 12 months of age and should be strongly considered in children 12 to 18 months of age because typical signs of meningitis may be absent in these age-groups. Seizure may be the first presentation of meningitis. LP should also be performed in patients with complex febrile seizures or a concerning physical or neurologic finding.

In patients between 18 months and 5 years of age for whom the history is consistent with a simple febrile seizure, there is no clinical concern for CNS infection, if the neurologic examination findings are normal then further neurologic evaluation is not indicated, although further fever evaluation may be warranted based on age and immune and vaccination status (see Chapter 14, Fever).

Patients older than 5 years require a full evaluation (see the section Seizures without an Identifiable Cause).

Comments and Treatment Considerations
After the first febrile seizure, approximately 33% of patients will have at least one recurrence and about 9% will have three or more episodes. The younger the patient at first presentation, the greater the likelihood of recurrence. Most recurrences (75%) will also happen within 1 year. The exact risk of developing epilepsy after a febrile seizure is unknown, but most studies indicate that it is <5%. Risk factors for developing epilepsy after a febrile seizure include abnormal development before the episode, a family history of afebrile seizures, and a complex first febrile seizure.

The treatment of a patient who presents during a febrile seizure is identical to that for those with other seizure types (see the earlier section Status Epilepticus). The primary goal is the establishment of a clear airway, and secondary efforts are then directed at termination of the seizure if prolonged. Simple

Table 32–1	Diazepam Rectal Gel (Diastat) Dosing
Age	Dose
<6 mo	Not recommended
6 mo to 2 yr	Safety and efficacy unknown
2-5 yr	0.5 mg/kg/dose
6-11 yr	0.3 mg/kg/dose
≥12 yr	0.2 mg/kg/dose

febrile seizures are usually brief and the typical patient presents for evaluation with seizure activity having spontaneously ended.

Patients who have a simple febrile seizure may be safely discharged to home. Parents should be reassured that febrile seizures are quite common and that most patients have no further episodes. They do need to be cautioned about the chance that a recurrence may happen and should be given simple instructions on what to do should another seizure occur. They can also be instructed on the proper use of antipyretics, although several studies have failed to document that acetaminophen or ibuprofen is effective in reducing the recurrence rate as many febrile seizures occur during the initial rapid increase in body temperature associated with viral illness. Acetaminophen should be dosed at 15 mg/kg/dose (max 1000 mg/dose) PO/PR q4-6h not to exceed 75 mg/kg/day or 4 g/day, whichever is less. Ibuprofen is generally dosed at 10 mg/kg/dose (max 800 mg/dose) PO q6h, not to exceed 40 mg/kg/day. Aspirin is not recommended as an antipyretic for the prevention of febrile seizures because of the risk of Reye's syndrome. Some children with recurrent or complex febrile seizures may also benefit from the home use of rectal diazepam (Diastat); see Table 32-1 for dosing. Finally, any identified source of the fever should be properly treated.

 ## SUBTHERAPEUTIC ANTICONVULSANT LEVELS

Subtherapeutic anticonvulsant levels are one of the leading causes of seizure in a patient with a known seizure disorder who presents for medical evaluation. A thorough history of medication use and anticonvulsant levels must be obtained in any patient who presents with a seizure. Treatment requires adjustment of dosing and/or replacing missed doses after consultation with the child's neurologist.

 ## SEIZURES WITHOUT AN IDENTIFIABLE CAUSE

Many children will have a history of a nonfebrile seizure or a brief seizure that did not affect oxygenation or ventilation and did not require anticonvulsant therapy. The physician must rule out any concerning etiologies that would require immediate identification and therapy, particularly possible infection or trauma, discussed in the preceding sections. A neurologically normal patient with normal laboratory and imaging study findings (if obtained) may be able to be discharged home without anticonvulsants to follow-up with a neurologist for further evaluation EEG, and possible MRI. Many practitioners are not obtaining an initial head CT unless needed to rule out an emergent diagnosis if an MRI can be obtained in a relatively short period of time and provide greater anatomic detail. Most parents will require a significant amount of reassurance and education on what to do should another seizure occur. When in doubt about safety for discharge, a consultation with a neurologist should be sought. Some families will require admission for observation because of parental anxiety.

 ## NONSEIZURE PAROXYSMAL EVENTS

A number of childhood paroxysmal events are often mistaken for seizure activity. Every attempt should be made to differentiate these events from seizures to ensure appropriate diagnosis, correct treatment, and accurate prognosis. Each "episode" should be evaluated by examining the preceding events, the episode itself, and the nature and duration of the postictal impairment.

SYNCOPE

A large percentage of patients with syncope exhibit some sort of convulsive movement that may be confused with true seizure activity. Although vasovagal episodes or orthostatic hypotension are the most common causes for syncope, these patients must be evaluated for possible underlying cardiac disease and if any doubt exists for seizure (see Chapter 33, Syncope).

BREATH-HOLDING SPELLS

Breath-holding spells are quite common, affecting 4% to 5% of all children, and may be confused with seizures. (see Chapter 4, Apnea).

MOVEMENT AND OTHER NONSPECIFIC DISORDERS

Paroxysmal choreoathetosis is often associated with a positive family history and exacerbated by intentional movement. Tic disorders can manifest by twitching, blinking, head shaking, or other repetitive motions. These are usually suppressible and are not associated with any loss of consciousness. Shudder attacks are whole-body tremors similar to essential tremor in adults. Benign myoclonus of infancy can look like seizures but are associated with a completely normal EEG. Somnambulism, night terrors (preschool-aged children), and narcolepsy (typically in adolescents) can often be diagnosed based on the history alone. Infants with gastroesophageal reflux may exhibit torticollis or dystonic posturing (Sandifer's syndrome). Atypical migraines and pseudoseizures are often diagnosed after other etiologies are excluded.

REFERENCES

Annegers JF, Hauser WA, Beghi E, et al: The risk of unprovoked seizures after encephalitis and meningitis, *Neurology* 38(9):1407-1410, 1988.

Chiang VW: Seizures. In Fleisher GF, Ludwig S, editors: *Textbook of pediatric emergency medicine*, 4th ed, Philadelphia, 2000, Lippincott Williams & Wilkins.

Green SM, Rothrock SG, Clem KJ, et al: Can seizures be the sole manifestation of meningitis in febrile children? *Pediatrics* 92(4):527-534, 1993.

Lowenstein DH, Alldredge BK: Status epilepticus, *N Engl J Med* 338:970-976, 1998.

Provisional Committee on Quality Improvement: Subcommittee on Febrile Seizures, Practice Parameter: The neurodiagnostic evaluation of the child with a first simple febrile seizure, *Pediatrics* 97(5):769-771, 1996.

Rosman NP: Evaluation of the child with febrile seizures. In Baram TZ, Shinnar S, editors: *Febrile seizures*, Boston, 2002, Academic Press.

Schutzman SA: Injury: head. In Fleisher GF, Ludwig S, editors: *Textbook of pediatric emergency medicine*, 4th ed, Philadelphia, 2000, Lippincott Williams & Wilkins.

Vining EP: Pediatric seizures, *Emerg Med Clin North Am* 12:973-988, 1994.

Volpe JJ: Neonatal seizures. In Volpe JJ, editor: *Neurology of the newborn*, 4th ed, Philadelphia, 2000, WB Saunders.

Whitley RJ, Kimberlin DW: Viral encephalitis, *Pediatr Rev* 20(6):192-198, 1999.

CHAPTER 33

Syncope

SARA SCHUTZMAN

Syncope is a transient, usually brief, nontraumatic loss of consciousness and postural tone caused by an impairment in cerebral perfusion or substrate delivery (oxygen or glucose). More common in older children and teens, syncope occurs in approximately 15% of children by the end of adolescence and accounts for approximately 0.1% to 1.0% of ED visits. Most episodes of syncope are due to benign etiologies; however, it rarely may be due to an underlying process that puts the patient at risk for sudden death (Table 33-1).

Clinicians can usually determine the most likely cause of syncope based on the history, physical examination, and a few simple tests. The history should include a description of the circumstances, any prodrome, the episode itself, and the recovery period, as well as a complete medical and family history. Syncope occurring during exercise or with no apparent cause (especially while seated or supine) and those with either no prodrome or chest pain/palpitations are more concerning for serious underlying pathology (see Chapter 34, Tachycardia). History of neurologic or cardiac problems and family history of sudden death are of obvious concern.

A complete physical examination with particular attention to cardiac and neurologic examination is mandatory. All patients should have a screening ECG and vital signs. Postpubertal females should take a pregnancy test. The clinician should strongly consider checking hematocrit, glucose concentration, and orthostatic blood pressure. Further diagnostic testing is guided by the results of the history and physical. When there are diagnostic questions after this initial evaluation, or when syncope is recurrent, referrals for specialized testing may be indicated.

Table 33-1 Differential Diagnosis of Syncope

True Syncope
- Vascular/reflex
  - Vasovagal (a.k.a., vasodepressor, neurocardiogenic), orthostatic hypotension, situational (cough/micturition), hyperventilation, Valsalva, pregnancy, anemia/volume loss, breath-holding, pulmonary embolus
- Cardiac
  - Structural, dysrhythmia
- Neurologic
  - Migraine, tumor/increased intracranial pressure, cerebrovascular accident/transient ischemic attack
- Toxic/metabolic
  - Hypoxemia, hypoglycemia, carbon monoxide, drug

Seizure

Hysterical Pseudosyncope

 CARDIOGENIC SYNCOPE

Although uncommon, cardiac causes for syncope are potentially lethal and must be ruled out in any patient with syncope. Although one study of patients coming to the ED with syncope found no patients had a cardiac cause (N = 40), two larger studies of patients referred to cardiology and/or neurology clinic found 5% to 6% had a cardiac etiology of syncope. Ritter et al. (2000) found that 21 of 22 patients with cardiac syncope had a concerning history, abnormal physical examination findings, a positive family history, or abnormal ECG findings. Cardiac causes include the following:

Dysrhythmias
- Tachydysrhythmia
  - Supraventricular tachycardias (SVTs) (though frank syncope unusual in this case)
  - Ventricular tachycardia: Etiologies include the following:

- Prolonged QT interval: This may be congenital or acquired; if familial, may be associated with congenital deafness. Acquired causes include myocarditis, stroke, electrolyte imbalance, and drugs (tricyclic antidepressants, phenothiazines, class I antiarrhythmics).
- Catecholamine or drug induced
- Postsurgical or other conduction system disease
- Bradycardia
  - Heart block
  - Sinus node disease (including postoperative)
  - Vagotonia

Structural Heart Disease

Ineffective cardiac output may result from the following:
- Outflow obstruction
  - Hypertrophic obstructive cardiomyopathy
  - Aortic stenosis
  - Pulmonic stenosis
  - Atrial myxoma
  - Pulmonary hypertension
- Anomalous coronary artery
- Other congenital heart disease
- Cardiomyopathy/myocarditis
- Pericarditis with tamponade

Symptoms

- Occurs during exercise or in a seated/recumbent position
- Either no prodrome or associated chest pain or palpitations
- Patients may report weakness, fatigue, or dyspnea
- May have more prolonged loss of consciousness (>5 minutes)
- May have family history of sudden death, dysrhythmia, or congenital deafness
- May have history of drug ingestion or abuse

Signs

- If abnormal cardiac structure or function, the patient may exhibit an abnormal heart rate (HR), blood pressure (BP), or have a cardiac murmur, rub, or gallop

- If a dysrhythmia is present, the patient will have an obvious abnormal rate, but if the preceding dysrhythmia has resolved, examination findings may be normal

Workup

- Complete history and physical examination including orthostatic vital signs.
- ECG: Normal findings do not exclude cardiac disease. Abnormalities concerning for cardiac etiology include abnormal HR, rhythm, intervals, and voltages. A QT and a corrected QT (QTc) interval must be calculated and then corrected for variation caused by HR.

$$QTc = \frac{\text{Measured QT (sec)}}{\sqrt{\text{R-R interval (sec)}}}$$

Normal QTc values are as follows:
$\leq$0.45 second in infants younger than 6 months
$\leq$0.44 second in children
$\leq$0.425 second in adolescents and adults

- Consider CXR, particularly if concerns for structural disease. Look for cardiomegaly, an abnormally shaped heart/great vessel, or abnormal pulmonary blood flow.
- Consider echocardiogram if high suspicion for structural abnormality.
- Labs to evaluate drugs/electrolytes should be obtained as warranted.
- Human chorionic gonadotropin (hCG) in postpubertal females.

Comments and Treatment Considerations

If the history or examination findings are concerning, a normal ECG does not rule out a cardiac cause of syncope. Further evaluation may include Holter monitoring, echocardiography, stress test, event recorders, or electrophysiologic testing. Concern for a cardiac etiology of syncope should prompt consultation with a cardiologist. Patients with syncopal episodes and a prolonged QTc interval should be discussed immediately and then referred to a cardiologist. Further evaluation and treatment will obviously be individualized (see Chapter 34, Tachycardia).

 ## NEUROLOGIC/INTRACRANIAL

Though not truly a syncopal episode, seizure is one of the most common causes of loss of consciousness, and children with seizures are commonly brought to the ED for evaluation of "passing out." In two studies of children evaluated for syncope, 8% had seizures. Seizures may be distinguished from syncope by differences in the history (prodrome uncommon, frequent tonic-clonic activity, unconsciousness often >5 minutes, and prolonged postictal/confusional phase), although this may be difficult with unwitnessed episodes (see Chapter 32, Seizures).

Neurologic and CNS causes of true syncope are rare and include syncopal migraine, stroke, increased ICP, and subarachnoid hemorrhage (see Chapter 17, Headache).

 ## TOXIC/METABOLIC

Drugs (nonprescription, prescription, and illicit) may cause syncope for a variety of reasons. Diuretics and antihypertensives can affect the vasomotor tone or volume status of patients and may cause orthostatic syncope. Tricyclics, fluoroquinolones, and phenothiazines are only a few of the drugs that may prolong the QT interval. Sympathomimetics may cause SVT. Cocaine can cause direct toxic effects on the cardiovascular system, eliciting hypertension, SVT, and ventricular dysrhythmias (see Chapter 35, Toxic Ingestion, Approach To).

Metabolic causes of syncope include hypoglycemia and hypoxemia (including carbon monoxide poisoning and asphyxiant-related hypoxia). Syncope from hypoglycemia is rare and is typically preceded by symptoms that may include weakness, hunger, sweating, agitation, and confusion (see Chapter 30, Respiratory Distress, and Chapter 32, Seizure).

ORTHOSTATIC HYPOTENSION

Orthostatic hypotension can result from decreased circulating blood volume (from anemia/hemorrhage or volume deficit caused by vomiting, diarrhea, sweating, inadequate intake, and/or hyperglycemia), drugs (vasodilators, diuretics, or those affecting the autonomic nervous system), venous pooling, prolonged recumbency, or rarely autonomic neuropathy. In a study of pediatric patients coming to the ED with syncope, orthostatic hypotension caused 20% of episodes (15% caused by dehydration and 5% caused by anemia).

Symptoms
- Typically occurs immediately after rising from a sitting or supine position
- Symptoms that may occur before loss of consciousness include:
  - Light-headedness
  - Weakness
  - Visual changes
  - Diaphoresis
  - Nausea
  - Epigastric discomfort

Signs
- If anemic or dehydrated, the patient may have pallor, signs of dehydration, or poor perfusion

Workup
- Orthostatic vital signs (HR and BP when supine, seated, and standing) are considered positive if there is a >20 mm Hg decrease in systolic BP moving from supine to seated to standing or an abnormal increase in HR+++.
- ECG.
- hCG in postpubertal females.
- Hematocrit.
- Glucose.
- Electrolytes may be warranted with history of volume loss or signs of dehydration.

Comments and Treatment Considerations

Patients with anemia should undergo evaluation for the etiology with treatment based on the cause and degree of anemia (see Chapter 6, Bleeding and Bruising). Patients with volume depletion should be rehydrated (orally or intravenously, depending on degree and situation) and evaluated for the underlying cause (see Chapter 20, Hypotension/Shock, and Chapter 38, Vomiting). Consider ruptured ectopic pregnancy in pregnant females with unexplained syncope.

 HYPERVENTILATION

Hyperventilation may be volitional or due to anxiety and causes hypocapnia (resulting in cerebral vasoconstriction) and respiratory alkalosis (causing a decrease in serum ionized calcium). Hyperventilation generally causes weakness and light-headedness rather than frank syncope.

Symptoms
- History of breathing fast or heavy, typically in the setting of feeling anxious
- Light-headedness, paresthesias, or carpopedal spasm; frank syncope less common
- Other symptoms include breathlessness, chest pain, palpitations, blurred vision, and/or tremors/muscle pain

Signs
- If episode ongoing, patient will be breathing faster and/or deeper than normal
- May have carpopedal spasm, if ongoing hyperventilation
- Normal examination findings if hyperventilation has resolved

Workup
- Complete history and physical examination.
- ECG and pregnancy test with consideration for hematocrit, glucose, electrolytes, and calcium if indicated to rule out organic causes of syncope.

- When a diagnosis with psychological implications is being considered, the physician may elect to order supportive laboratory tests. A blood gas determination that demonstrates a respiratory alkalosis can be useful but is generally not needed.

Comments and Treatment Considerations

If still hyperventilating, the patient can breathe into a paper bag, thereby inspiring air enriched with CO_2. Emphasizing to the patient his or her control over the symptoms and reassuring them that nothing is wrong can be beneficial. Further counseling may be necessary to discover the sources of psychological disturbance.

 ## *NEUROCARDIOGENIC (VASOVAGAL) SYNCOPE (VASODEPRESSOR SYNCOPE OR "SIMPLE FAINT")*

Symptoms
- A history of identifiable triggering events, including pain, emotional stress, or anxiety
- Occurs while upright, often exacerbated by hot/crowded conditions
- May have history of similar episodes
- Presyncopal or prodromal symptoms lasting a few seconds to a few minutes includes light-headedness, dizziness, headache, visual changes, diaphoresis, weakness, nausea/epigastric distress, and/or pallor
- Period of loss of consciousness typically brief (<1 to 2 minutes)
- Patient without prolonged confusion/recovery phase

Signs
- The physical examination findings are most often normal
- Decreased HR and low BP are noted if the patient is still symptomatic

Workup
- Complete history and physical examination (including orthostatic vital signs).

- ECG.
- hCG in postpubertal females.
- Hematocrit and glucose as indicated.

Comments and Treatment Considerations

In one ED study, neurocardiogenic syncope caused 50% of all syncopal episodes. It may be differentiated from seizure and cardiac etiologies based on the typical history and a benign examination and screening test results. Head-upright tilt-table testing may be useful for recurrent episodes or if the diagnosis is in question. Treatment usually consists of reassurance and recommendations to avoid situations that predispose to syncope. For the rare child with recurrent vasodepressor syncope, pharmacologic prophylaxis may be needed.

BREATH-HOLDING SPELLS

Breath-holding spells occur in infants and young children, may be cyanotic or pallid, and tend to have a classic history. Infants and young children who have syncope without a history consistent with these spells should undergo a more extensive evaluation for other more serious causes of syncope (see Chapter 4, Apnea).

HYSTERICAL (PSEUDOSYNCOPE)

Hysterical syncope is a feigned faint. It typically occurs in an adolescent and in front of an audience. Patients can describe the event, suggesting a lack of complete loss of consciousness.

Symptoms
- No overt or objective prodromal symptoms
- May have history of eye fluttering behind half-closed eyes
- Pallor not observed
- Fall is typically gentle "swoon"; self-protective behaviors are preserved, so unlikely to have injuries

Signs
• Normal physical examination

Workup
• Complete history and physical examination.
• Screening studies as indicated (notably ECG, pregnancy test, and drug testing).

Comments and Treatment Considerations
Hysterical syncope should be a diagnosis of exclusion (typical history and normal examination/screening study results). If more significant stressors or psychopathology is suspected, psychological evaluation and counseling may be warranted.

REFERENCES
Delgado CA: Syncope. In Fleisher GR, Ludwig S, editors: *Textbook of pediatric emergency medicine*, 4th ed, Philadelphia, 2000, Lippincott Williams & Wilkins.

DiMario FJ: Breathholding spells in childhood, *Curr Probl Pediatr* 29:281-299, 1999.

Farah MM, Zorc JJ: Behavioral emergencies. In Fleisher GR, Ludwig S, editors: *Textbook of pediatric emergency medicine*, 4th ed, Philadelphia, 2000, Lippincott Williams & Wilkins.

Hanna DE, Hodgens JB, Daniel WA: Hyperventilation syndrome, *Pediatr Ann* 15:708-712, 1986.

Hannon DW, Knilans TK: Syncope in children and adolescents, *Curr Probl Pediatr* 23:358-384, 1993.

Lerman-Sagie T, Rechavia E, Strasberg B, et al: Head-up tilt for the evaluation of syncope of unknown origin in children, *J Pediatr* 5:676-679, 1991.

Lombroso CT, Lerman: Breathholding spells (cyanotic and pallid infantile syncope), *Pediatrics* 39:563-581, 1967.

McHarg ML, Shinnar S, Rascoff H, Walsh CA: Syncope in childhood, *Pediatr Cardiol* 18:367-371, 1997.

Pratt JL, Fleisher GR: Syncope in children and adolescents, *Pediatr Emerg Care* 5:80-82, 1989.

Ritter S, Tani L, Etheridge SP, et al: What is the yield of screening echocardiography in pediatric syncope? *Pediatrics* 105(5):e58, 2000.

CHAPTER 34

Tachycardia

MARY CHRISTINE BAILEY

Tachycardia in childhood is most commonly a sinus tachycardia. Although malignant dysrhythmias are less common in children than in adults, they require prompt intervention and can prove deadly if not recognized and treated aggressively.

The first goal in evaluating a child with tachycardia is to determine whether the rapid heart rate (HR) is due to a physiologic hyperdynamic state or secondary to a dysrhythmia. Once this determination is made, treatment will be based on the etiology of the tachycardia. In children with dysrhythmias, early consultation with a cardiologist is generally warranted.

Because the normal HR varies with age in children, it is important to know the normal HR ranges for a specific age-group to determine whether tachycardia is present (Table 34-1).

 ## VENTRICULAR TACHYCARDIA

Ventricular tachycardia (VT) has been shown to be present in up to 17% of children older than 8 years who suffer cardiac arrest. In the pediatric patient not in arrest, signs and symptoms of VT can be very subtle. Any wide-complex tachycardia should be considered ventricular in origin until proven otherwise. Electrophysiologic studies have suggested that it is nearly impossible to definitively diagnose a wide-complex tachycardia as being supraventricular in origin. Erroneously treating VT as a supraventricular tachycardia (SVT) with aberrant conduction can be deadly.

VT may be associated with hypertrophic cardiomyopathy, myocarditis, or postsurgical repair of congenital heart disease (CHD). Many drugs can cause VT, including tricyclic antidepressants, cocaine, and amphetamines. Torsades de

Table 34-1   Normal Heart Rate Range by Age

Age-Group	Heart Rate Range (beats per minute)
Newborn	100-160
Infant	120-160
Toddler	80-150
Child older than 6 yr	60-120

pointes is a specific type of VT that is marked by varying amplitude of the QRS complex. Torsades de pointes is associated with certain drug ingestions, especially tricyclic antidepressants, and as part of an inherited conduction abnormality referred to as the *long QTc syndrome*. Long QTc syndrome should always be considered in children with seizures or syncope (see Chapter 33, Syncope).

Symptoms

Although many children with brief episodes of VT will be asymptomatic, concerning symptoms when present include the following:
- Syncope or near syncope, especially if associated with exercise, should always be considered secondary to a dysrhythmia, particularly torsades, until proven otherwise (see Chapter 33, Syncope)
- Seizures can be the first presenting symptom of torsades de pointes
- Shortness of breath, poor feeding, lethargy, and restlessness can be seen in children with congestive heart failure (CHF) caused by VT
- Palpitations that are irregular or sustained are often associated with an underlying dysrhythmia
- Chest pain may be reported by the older patient

Signs

Signs are most commonly related to resultant CHF and include the following:
- Pallor with poor perfusion
- Cyanosis

- Tachypnea, dyspnea, wheezing, and retractions
- Hepatomegaly

Workup

- ECG is always indicated and may exhibit a recognizable rhythm pattern. The corrected QT (QTc) interval should be measured and is abnormal if >0.45 second (Fig. 34-1) in patients of any age. It can be determined by the formula:

$$QTc = \frac{\text{Measured QT (sec)}}{\sqrt{\text{R-R interval (sec)}}}$$

- A rhythm strip and continuous bedside monitoring is helpful in patients with unstable or potentially unstable rhythms.
- Potassium, magnesium, calcium, and electrolytes should be measured because metabolic derangements can result in ventricular arrhythmias. Hypokalemia, hyperkalemia, hypomagnesemia, acidemia, and hypocalcemia all need to be considered.
- Toxicology screen may identify some of the drugs that can induce arrhythmias.
- Consider tamponade, tension pneumothorax, and thromboembolism if indicated (see Chapter 8, Chest Pain, and Chapter 30, Respiratory Distress).

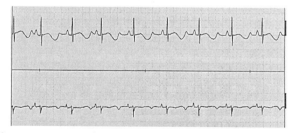

Fig. 34-1 Portion of a 24-hour ambulatory monitor recording from a patient with long QT syndrome and multifaceted T waves with a short ST segment. (From Gillette P, Garson A: *Clinical pediatric arrhythmias,* 2nd ed, Philadelphia, 1999, WB Saunders.)

- CXR can show signs of CHF, abnormal heart shape suggestive of CHD, or an enlarged heart consistent with hypertrophic cardiomyopathy or myocarditis.

Comments and Treatment Considerations

The rapidity with which treatment must be instituted depends on the patient's diagnosis and circulatory status.

Pulseless VT/VF

- ABCs, cardiopulmonary resuscitation, 100% oxygen by bag-mask ventilation (do not delay defibrillation for intubation).
- Defibrillate three times, checking the rhythm after each shock without removing paddles from patient's chest.
  - First shock: 2 J/kg (max 200 J).
  - Second shock: 2-4 J/kg (max 300 J).
  - Third and all subsequent shocks: 4 J/kg (max 360 J).
- If persistent pulseless VT/ventricular fibrillation (VF)
  - Establish IV/IO access and give epinephrine 0.01 mg/kg (0.1 ml/kg of 1:10,000 solution) then repeat shock.
  - If access not available, give epinephrine via endotracheal tube (ETT) at a dose of 0.1 mg/kg (0.1 ml/kg of 1:1000 solution diluted in 3-5 ml of NS). Follow with several positive pressure breaths to ensure adequate dispersion.
- If pulseless VT or VF continues or recurs after the above treatment, give one of the following:
  - Amiodarone 5 mg/kg bolus (max 300 mg/dose) followed by a shock.
  OR
  - Lidocaine 1 mg/kg bolus followed by shock.
  - Identify and treat possible etiologies of arrhythmia (Table 34-2).

Table 34-2   Potentially Treatable Causes of Arrhythmias

• Hypoxemia	• Tamponade
• Hypovolemia	• Tension pneumothorax
• Hyperthermia	• Toxins/poisons/drugs
• Hyperkalemia/hypokalemia and other metabolic disorders	• Thromboembolism

Torsades de pointes or documented hypomagnesemia

Treatment of choice is magnesium sulfate as an IV/IO bolus of 25 to 50 mg/kg over 10 to 20 minutes. May repeat to a maximum total dose of 2 g. Be prepared to manage the airway because respiratory depression can be a side effect of a large, rapid magnesium load.

Stable VT: If the child is alert with palpable pulses

- Early consultation with a cardiologist is recommended.
- Focus on determining and correcting the etiology of the tachycardia (see Tables 34-2).
- Consider cardioversion with 0.5 to 1 J/kg with sedation.
- Consider medical therapy with:
  Amiodarone 5 mg/kg (max 300 mg/dose) over 20-60 minutes.
  OR
  Procainamide: 15 mg/kg IV over 30-60 minutes (do not use with amiodarone).
  OR
  Lidocaine: 1 mg/kg over 2-4 minutes.

 ## ATRIAL TACHYCARDIA

Atrial dysrhythmias other than SVT are extremely rare in children and are seen primarily in children who have had repair of CHD. Consider in any child who has undergone repair of CHD or if adenosine fails to convert SVT. Consultation with a pediatric cardiologist is recommended.

SUPRAVENTRICULAR TACHYCARDIA

SVT is the most common arrhythmia in children. The term *SVT* describes a group of tachyarrhythmias with similar ECG features but different mechanisms. Sixty percent of children with SVT have structurally normal hearts and no predisposing factors. Infants presenting in the first few months of life with the first episode of SVT will often go unrecognized. CHF may ensue with resultant symptoms such as poor feeding, restlessness, listlessness, or fussiness.

A rhythm strip or continuous bedside cardiac monitoring can usually identify SVT. The hallmark is a HR >220 beats per minute in an infant and >180 beats per minute in an older child and a monotonous rhythm with no beat-to-beat variation in rate.

Symptoms

- Dizziness, palpitations, fatigue, and chest pain may be described by the older child
- The sensation of pounding in the neck can also be reported by the older patient (particularly common in atrioventricular node reentrant tachycardia caused by cannon waves)

Signs

- Pallor, sweating, dyspnea, and/or tachypnea, especially in infants and younger children
- Tachycardia may be described by the older patient

Workup

- ECG will reveal a narrow an-complex tachycardia with a HR >220 beats per minute in infant and >180 beats per minute in an older child. P waves will be absent or abnormal. A rhythm strip shows a monotonous rhythm with no beat-to-beat variability. A delta wave (slurred upstroke of the R wave) and a short PR interval can be seen in the Wolff-Parkinson-White type of SVT (Figs. 34-2 and 34-3).
- CXR is indicated for first episode of SVT.

Comments and Treatment Considerations

Initial management choices are dictated by the stability of the patient and the distance from a pediatric cardiologist. Patients with unstable SVT require emergent therapy.

After conversion to a normal rhythm, pediatric cardiology consultation is recommended to determine the patient's electrophysiology. Asymptomatic patients with recurrent SVT may be safely discharged home after vagal or medical cardioversion and discussion with their cardiologist.

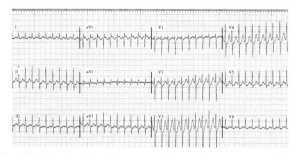

Fig. 34-2 Twelve-lead electrocardiogram in a patient with atrioventricular node reentrant tachycardia. Note that P waves are not discernible because they are buried in the QRS complex. (From Gillette P, Garson A: *Clinical pediatric arrhythmias,* 2nd ed, Philadelphia, 1999, WB Saunders.)

SVT Therapy

- Unstable SVT: CHF with poor perfusion, decreased pulses, altered mental status, increased work of breathing, or hypotension
  - Synchronized cardioversion: 0.5 J/kg. If persistent SVT, repeat cardioversion at 1 J/kg increments until effective or 4 J/kg is reached.
  - Support the ABCs and treat underlying or associated issues, especially hypoxia and acidosis (see Table 34-1).
- Stable SVT
  - Attempt vagal maneuvers first. In infants, applying ice to the face for 15 to 30 seconds will induce the diving reflex. An older child can be asked to bear down as if they were trying to stool or have them blow as hard as they can into a straw that is crimped or occluded at the end.
  - Adenosine is the drug of choice for initial medical therapy for SVT in the stable patient. The first dose should be given at 0.1 mg/kg (max 6 mg/dose) simultaneously with a rapid 5 ml 0.9% NS push. If

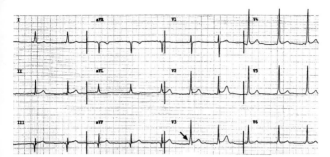

Fig. 34-3 Wolff-Parkinson-White syndrome. Note delta wave *(arrows)*. (From David M, Votey, S, Greenough PG: *Signs and symptoms in emergency medicine*, St. Louis, 1999, Mosby.)

conversion to normal sinus rhythm does not occur, give a second dose of adenosine at 0.2 mg/kg (max 12 mg/dose) simultaneously with a rapid 5 ml 0.9% NS push. Secondary to the extremely short half-life of adenosine, the more central the location of venous access the better. Therefore, an antecubital vein is preferable to a hand, scalp, or lower extremity vein when giving adenosine.

- If adenosine fails to convert the stable patient with SVT, consultation with a pediatric cardiologist may be helpful. Other options may include cardioversion with sedation, amiodarone, digoxin, procainamide, or a β-blocker. Verapamil is not used in children <2 years of age because it has been reported to cause apnea and cardiovascular collapse.

SINUS TACHYCARDIA

Most children with tachycardia will have sinus tachycardia, although differentiating sinus tachycardia from SVT may be difficult. Children increase their cardiac output primarily through increases in HR rather than stroke volume, and as a result almost any stress state from emotional to organic disease can cause sinus tachycardia. Fear, fever, sepsis, dehydration, and respiratory distress are common causes of sinus tachycardia. Rare pediatric causes of tachycardia include thyrotoxicosis and pheochromocytoma.

Given that sinus tachycardia is such a nonspecific symptom, it is imperative to obtain a careful history and physical examination to help dictate further evaluation and to rule out any potentially life-threatening etiologies such as cardiac tamponade, pneumothorax, toxins, drugs, and thromboembolism (see Chapter 8, Chest Pain, and Chapter 30, Respiratory Distress).

Signs

- Fever
- Pallor
- Tachypnea and other signs of respiratory distress
- Poor perfusion and other signs of dehydration or shock

Workup

Sinus tachycardia is often suspected on the basis of the clinical evaluation of the patient. The rest of the workup of sinus tachycardia is directed at uncovering the cause of the patient's hyperdynamic state.

- An ECG to rule out SVT looking for P waves and beat-to-beat variability (seen in sinus tachycardia but not in SVT).
- Glucose: Hypoglycemia or hyperglycemia can be associated with sinus tachycardia.
- A CXR can be useful to look for underlying pulmonary or cardiac pathology.
- CBC can help identify possible infection and anemia.
- ABG analysis will reveal acidosis and level of hypoxia.
- Thyroid function tests can be considered for any findings consistent with thyrotoxicosis; elevated free T_4 and decreased TSH values are expected.
- A 24-hour urine collection for catecholamines is necessary for the diagnosis of pheochromocytoma. Admission will be necessary to confirm the diagnosis and institute treatment.

Comments and Treatment Considerations

Treatment will depend on the underlying cause of the tachycardia. Ill-appearing children should be promptly assessed for underlying causes of the sinus tachycardia as directed by history and physical examination findings and treated appropriately based on etiology.

If sinus tachycardia cannot be differentiated from SVT, the child should be presumed to have SVT until proven otherwise. Patients with probable SVT will not routinely have associated signs and symptoms of other disorders; P waves on ECG will be abnormal or absent and HR will not vary with activity.

Tachycardia associated with excessive sweating, respiratory distress, nausea, abdominal pain, fatigue, anxiety, weight loss, diarrhea, and heat intolerance should prompt the consideration of thyrotoxicosis, especially if the patient's temperature exceeds 38.5° C. For the patient with suspected thyroid storm, β-blockade with propranolol dosed at 0.5 to 2 mg/kg/day PO divided tid-qid (max 40 mg/dose) may be started for symptomatic control while waiting for additional advice from a pediatric endocrinologist. IV propranolol dosed at 0.025 mg/kg/dose (max total dose 3 mg) can be used in patients unable to tolerate oral medication. A more symptomatic patient may require an esmolol infusion dosed at 500 mcg/kg bolus IV over 1 minute, followed by 50 to 100 mcg/kg/min titrated to effect to a maximum of 200 mcg/kg/min. Active cooling measures may be needed for patients with excessive heat production. Appropriate consultation should be sought.

Headache, diaphoresis, and palpitations compose the classic triad of pheochromocytoma. Given the rarity of this diagnosis, endocrinology should be consulted emergently.

REFERENCES

Davis AM et al: Clinical spectrum, therapeutic management and follow-up of ventricular tachycardia in infant and young children, *Am Heart J* 131:186, 1996.

Dysrhythmias. In Barkin RM, Rosen P, editors: *Emergency pediatrics*, 5th ed, St. Louis 1999, Mosby.

Hale DE: Endocrine emergencies. In Fleisher GR, Ludwig S, editors: *Textbook of pediatric emergency medicine*, 3rd ed, Philadelphia, 1993, Lippincott Williams & Wilkins.

LaFranchi S: Disorders of the thyroid gland. In Behrman R, Kliegman R, Jenson H, editors: *Nelson textbook of pediatrics*, 16th ed, Philadelphia, 2000, WB Saunders.

Levy S: Factors predisposing to the development of atrial fibrillation, *Pacing Clin Electrophysiol* 20:2070, 1997.

Liberthson RR: Sudden death from cardiac causes in children and young adults, *N Engl J Med* 334:1039, 1996.

Mogayzel C, Quan L, et al: Out of hospital ventricular fibrillation in children and adolescents: causes and outcomes, *Ann Emerg Med* 25:484, 1995.

Pfammatter J-P, Paul T: Idiopathic ventricular tachycardia in infancy and childhood, *J Am Coll Cardiol* 33:2067, 1999.

Ralston M et al: Use of adenosine for diagnosis and treatment of tachyarrhythmias in pediatric patients, *J Pediatr* 124:139, 1994.

Schwartz PJ et al: Diagnostic criteria for the long QT syndrome: an update, *Circulation* 88:782, 1993.

Singhai A, Campbell D: Thyroid storm, *eMed J* 2:1, 2001.

Strasburger JF: Cardiac arrhythmias in childhood. Diagnostic considerations and treatment, *Drugs* 42:974, 1991.

Yabek SM: Ventricular arrhythmias in children with an apparently normal heart, *J Pediatr* 119:1, 1991.

Zritsky AL et al, editors: *Instructor's manual: pediatric advanced life support*, Washington, DC, 2001, American Heart Association.

CHAPTER 35

Toxic Ingestion, Approach to

JENNIFER AUDI AND MICHAEL J. BURNS

An estimated 5 million poison exposures occur annually in the United States and account for 5% to 10% of all ED visits. In 2002 more than 2.3 million poison exposures were reported to U.S. poison control centers and more than 50% of such exposures occurred in children younger than 6 years. Most toxic exposures in pediatric patients are the result of unintentional ingestion of substances found in the home. Fortunately, the majority of such poison exposures are minor and do not produce signs and symptoms, although a few ingestions such as acetaminophen (APAP) can be very dangerous and require treatment. In 2002 children younger than 6 years accounted for just 2.0% of all fatalities from poisoning. The substances most commonly involved in pediatric exposures include cosmetics and personal care products, cleaning substances, analgesics, foreign bodies, topical agents, plants, and cough and cold preparations. The substances most commonly implicated in childhood poisoning deaths are carbon monoxide (CO), analgesic agents, and hydrocarbons. There is a second peak in the incidence of toxic ingestions in adolescence as a result of experimentation with or use of illicit drugs and suicidal attempts or gestures.

The physician will frequently be challenged by toxicologic issues in children and should therefore be familiar with and skilled in the diagnosis and management of poisoning in this patient population. Rapid assessment of the severity of the exposure is required to make a diagnosis and provide sound initial treatment, often without the results of complete history or extensive laboratory tests. Therefore a systematic and consistent approach to the evaluation and treatment of the poisoned patient is necessary. Evaluation involves recognition that poisoning has occurred, identification of the agents involved, assessment of severity, and prediction of toxicity. Treatment involves the provision of supportive care, prevention of poison absorption, and when necessary the administration of antidotes and enhancement of poison elimination. The tempo, sequence, methods, and priorities of treatment are determined by the agent(s) involved and the presenting and predicted severity of poisoning. The local poison center is an excellent resource. A general approach to the poisoned patient is discussed, followed by issues specific to common ingestions.

GENERAL APPROACH TO ALL PATIENTS WITH POSSIBLE INGESTION
Initial Emergent Considerations

It is imperative to remember that children are often more sensitive to the effects of toxic exposures compared with adults. In addition, children have limited glycogen stores, producing a greater susceptibility to the hypoglycemic effects of toxins, particularly β-adrenergic antagonists, ethanol, and sulfonylureas.

- ABCs as necessary.
- Maintain inline cervical immobilization in those with suspected coexisting trauma.
- Intravenous access, O_2 supplementation.
- ECG with particular attention to conduction disturbances and dysrhythmias.
- Rapid initial screening physical examination, including vital signs, pulse oximetry, rectal temperature, mental status, and pupillary assessment.
- For those with altered mental status
  - Immediate Dextrostick. If unavailable, empiric glucose administration as D25W at 2-4 ml/kg IV is warranted.
  - Consider naloxone administration. The dose of naloxone is dependent on the opiate agonist present and the degree of reversal required. Doses typically range from 10 to 100 mcg/kg IV (max 2 mg initial dose). Full reversal dose of 100 mcg/kg should be used when a patient is unresponsive with no history of opioid dependence. If ETT placement becomes necessary, use 2 to 10 times the intravenous dose diluted in 3 to 5 ml

of normal saline, followed by several positive pressure breaths. Repeated or larger doses (up to 8 to 10 mg) may be necessary for certain synthetic opioids (e.g., propoxyphene and methadone) that have a longer half-life or greater potency at opioid receptors than naloxone. Naloxone administration has been associated with hypertension, tachycardia, ventricular arrhythmias, pulmonary edema, and seizures, especially in opioid-dependent patients.

- Use of flumazenil is *not* recommended for routine use but may obviate the need for endotracheal intubation in the nonhabituated pediatric patient with isolated benzodiazepine overdose and no history of seizure activity. Consider flumazenil only in those patients with known benzodiazepine ingestion who have CNS or respiratory depression and ECG reveals QRS < 100 ms (i.e., making a severe tricyclic antidepressant [TCA] ingestion unlikely). Flumazenil is dosed at 0.01 mg/kg/dose IV (max 0.2 mg initial dose) with subsequent doses given every minute to a maximum of 0.05 mg/kg or 1 mg, whichever is less. Flumazenil may precipitate seizures in those with mixed ingestion, especially if one of the other substances ingested are known to lower the seizure threshold, such as isoniazid (INH), cocaine, lithium, and monoamine oxidase inhibitors (MAOIs). In addition, patients with underlying seizure disorder, particularly those who are dependent on benzodiazepines for seizure control, or those treated with a complete coma-reversing dose (i.e., acute benzodiazepine withdrawal) are more likely to experience a seizure secondary to flumazenil.
- Endotracheal intubation is recommended for those who remain in severe respiratory distress or have depressed mental status and are unable to protect their airway.
- Initiate patient decontamination. This is discussed in detail later in the chapter. Gastric lavage may be considered but is rarely indicated for most toxic ingestions (see the section Comments and Treatment Considerations).
- Detailed history and physical exam (see section on Symptoms and Signs on p. 506).

- Directed toxicologic laboratory evaluations (see section on Workup, p. 532).
- Call a poison control center for treatment and decontamination recommendations (1-800-222-1222).
- Antidote administration as indicated (Table 35-1).
- Gastrointestinal elimination methods and enhanced elimination techniques, also discussed later in detail (Table 35-2 and 35-3).

Symptoms and Signs

A group of signs and symptoms often associated with a particular poison or type of poison is referred to as a *toxidrome*. Familiarity with the common toxidromes is important to the practicing physician and allows for clinical toxin-pattern recognition (Table 35-4). Munchausen by proxy and child abuse should also be considered in a child younger than 1 year who may not have the physical capacity to self-administer a poison. Child abuse or neglect should also be considered in children who present with recurrent poisonings or have a history of trauma.

History

- May be unreliable when obtained from patient; corroborate with family, friends, police, prehospital personnel, PCP, and pharmacist.
- Thoroughly search exposure environment for pill bottles and available household products, suicide note, drug paraphernalia (the latter two most commonly in adolescents).
- Inquire about pet medications or those family members who may care for the child (grandparents, aunts, uncles).
- Obtain source, nature, time, route, amount, and location of and reason for exposure.
- Inquire specifically about over-the-counter (OTC) drugs.
- Inquire about treatment rendered before arrival.
- Assess intent of exposure (accidental, suicide attempt, recreational misadventure, or victim of intentional poisoning by another).
- Obtain information about the child's medical and psychiatric history.
- Correlate history with PE and ancillary testing findings.

Table 35-1 Common Antidotes*

Poison	Antidote(s)	Dose
Acetaminophen	N-Acetylcysteine (Mucomyst 20%; Acetadote)	Initial oral dose: 140 mg/kg PO × 1, then 70 mg/kg/dose PO q4h × 17 doses Initial IV dose: 140 mg/kg IV × 1, then 70 mg/kg/dose IV q4h × 12 doses*
Anticholinergic agents†	Physostigmine (Antilirium)	Initial dose: **Children:** 0.01-0.03 mg/kg/dose, up to 2 mg slow IV over 5 min **Adult:** 0.5-2 mg slow IV over 5 min; may need to repeat if life-threatening toxicity reemerge
Arsenic‡	See Mercury	

*Multiple possible intravenous treatment regimens exist; consult toxicologist for recommendations. Consultation with a toxicologist should be sought for any ingestion in which the practitioner is unfamiliar with therapy.
†Risks may outweigh benefits; consultation with a toxicologist is recommended before therapy.
‡Consultation with a toxicologist is recommended.

Continued

Table 35-1   Common Antidotes—cont'd

Poison	Antidote(s)	Dose
Benzodiazepines[†]	Flumazenil (Romazicon)	Initial dose: 0.01 mg/kg/dose IV (max 0.2 mg/dose) over 30-60 sec, repeat every minute as needed to a total max dose of 0.05 mg/kg or 1 mg (whichever is less)
β-Blockers	Atropine	Atropine 0.02 mg/kg IV (min 0.1 mg, max 1 mg); may repeat
	Glucagon	Glucagon initial dose: **Children:** 50-150 mcg/kg IV bolus over 1 min initially, followed by continuous infusion 0.07 mg/kg/hr IV **Adult:** 5-10 mg IV bolus, then 1-5 mg/hr titrated to a max of 10 mg/hr IV infusion.
	Isoproterenol + dopamine	Isoproterenol 0.05-0.5 mcg/kg/min plus dopamine 5-20 mcg/kg/min, titrate to blood pressure
Calcium channel blockers	Calcium	Calcium chloride 10% injection (must be further diluted before injection): **Children:** 20 mg/kg (0.2 ml/kg) IV over 5 min initially, may repeat **Adult:** 1-2 g (10-20 ml) IV over 5 min; repeat up to four times

Glucagon	**Children:** Glucagon 50-150 mcg/kg IV bolus over 1 min initially, followed by continuous infusion 0.07 mg/kg/hr IV **Adult:** glucagon 5-10 mg IV bolus, then 1-5 mg/hr titrated to a max of 10 mg/hr IV infusion
Insulin + dextrose	Initial dose: Insulin load: 0.5-1 unit/kg IV bolus, then 0.5-1 units/kg/hr, with concurrent dextrose (D10W) infusion to maintain euglycemia. **NOTE: This dose is 10 times greater than the insulin dose used to treat DKA.***
Carbon monoxide	Oxygen ± hyperbaric chamber	100% oxygen by ventilator or NRB high-flow oxygen by tight-fitting face mask
Crotaline Snakebite*	Wyeth polyvalent Crotalidae antivenin (equine origin)	See Chapter 5, Bites, Tables 5-4 and 5-5, pp. 76-77

Continued

†Risks may outweigh benefits; consultation with a toxicologist is recommended before therapy.
*Consultation with a toxicologist is recommended.

Table 35-1 Common Antidotes—cont'd

Poison	Antidote(s)	Dose
	CroFab polyvalent Crotalinae antivenin (ovine origin)	
Cyanide	Amyl nitrate pearls	Amyl nitrate: one ampule by inhalation for 15 sec every 3 min until IV access is obtained
	Sodium nitrite (3% solution)	Sodium nitrite: **Children:** 0.33 ml/kg IV, max 10 ml, no faster than 2.5 ml/min; may repeat 50% of dose in 30 min, monitoring methemoglobin levels **Adult:** 10 ml (300 mg) IV over 4 min
	Sodium thiosulfate (25% solution)	Sodium thiosulfate: **Children:** 1.65 ml/kg IV, max 50 ml, over 10 min; may repeat 50% of dose in 30 min, monitoring methemoglobin levels **Adult and children >25 kg:** 50 ml (12.5 g) IV over 10 min
Digitalis	Digoxin immune Fab (Digibind)	Equations to calculate number of vials needed: (# mg ingested × 0.8) ÷ 0.6 = # vials needed OR

Total Body Load (TBL) = serum conc (5.6 L/kg)(wt)
If <6 hr, # vials = TBL/0.8
If >6 hr, # vials = TBL/0.6
OR
Empiric dose: 10 vials (acute poisoning); 1-3 vials (chronic)
Reconstitute each vial of Digibind with 4 ml of sterile water and then dilute in NS to 1 mg/ml and administer IV via a 0.22-micron filter over 15-30 min, may give IV push in cardiac arrest

Ethylene glycol	Ethanol 10% in D5W ± Hemodialysis	Ethanol initial load: 8-10 ml/kg IV (max 200 ml) of 10% ethanol over 30 min, then 0.8-2 ml/kg/hr IV infusion (titrate drip to serum ethanol 100-150 mg/dl); double to triple infusion rate during hemodialysis
	Fomepizole (Antizol) ± hemodialysis	Fomepizole initial load: 15 mg/kg IV over 30 min, then 10 mg/kg/dose IV q12h × 4 doses, then 15 mg/kg IV q12h until ethylene glycol concentration <20 mg/dl (give 10 mg/kg/dose IV q4h during HD)
Gold*	See Mercury	

*Consultation with a toxicologist is recommended.

Continued

Table 35-1	Common Antidotes—cont'd	
Poison	**Antidote(s)**	**Dose**
Heparin	Protamine sulfate	1 mg neutralizes 90-115 units of heparin. Initial dose: Time since IV heparin dose <30 min, use 1 mg/100 Units of heparin; 30-60 min use 0.5-0.75 mg/100 Units of heparin; 60-120 min use 0.375-0.5 mg/100 Units of heparin; >120 min use 0.25-0.375 mg/100 Units of heparin If subcutaneous heparin, use 1-1.5 mg of protamine per 100 Units of heparin; give a portion of the dose (i.e., 25-50 mg) IV then infuse remainder over 8-16 hr
Hydrofluoric acid	Calcium gluconate	Topical calcium gluconate gel 2.5-3% applied for 1-2 days; may be compounded or obtained via orphan drug status from Calgonate Corporation or Intradermal or subcutaneous calcium gluconate 5% injection at burn site—0.5 ml/cm² burn area; intraarterial calcium gluconate 10% injection should be used on digits: 10-20 ml in 40 ml NS over 4 hr; repeat as necessary until pain relief

Iron	Deferoxamine (Desferal)	15 mg/kg/hr IV infusion (max 6000 mg/day), dilute to 10 mg/ml in D5W, NS or LR; deferoxamine may also be given IM at 50 mg/kg/dose q6h, max 6000 mg/day
Isoniazid	Pyridoxine (vitamin B_6)	1 g pyridoxine for every gram of isoniazid ingested or empiric 5 g IV over 10 min if amount ingested unknown; may repeat every 5-20 min as needed
Lead*	Dimercaprol (BAL—British antilewisite) in peanut oil + calcium disodium EDTA (acute poisoning with encephalitis or level >70 mcg/dl)	Dimercaprol 4 mg/kg initial dose IM followed by 3-4 mg/kg/dose IM q4h for 2-7 days plus calcium disodium EDTA 25-50 mg/kg/day as continuous IV infusion
	2,3-Dimercaptosuccinic acid (DMSA)-succimer (Chemet)	Succimer 30 mg/kg/day PO divided q8h × 5 days, then 20 mg/kg/day PO divided q12h × 14 days (available in 100-mg capsules); repeat therapy prn after 2-week drug-free interval

*Consultation with a toxicologist is recommended.

Continued

Table 35-1 Common Antidotes—cont'd

Poison	Antidote(s)	Dose
	D-Penicillamine	D-Penicillamine 15-30 mg/kg/day PO divided tid-qid (max 1.5 g/day); begin at 25% of dose and titrate over 2-3 wk
Low-molecular-weight heparin (enoxaparin)	Protamine sulfate	1 mg of protamine neutralizes 1 mg of LMWH Initial dose: If LMWH dose <4 hours, use 1 mg of protamine per 1 mg LMWH, may repeat 0.5 mg protamine per 1 mg LMWH if aPTT still prolonged 2-4 hr after first dose
Mercury*	Dimercaprol (BAL—British antilewisite) in peanut oil	Initial dose: 2.5-6 mg/kg/dose IM q4-6h × 10 days (follow regimen specific to toxicity)
Methanol	See ethylene glycol	
Methemoglobinemia	Methylene blue (1% solution)	Methylene blue initial dose: 1-2 mg/kg/dose IV over 5 min; may repeat in 1 hr (max 7 mg/kg)

Opiates	Naloxone (Narcan)	Naloxone initial dose: 10-100 mcg/kg IV (max 2 mg/dose) depending on degree of reversal needed (opioid-dependent patients should receive 1-10 mcg/kg [adult 0.1 mg] IV every 30-60 sec until clinical response); synthetic opiates may require up to 10 mg for initial reversal dose
Organophosphates Nerve agents Carbamates[†]	Atropine	Initial dose: **Children:** 0.05 mg/kg/dose IV (max 2 mg/dose); repeat q3-5min until secretions clear **Adults:** 0.5-2 mg IV; repeat q3-5min until sweat and secretions clear
	Pralidoxime (2-PAM) (Protopam)	Initial dose: **Children:** 25-50 mg/kg IV/IM initially, may repeat in 1-2 hr (max 2 g/dose), then every 10-12 hr **Adult:** 1-2 g IV no faster than 200 mg/min, may repeat in 1-2 hr and then every 10-12 hr or IV infusion of 3-4 mg/kg/hr for 24-72 hr/until clinical toxicity resolves

Continued

LMWH, Low-molecular-weight heparin.
*Consultation with a toxicologist is recommended.
[†]The use of 2-PAM for carbamate poisoning is controversial.

Table 35-1   Common Antidotes—cont'd

Poison	Antidote(s)	Dose
Sulfonylureas	Octreotide (Sandostatin) + dextrose	Octreotide initial dose: **Children:** 1-2 mcg/kg/dose SC/IV initially, then repeat dose (max 50 mcg) SC/IV q12h until euglycemia maintained without supplemental dextrose **Adult:** 50-100 mcg SC/IV, then 50 mcg q12h until euglycemia maintained without supplemental dextrose
	Glucagon	Glucagon: **Children:** 50 mcg/kg IV/IM/SC bolus (max 2 mg/dose) **Adult:** 1-2 mg IV/IM/SC bolus
	Diazoxide	Diazoxide: Consult toxicologist.

| Tricyclic antidepressants | Sodium bicarbonate 8.4% (1 mEq/ml) | Initial dose:
Children: 1-2 mEq/kg IV bolus (max 100 mEq/dose), then IV infusion to maintain blood pH 7.45-7.55 and $P_{CO_2} \approx 30$ mm Hg
Adult: 1-2 ampules (50-100 mEq) IV bolus, then IV infusion to maintain blood pH 7.45-7.55 and $P_{CO_2} \cong 30$ mm Hg
Usual IV solution: 75-150 mEq sodium bicarbonate in 1 L D5W infused at three times maintenance IVF rate |

Table 35-2 Gastrointestinal Decontamination Methods

Method	Indications	Contraindications	Dosing / Technique	Complications
Activated charcoal (AC)	Consider for all poison ingestions unless clearly nontoxic or known heavy metal, alcohol, glycol, caustic or hydrocarbon	Bowel obstruction or perforation Depressed mental status and unprotected airway (intubate first) Relative: corrosive and low-viscosity hydrocarbon ingestions Do not use more than one sorbitol-containing AC dose in children	1 g/kg AC or 10:1 (g:g) AC to toxicant (max 60 g/dose); given as a slurry in 100 ml of water orally or via gastric tube; may enhance palatability by mixing AC with cherry or chocolate artificial sweetener	Nausea and vomiting Abdominal cramps Diarrhea (with sorbitol) Constipation (aqueous suspensions) Aspiration
Gastric lavage	Consider for obtunded patient or patient with life-threatening	Corrosive ingestion Low-viscosity hydrocarbon ingestion	Left lateral decubitus or supine 24-28 Fr tube (pediatric); 36-40 Fr tube	Aspiration Esophageal perforation Tracheal lavage

Method	Procedure/Dose	Contraindications	Complications
	ingestion and can be performed within 60 min of ingestion Consider for life-threatening ingestion of agent not bound by AC. (adults) Gravity instillation and drainage of up to 5 L of tap water or NS.	Depressed mental status and unprotected airway (intubate first) Patient noncompliance Esophageal or gastric pathology Foreign body or battery ingestion Cardiac dysrhythmias	GI bleeding Hypoxia and hypercapnia Laryngospasm Fluid and electrolyte disturbance
Syrup of ipecac*	Home or prehospital setting Alert patient within 15-60 min of ingestion NOTE: usage is controversial, consult poison center	CNS depression Corrosive ingestion Low-viscosity hydrocarbons Agent which may rapidly compromise airway Debilitated patients Third trimester pregnancy	0-6 mo: do not use 6-12 mo: 10 ml 12 mo to 12 yr: 15 ml >12 yr: 30 ml May repeat once in 20 min if not effective	Limited efficacy Protracted vomiting Delays administration of AC or antidotes Lethargy Aspiration

*This method of GI decontamination is no longer recommended by the American Academy of Pediatrics.

Continued

Table 35-2 Gastrointestinal Decontamination Methods—cont'd

Method	Indications	Contraindications	Dosing / Technique	Complications
Whole bowel irrigation (WBI)	Consider for toxic foreign bodies (e.g., cocaine and heroin drug packets), extended-release drug preparations, heavy metals (e.g., As, Fe, Li, Hg, Zn), and suspected drug concretion	Bowel obstruction, perforation, bleeding, or ileus Depressed mental status and unprotected airway (intubate first)	PEG-3350 (e.g., Colyte, GoLYTELY) NGT administration recommended 1-6 yr: 40 ml/kg/hr to max of 500 ml/hr 6-12 yr: 1 L/hr >12 yr: 1-2 L/hr (until clear rectal effluent)	Nausea and vomiting Abdominal cramps and bloating Electrolyte disturbances Aspiration
Cathartics	Optional adjunct to AC (give single dose only) Most experts do not recommend cathartic use	Bowel obstruction, perforation, ileus Electrolyte imbalance Hypotension Mg cathartics in those with renal	Sorbitol (35%): 4.3 ml/kg for children (max 2 g/kg sorbitol) given with AC 1 g/kg; sorbitol	Nausea, vomiting, diarrhea Abdominal cramps and bloating Dehydration, hypotension,

	Indications	Contraindications	Dose	Complications
	(i.e. sorbitol) in children receiving AC	failure	70% at 4.3 ml/kg for adults with 1 g/kg of AC Mg citrate: 4 ml/kg PO × one dose (max 300 ml/dose) Magnesium Sulfate: 250 mg/kg PO × 1 dose	hypernatremia, hypermagnesemia
Endoscopy surgery	Pharmacobezoars Heavy metals in stomach Surgery for those with suspected ruptured cocaine packets	Endoscopy should *not* be used to remove intact drug packets (high risk for iatrogenic rupture)		Viscus perforation Aspiration
Dilution	Corrosive ingestion NOTE: Usage is controversial; consult poison center.	Vomiting patient	5 ml of milk or water per kilogram (up to 250 ml)	Vomiting and increased toxic exposure

Table 35-3   Enhanced Elimination Techniques

Technique	Dosing Technique Requirements	Complications	Agents for which Effective
Multiple-dose aqueous activated charcoal	0.5-1 g/kg (max 60 g/dose) q2-6h Requires bowel sounds	Nausea, vomiting, diarrhea, constipation, bowel obstruction and infarction, aspiration	Carbamazepine, phenobarbital, theophylline, quinine, nadolol, dapsone, meprobamate, salicylates, valproate, SR and EC preparations, agents undergoing enterohepatic recirculation
Forced diuresis	Isotonic fluid (e.g., NS) at 500 ml/hr in adults; this technique not recommended in children because of unacceptably high risk of complications	Fluid overload, pulmonary edema, cerebral edema, acid-base and electrolyte disturbances, drug-induced SIADH	Barium, bromides, chromium, cisplatin, iodide, fluoride, calcium, lithium, potassium

Urinary alkalinization	Initial 1-2 mEq/kg sodium bicarbonate IV bolus (max 100 mEq/dose), then D5W plus 50-150 mEq sodium bicarbonate per liter at 2-3 times maintenance IVF Goal: urine flow 3 ml/kg/hr and urinary pH ≥ 7.5	Fluid overload, pulmonary edema, cerebral edema, hypernatremia, hypokalemia, alkalemia, ionized hypocalcemia	Chlorpropamide, salicylates, barbiturates, methotrexate, fluoride, sulfonamides
Peritoneal dialysis	Although easier and less hazardous than hemodialysis, PD is usually not acceptable in overdose situations as the mesenteric blood flow cannot be adjusted; may be helpful in small children; see hemodialysis requirements	Bleeding, infection	Alcohols and glycols, barbiturates, bromide, ethchlorvynol, inorganic mercury, lithium, salicylates, theophylline (hemoperfusion better)

IVF, Intravenous fluid; *NS*, normal saline; *PD*, peritoneal dialysis; *SIADH*, syndrome of inappropriate secretion of antidiuretic hormone.

Continued

Table 35-3   Enhanced Elimination Techniques—cont'd

Technique	Dosing Technique Requirements	Complications	Agents for which Effective
Hemodialysis	Requires poison with: MW <500 daltons low protein binding High water solubility Low endogenous clearance Small Vd	Hypotension, bleeding, hypothermia, air embolus, central venous access complications	Barbiturates, bromides, chloral hydrate, alcohols, lithium, procainamide, theophylline (hemoperfusion better), salicylates, atenolol, sotalol
Hemoperfusion	Requires drug to be bound by activated charcoal	Charcoal embolization, hypocalcemia, hypoglycemia, thrombocytopenia, leukopenia, hypotension, bleeding, hypothermia	Barbiturates, meprobamate, glutethimide, phenytoin (may be useful), carbamazepine, valproate, theophylline, disopyramide, paraquat, procainamide, *Amanita* mushrooms, methotrexate

Hemofiltration	Can be run continuously	Clotting of filter, bleeding	Aminoglycosides (only valuable in renal failure), vancomycin, metal chelate complexes, procainamide
Exchange transfusion	Double- or triple-volume exchanges usually performed	Transfusion reactions, ionized hypocalcemia, hypothermia	Arsine, sodium chlorate, methemoglobinemia, sulfhemoglobinemia, neonatal drug toxicity

Table 35-4 Toxidromes

Toxidrome	Symptoms	Signs	Examples of Toxic Agents
Sympathomimetic	Agitation Hallucinations Headache Nausea Vomiting Palpitations Paranoia Tremors	CNS: Agitation, hyperalert, delirium, seizures, coma VS: Hypertension, widened pulse pressure, tachycardia, tachypnea, hyperpnea, hyperthermia Pupils: Mydriasis Other: Diaphoresis, tremors, hyperreflexia, flushed or pale skin	Cocaine, amphetamines, ephedrine, pseudoephedrine, phenylpropanolamine, theophylline, caffeine, albuterol, methylphenidate, pemoline
Anticholinergic	Agitation Hallucinations Mumbling speech Unresponsive	CNS: Agitation, delirium, hypervigilance, mumbling speech, hallucinations, coma Peds: CNS excitation predominates VS: Hyperthermia, tachycardia, hypertension, tachypnea Pupils: Mydriasis Other: Dry flushed skin, dry mucous membranes, decreased bowel sounds, urinary retention,	Antihistamines, TCAs, cyclobenzaprine, orphenadrine, antiparkinsonian agents, antispasmodics, phenothiazines, atropine, scopolamine, belladonna alkaloids (e.g., Jimson weed)

Hallucinogenic	Hallucinations Perceptual distortions Depersonalization synesthesia Agitation	myoclonus, choreoathetosis, picking behavior, seizures (rare) Mnemonic: "Hot as a hare, blind as a bat, dry as a bone, red as a beet, mad as a hatter, the bowel and bladder lose their tone and the heart goes on alone" CNS: Hallucinations, depersonalization, agitation VS: Hyperthermia, tachycardia, hypertension, tachypnea Pupils: Mydriasis (usually) Other: Nystagmus	Phencyclidine, dextrome- thorphan, LSD, mesca- line, psilocybin, other tryptamins, designer amphetamines (e.g., MDMA, MDEA, STP, DOM)
Opioid	Lethargy Confusion Unresponsive	CNS: Lethargy, coma, confusion Pupils: Miosis (usually) VS: Hypothermia, bradycardia, hypotension, hypopnea, bradypnea	Heroin, morphine, meperidine, methadone, oxycodone, hydrocodone, fentanyl, hydromorphone,

Continued

Table 35-4 Toxidromes—cont'd

Toxidrome	Symptoms	Signs	Examples of Toxic Agents
		Other: Hyporeflexia, pulmonary edema, needle marks	diphenoxylate, loperamide, propoxyphene, pentazocine
Sedative-hypnotic	Confusion Unresponsive Slurred speech	CNS: Lethargy, coma, confusion, dysarthria, ataxia, CNS excitation in children VS: Hypothermia, bradycardia, hypotension, hypopnea, bradypnea Pupils: Miosis (usually) Other: Hyporeflexia, nystagmus	Benzodiazepine barbiturates, carisoprodol, meprobamate, glutethimide, alcohols, zolpidem
Cholinergic	Confusion Unresponsive Shortness of breath Cramps Nausea Vomiting	CNS: Agitation, coma, confusion, seizures VS: Bradycardia, hypertension or hypotension, tachypnea or bradypnea Pupils: Miosis (not universal)	Organophosphate and carbamate insecticides, nerve agents, nicotine, pilocarpine, physostigmine, edrophonium,

Continued

	Diarrhea Weakness Seizures Drooling	Other: Salivation, urinary and fecal incontinence, diarrhea, emesis, diaphoresis, lacrimation, GI cramps, bronchoconstriction, muscle fasciculations, weakness Mnemonic: DUMBELS (defecation, urination, miosis, bronchospasm, excessive salivation, lacrimation, seizures)	bethanechol, urecholine, neostigmine, pyridostigmine
Serotonin syndrome	Lethargy Confusion Agitation Tremulous	CNS: Agitation, lethargy, coma, confusion, delirium VS: Hyperthermia, tachycardia, hypertension, tachypnea Pupils: Mydriasis Other: Tremor, myoclonus, hyperreflexia, clonus, diaphoresis, flushing, trismus, rigidity, diarrhea	MAOIs alone or with SSRIs, meperidine, dextromethorphan, TCAs, L-tryptophan, trazodone, nefazodone, linezolid

MAOI, Monoamine oxidase inhibitors; *SSRI*, selective serotonin reuptake inhibitor; *TCA*, tricyclic antidepressant.

Table 35-4 Toxidromes—cont'd

Toxidrome	Symptoms	Signs	Examples of Toxic Agents
Tricyclic antidepressants	Confusion Agitation Unresponsive Slurred speech	CNS: Lethargy, coma, confusion, seizures VS: Hyperthermia, tachycardia, hypertension then hypotension, hypopnea Pupils: Mydriasis Other: Dry skin, myoclonus, choreoathetosis, cardiac arrhythmias and conduction disturbances	Amitriptyline, nortriptyline, imipramine, clomipramine, desipramine, doxepin, trimipramine
Sympatholytic	Lethargy Confusion Unresponsive	CNS: Lethargy, confusion, coma, seizures (uncommonly) VS: Bradycardia, hypotension, bradypnea, hypopnea Pupils: Miosis (often) Other: Hypoglycemia	α-Adrenergic antagonists (e.g., prazosin) β-Blockers (e.g., propranolol) Calcium channel blockers (e.g., verapamil, diltiazem) α_2-Adrenergic agonists (e.g., clonidine and imidazolines)

| **Digitalis, other cardiac glycosides, and cardioactive steroids** | Anorexia
Nausea
Vomiting
Diarrhea
Lethargy
Weakness
Dizziness
Vertigo
Visual disturbances (xanthopsia/chromatopsia)
Syncope | CNS: Normal or lethargy and confusion
VS: Bradycardia, hypotension
Pupils: Normal
Other: Cardiac arrhythmias and conduction disturbances | Digoxin, digitoxin,
Digitalis purpurea (foxglove), *Digitalis lantana*, *Nerium oleander* (oleander), *Thevetia peruviana* (Yellow oleander), *Convallaria majalis* (Lily of the Valley), *Urginea maritima* (red squill), Chan su and bufadienolides |
| **Extrapyramidal**
Dystonia
Akathisia
Parkinsonism | Anxious
Inability to talk | CNS: Alert and oriented, anxious, dysarthria, mutism
VS: Normal
Pupils: Normal
Other: Oculogyric crisis, facial grimacing, torticollis, buccolingual spasm, tremor, rigidity, involuntary movements, opisthotonus, bradykinesia, masked facies, akathisia | Antipsychotics (e.g., haloperidol, phenothiazines, molindone)
Antiemetics (e.g., droperidol, prochlorperazine, metoclopramide) |

CNS, Central nervous system; *GI,* gastrointestinal; *MAOI,* monoamine oxidase inhibitors; *SSRI,* selective serotonin reuptake inhibitor; *TCA,* tricyclic antidepressant; *VS,* vital signs.

Physical Examination

VS, mental status, skin findings, and pupillary signs are most useful and allow for patient classification into a state of physiologic stimulation or depression.

- Physiologic stimulation (increased pulse, BP, RR, temperature, agitation, seizures, and mydriasis) commonly occurs from the following:
  - Sympathomimetics
  - Anticholinergics
  - Central hallucinogens
  - Drug withdrawal states
- Physiologic depression (decreased pulse, BP, RR, temperature, lethargy, coma, and miosis) commonly occurs from the following:
  - Sympatholytics
  - Cholinergics
  - Opiates
  - Sedative/hypnotics and alcohols
  - Simple asphyxiants (e.g., inert gases)
- Mixed physiologic effects may occur from the following:
  - Polydrug overdoses
  - Metabolic poisons (e.g., hypoglycemic agents, salicylates, cyanide)
  - Heavy metals (e.g., arsenic, iron, lead, lithium, mercury)
  - Membrane-active agents (e.g., volatile inhalants, antiarrhythmics, local anesthetic agents)
  - Agents with multiple mechanisms of action (e.g., TCAs)
  - Cellular asphyxiants (e.g., CO, cyanide, hydrogen sulfide)
- The absence of VS or mental status abnormalities may indicate that a nontoxic exposure has occurred or that insufficient time has passed from exposure to the onset of clinical effects.

Workup

- Ancillary studies may be useful to confirm, establish, or refute a poisoning diagnosis. Tests ordered should be guided by history and PE.
- ECG is recommended for all symptomatic or intentional poisonings as well as those involving cardiotoxic agents.

ECG provides clues for diagnosis (e.g., sinus tachycardia and QRS prolongation for TCA poisoning).

- Symptomatic patients or those with unreliable or unknown history should minimally have measurements of serum electrolytes (calculate anion gap), BUN, SCr, glucose, UA.
- Routine urine pregnancy testing is recommended in Tanner stage IV and V females.
- ABG, cooximetry, serum osmolality, and lactate measurements are recommended in patients with acid-base, cardiovascular, neurologic, or respiratory disturbances.
- If anion gap metabolic acidosis is present, it should prompt measurement of serum Ca^{2+}, SCr, glucose, ketones, lactate, osmolality, salicylates, solvents (e.g., toxic alcohols such as methanol and ethylene glycol), and examination of the urine for crystals.

The anion gap is calculated as follows (normal <16 mEq/L):

Anion gap = $(Na^+ + K^+) - (Cl^- + HCO_3^-)$

- Causes of an increased anion gap include the following:
  - Decreased unmeasured cation
    - Hypocalcemia
    - Hypomagnesemia
  - Increased unmeasured anion
    - Organic anions: lactate, ketones
    - Inorganic anions: phosphate, sulfate
    - Proteins: hyperalbuminemia
    - Exogenous anions
    - Salicylate
    - Formate (metabolite of methanol)
    - Glycolate (metabolite of ethylene glycol)
    - Nitrate
    - Penicillins
- Laboratory error
  - Falsely increased serum sodium
  - Falsely decreased serum chloride or bicarbonate
- Liver function tests (LFTs) and PT (INR) should be performed in all patients with acetaminophen or other hepatotoxic agent ingestions.

- Toxic screening should minimally include serum measurements of acetaminophen and salicylate in those with intentional poisoning or uncertain history.
- Comprehensive toxic screening is rarely necessary or indicated, particularly when patients are asymptomatic or have clinical findings consistent with history. Drugs of abuse (i.e., immunoassay) screening of serum and/or urine are usually also unnecessary.
- At times, quantitative levels of toxins are required to determine or predict the severity of poisoning and guide treatment (Table 35-5).

Comments and Treatment Considerations

Management strategies are dictated by the poison involved, presenting and predicted severity of illness, and time of presentation in relation to time of exposure. Supportive care in conjunction with decontamination procedures is sufficient for most patients. Some patients who have taken only a small amount of a substance may require admission for observation given delayed absorption (if extended-release or taken in conjunction with another substance that may alter gastric emptying time) or seriousness of ingestion of even a small amount (Table 35-6).

Poison Decontamination

- The sooner decontamination is performed, the more effective it is at preventing poison absorption.
- Dermal and ocular exposures should be treated with the immediate removal of any contaminated clothing and particulate matter, followed by copious irrigation of exposed areas with NS or tap water.
- Inhalation exposures should be mitigated by immediately removing the patient from contaminated area and administering supplemental oxygen.
- GI decontamination is recommended for poison ingestions unless the exposure was clearly nontoxic.
  Recommendations are largely based on theoretical grounds, however, because insufficient data exist to support or

Table 35-5   Drugs for which Quantification May Be Useful

Acetaminophen
Carboxyhemoglobin
Methemoglobin
Digoxin (serial levels)
Lithium
Theophylline (serial levels)
Salicylates (serial levels)
Paraquat
Iron
Methanol
Ethanol
Ethylene glycol
Antiepileptic agents (serial levels)
   Carbamazepine
   Phenobarbital
   Phenytoin
   Valproic acid
Heavy metals (24-hr urine)
   Lead
   Mercury

exclude the use of GI decontamination more than 1 hour after poison ingestion (see Table 35-2).
- Activated charcoal (AC) administration alone is the preferred means of GI decontamination for most poison ingestions.
- AC does not effectively adsorb heavy metals, inorganic ions, corrosives, boric acid, hydrocarbons, alcohols, and essential oils
- Gastric lavage may be useful and, thus, considered (in addition to AC) after life-threatening ingestions (e.g., obtunded patients, lethal toxin not bound by AC) for which it can be performed within 60 minutes of ingestion.

Table 35-6   Special Cases*

Over-the-Counter/Household Exposures	Prescription Medications
Iron (>20 mg/kg elemental Fe)	Sulfonylureas[†] (small glycogen stores increase risk of hypoglycemia)
Camphor (100 mg/kg)	
Cocaine (prolonged observation if drug packet ingested[†])	β-Adrenergic antagonists[†]
	Calcium channel antagonists[†] (sustained-release characteristics associated with delayed and prolonged toxicity)
Methyl salicylate (topical rub, 7-8 g salicylate/tsp, oil of wintergreen)[†]	
Diphenhydramine (25 mg/kg)	
Lomotil (diphenoxylate/atropine)[†] 1-1.5 mg/kg; delayed-onset opioid anticholinergic and effects, respiratory depression/arrest in children	Clonidine and other imidazoline derivatives
	Tricyclic antidepressants (including topical preparation of doxepin; 10-15 mg/kg)
Ethanol, methanol, ethylene glycol[†]	Digoxin (1 mg) and other cardiac glycosides; few oleander or foxglove leaves
Caustics	
Hydrocarbons (e.g., petroleum distillates)	Theophylline (7-8 mg/kg)
Benzocaine	Antimalarials (chloroquine, hydroxychloroquine, 20 mg/kg; quinine, 80 mg/kg)
	Opioids (methadone, codeine)[†]
	Monoamine oxidase inhibitors (15-25 mg/kg)[†]
	Antipsychotics (olanzapine, clozapine, phenothiazines)

*Toxins that cause significant effects in children in small doses; may cause significant toxicity or death after ingestion of one tablet or mouthful (teaspoon).

[†]Children who have ingested these agents should be admitted to the hospital for prolonged observation and monitoring even if they are asymptomatic because of the potential for delayed and life-threatening toxicity.

- Many experts advocate that whole-bowel irrigation (WBI) is useful for patients who have ingested heavy metals (e.g., arsenic, iron, lithium), drug packets ("body stuffer" or "body packer"), sustained-release or enteric-coated preparations, or those who are suspected to have drug concretions (pharmacobezoars).
- Syrup of ipecac is *not* recommended for hospital use.

Supportive Care

- Supportive care is frequently all that is necessary.
- *Hypertension*: Best treated initially with nonspecific sedation (e.g., benzodiazepines such as lorazepam dosed at 0.1 mg/kg IV q4h prn [max 4 mg/dose] or midazolam 0.05 to 0.1 mg/kg/dose IV q1-2h prn [max 10 mg/dose]). For further management of hypertension associated with a toxic exposure, consultation with a toxicologist is recommended. Avoid β-blockers alone in sympathomimetic states (e.g., cocaine), because they may precipitate unopposed α-adrenergic vasoconstriction.
- *Hypotension*: Often occurs because many poisons deplete endogenous catecholamine stores. Intravenous fluid is the first-line treatment (20 to 40 ml/kg intravenous crystalloid), and rarely vasopressors may be needed (e.g., dopamine and norepinephrine). Use antidotes and other specific treatments as indicated.
- *Agitation*: Generally best treated with benzodiazepines (see above dosing), supplemented as needed with neuroleptic agents such as haloperidol 0.025 to 0.075 mg/kg/dose (max 10 mg/dose) IV q6h, followed by half the initial dose IV/IM q2h prn for agitation. In anticholinergic syndrome, experienced practitioners may consider physostigmine dosed at 0.01 to 0.03 mg/kg/dose (max 2 mg/dose) IV slowly over 5 minutes in conjunction with a poison center specialist. The dose may need to be repeated every 30 to 60 minutes for recurrent agitation or life-threatening dysrhythmias. Caution should be used when administering physostigmine because of the potential for inducing severe bradycardia, asystole, or seizures. Physostigmine is contraindicated in patients with

prolonged PR and QRS intervals on the ECG (e.g., after TCA ingestions). Caution should be exercised before administration in patients with GI or genitourinary (GU) obstruction, asthma, diabetes, severe cardiovascular disease, and concurrent use of depolarizing neuromuscular blockading agents such as succinylcholine. Atropine should be available at the bedside.

- *Ventricular arrhythmias*: Standard doses of antiarrhythmics (lidocaine or amiodarone) recommended (see Chapter 34, Tachycardia). Sodium bicarbonate (1 to 2 mEq/kg/dose IV bolus) is indicated for wide-complex tachycardia resulting from TCAs and other membrane-active agents; antidotal treatment as indicated. Digoxin immune Fab (Digibind) is the drug of choice for digitalis-induced arrythmias. Fosphenytoin/phenytoin are potentially effective alternative therapies if Digibind is unavailable.

- *Bradyarrhythmias with hypotension*: Treatment is drug specific. Standard doses of atropine 0.02 mg/kg IV (min 0.1 mg, max 1 mg) are recommended. Administer calcium and glucagon to those with calcium channel blocker and β-blocker poisoning. Calcium can be given as calcium chloride 10% solution for injection, 20 mg/kg IV *diluted* every 10 minutes to a maximum initial dose of 1000 mg or as calcium gluconate 10% solution for injection, 60 to 100 mg/kg/dose IV (max 3000 mg initial dose). Digoxin Fab fragments should be given to those with digoxin or other cardioactive steroid poisoning (see Table 35-1 for dosing).

- *Seizures*: Always assess for hypoglycemia and treat accordingly. Benzodiazepines are good first-line agents (see Chapter 32, Seizures). However, the most important intervention is reversal of the toxin activity such as using pyridoxine for isoniazid-induced seizures (see Table 35-1 for dosing). Phenobarbital may be the second-line agent of choice for treating toxin-induced seizures, such as theophylline and tricyclic antidepressant ingestions, in which phenytoin administration could worsen arrhythmias and hypotension.

Antidotes

Antidotes are not commonly available for most toxic agents and are used in only about 1% of poison exposures. Common antidotes and their doses are listed in Table 35-1. It is appropriate to administer an antidote when the expected benefits of therapy outweigh its associated risk.

Enhanced elimination techniques

In approximately 1% of poison exposures it becomes necessary to accelerate the removal of absorbed toxins using enhanced elimination techniques. In a few selected cases an aggressive approach to elimination can be lifesaving. Enhanced elimination techniques should be considered when a patient fails or is unlikely to respond to maximal supportive care and the predicted benefit of the intervention outweighs its risks of complications. Consultation with a toxicologist is recommended. Children, especially infants, may not respond well to hemodialysis or hemoperfusion given the large volumes of blood required for the procedure. Exchange transfusion may be useful in neonates and infants (see Table 35-3).

 ## TOXIC TIME BOMBS

Certain poisons produce delayed toxic manifestations, usually secondary to toxic metabolites, and few, if any, early signs may be present after lethal dose ingestions of these agents (Table 35-7). Additionally, some of these agents may require only a small ingestion to cause significant toxicity or death. Both actual and predicted toxic effects determine patient disposition. If the history, PE, or initial laboratory testing results are suggestive of one of these ingestions, a prolonged period of observation or treatment is required, even if the patient is initially well appearing (see Table 35-6).

 ## ACETAMINOPHEN (TYLENOL)

Acetaminophen (APAP) is the most common cause of pharmaceutical-associated poisoning and death in the United States. Patients are often asymptomatic initially after APAP overdose and one should therefore consider obtaining a serum APAP

Table 35-7 Poisons with Delayed Clinical Toxicity

Acetaminophen
Pennyroyal oil
Carbon tetrachloride
Mushrooms
   Amanita (amatoxin)
   Lepiota (amatoxin)
   Gyromitra (gyromitrin)
   Cortinarius (orellanine/orelline)
Toxic alcohols
   Ethylene glycol
   Methanol
Sustained-release preparations
   Calcium channel blockers
   β-Blockers
   Lithium
   Theophylline
Enteric-coated preparations
   Aspirin
Monoamine oxidase inhibitors
Drug packet ingestion (heroin, cocaine)
Oral hypoglycemic agents
Lomotil
Methylene chloride (metabolized to carbon monoxide)
Paraquat/diquat
Cyanogenic glycosides
Warfarin/super warfarin
   Brodifacoum
Elapid snake envenomation
Antimetabolites
   Colchicine
   Methotrexate
   Alkylating agents
Fat-soluble organophosphate insecticides
Ergotamines
Heavy metals
   Lead
   Thallium
   Mercurys

concentration with all suspected ingestions. *N*-Acetylcysteine (NAC) should be empirically administered to patients who may have ingested a toxic amount of APAP ($\geq$150 mg/kg), for whom the estimated time since ingestion is near 8 hours or more, or if a delay while waiting for a level may/will result in treatment beginning >8 hours after ingestion.

Symptoms
- Early (first 24 hours): Initial toxicity is often mild, nonspecific, and often overlooked, consisting of anorexia, nausea, vomiting, and malaise
- Late (24 to 96 hours after ingestion): Develop symptoms of liver failure (e.g., recurrent nausea, vomiting, and malaise, abdominal pain, lethargy, confusion)

Signs
- Early: None
- Late (>24 hours): Right upper quadrant tenderness
- Signs of fulminant hepatic and multiorgan system failure (e.g., confusion, coma, tachypnea, jaundice, asterixis, coagulopathy) may ensue 24 to 96 hours after ingestion in those not treated or treated too late

Workup
- Serum APAP concentrations measured 4 to 24 hours after acute single overdose can be plotted on the modified Rumack-Matthew nomogram (Fig. 35-1) to predict the risk of subsequent hepatotoxicity and need for NAC antidotal treatment. It is important to note that this nomogram is not validated for extended-release preparations, when APAP has been ingested with an agent that decreases GI motility, or for chronic APAP ingestions.
- Perform baseline and daily BUN/SCr, LFTs, PT/INR.

Comments and Treatment Considerations
Those with a plasma concentration greater than the "possible hepatic toxicity" line on the Rumack-Matthew nomogram receive antidotal therapy with NAC in the United States (see Table 35-1 for dosing). NAC was previously only available as a

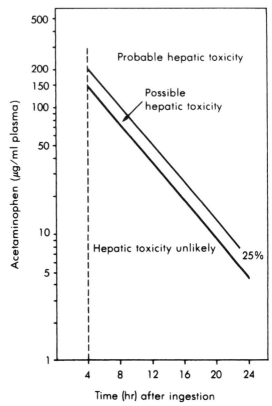

Fig. 35-1 Modified Rumack-Matthew nomogram. (From Rumack BH, Matthew H: *Pediatrics* 55:871, 1975.)

20% oral solution in the United States. The solution has an unpleasant taste and smell, best masked by dilution in cola or juice. Nausea and vomiting are common side effects of treatment with oral NAC, as well as symptoms of acute APAP ingestion. Antiemetic therapy recommendations include ondansetron (preferred) dosed at 0.1 mg/kg/dose (max 4 mg) IV/PO q8h prn or metoclopramide dosed at 0.5 to 1 mg/kg/dose (max 50 mg/dose) IV/PO q4-6h prn. Concurrent diphenhydramine dosed at 1 mg/kg/dose (max 50 mg/dose) IV/PO q4-6h is often recommended for prevention of metoclopramide-induced extrapyramidal side effects. A recently released IV preparation of NAC (Acetadote) may be given IV to patients who are unable to tolerate PO or nasogastric dosing. Intravenous administration is associated with an increased incidence of anaphylactoid and injection site reactions. Informed consent and consultation with a toxicologist is recommended. Intravenous administration is preferred in those patients with APAP-associated hepatic failure.

Treatment is almost 100% effective at preventing APAP toxicity if initiated within 8 to 10 hours of ingestion. Effectiveness progressively diminishes as delay in therapy beyond this time increases, although potential benefit has been seen following administration of NAC even after hepatotoxicity is evident. A decision to initiate or forgo antidotal treatment in those with multiple supratherapeutic ingestions or after ingestion of sustained-release preparations (e.g., Tylenol ER) or to abbreviate treatment in admitted patients (<72-hour treatment) should be made in conjunction with a medical toxicologist.

 IRON

Iron is one of the most common causes of accidental pediatric poisoning death. Children often present with lethargy and GI complaints. The ingestion of >20 mg/kg elemental iron produces significant gastroenteritis and the ingestion of >40 to 60 mg/kg is potentially lethal.

Symptoms

- Stage 1 (within 4 hours): abdominal pain, nausea, vomiting, diarrhea (direct corrosive effects to GI mucosa, may lead to GI tract bleeding)

- Stage 2 (6 to 24 hours): GI symptoms resolve, children may appear improved
- Stage 3 (6 to 24 hours): lethargy, seizures, coma
- Stage 4 (2 to 4 days): coma
- Stage 5 (2 to 8 weeks): nausea and vomiting (gastric outlet obstruction from strictures)

Signs
- Stage 1: abdominal tenderness, vomiting, diarrhea, hematemesis, melena
- Stage 3 to 4: lethargy, coma, seizures, hypotension, shock, hyperventilation, metabolic acidosis (from tissue hypoperfusion/ischemia, fluid third spacing, negative cardiac inotropic effects, and disrupted oxidative phosphorylation), hepatic failure, coagulopathy, anemia, renal failure, multiorgan system failure
- Stage 5: ileus, pyloric obstruction, intestinal scarring

Workup
- Serial measurements of electrolytes, glucose, and renal function. Serum glucose >150 mg/dl and WBC >15,000 may correlate with serum iron level >300 mcg/dl, but normal values do not rule out significant iron poisoning.
- Obtain serum iron level. Serum iron levels peak 2 to 6 hours after ingestion. Serum iron levels 300 to 500 mcg/dl can cause significant GI symptoms but only mild systemic toxicity; 500 to 1000 mcg/dl will lead to significant systemic toxicity; >1000 mcg/dl associated with high risk of mortality. A normal serum iron level beyond 6 hours does not rule out significant toxicity.
- Total iron binding capacity (TIBC) is easily confounded by other factors and is therefore of little value.
- Abdominal plain radiography is not a reliable means of diagnosis. Many preparations are not radiopaque; however, the presence of radiopacities on KUB confirms exposure.

Comments and Treatment Considerations
If the patient can tolerate oral therapy, GI decontamination with a single dose of milk of magnesia 60 ml/g of elemental iron

ingested or sodium bicarbonate 5 to 10 ml/kg of 2% to 5% solution may decrease solubility and prevent iron absorption. Iron concretions or bezoars are not amenable to gut decontamination and may require surgical removal. WBI is recommended in symptomatic patients with large ingestions by history or positive KUB scans. All symptomatic patients should be given 20 ml/kg IV crystalloid and maintenance IVF at twice normal rates. Iron poisoning is treated with chelation therapy, primarily with deferoxamine in patients with serum iron levels >500 mcg/dl or any symptomatic patient regardless of level. It is recommended that a toxicologist be consulted before starting chelation therapy.

Deferoxamine binds extracellular/serum iron as well as intracellular/cytoplasmic and mitochondrial free iron. The resulting ferrioxamine complex is excreted in the urine, usually causing a vin-rose discoloration. Urinary catheter placement to monitor for vin-rose urine is strongly recommended in symptomatic patients. Deferoxamine is contraindicated in patients with severe renal disease or anuria. Rapid infusion of deferoxamine can cause hypotension as a result of histamine release.

SALICYLATES

Salicylates are a common cause of poisonings in the United States. Salicylates are readily available in many OTC products such as aspirin, salicylic acid (Compound W), magnesium salicylate (Doan's pills), bismuth subsalicylate (Pepto-Bismol), Homo menthyl salicylate (sunscreen), and methyl salicylate (Ben-Gay or oil of wintergreen). Salicylate poisoning is frequently misdiagnosed, particularly when chronic poisoning exists. Symptoms and signs are often nonspecific and erroneous diagnoses such as sepsis, altered mental status, gastroenteritis, or congestive heart failure are frequently made.

Symptoms

- Mild/early poisoning (1 to 12 hours after acute ingestion): nausea, vomiting, abdominal pain, headache, tinnitus, dizziness, fatigue

- Moderate/intermediate poisoning (12 to 24 hours after ingestion): fever, sweating, deafness, lethargy, confusion, hallucinations, breathlessness
- Severe/late poisoning (>24 hours after acute ingestion or unrecognized untreated chronic ingestion): coma, seizures, fever

Signs

- Mild/early: lethargy, ataxia, mild agitation, hyperpnea, mild abdominal tenderness
- Moderate/intermediate: fever, asterixis, diaphoresis, deafness, pallor, confusion, slurred speech, disorientation, agitation, hallucinations, tachycardia, tachypnea, orthostatic hypotension
- Severe/late: dehydration, coma, seizures, hypothermia or hyperthermia, tachycardia, hypotension, respiratory depression, pulmonary edema, arrhythmias, papilledema

Workup

- Serum salicylate concentration, in conjunction with history (acute or chronic ingestion) and severity/phase of poisoning will determine appropriate treatment strategy.
- Obtain electrolytes, glucose, BUN/SCr, UA (particularly urine pH), ABG, salicylate concentration, LFTs, CBC, PT/INR, and calcium for those with severe poisoning.
- Acid-base disturbances: respiratory alkalosis (mild/early poisoning), respiratory alkalosis with metabolic acidosis (moderate/intermediate poisoning), and metabolic acidosis with or without respiratory acidosis (severe/late poisoning).
- The initial primary respiratory alkalosis is not typically seen in young children.

Comments and Treatment Considerations

History of salicylate ingestion may be difficult to elicit, especially in cases of chronic ingestion when the syndrome of confusion, hyperthermia, tachypnea, and dehydration may easily be confused with sepsis. Treatment requires GI decontamination (multidose AC, see dosing above); correction of acid-base, fluid, and electrolyte disturbances, as well as enhanced elimination with urinary alkalinization and/or hemodialysis (see Table 35-3). Alkalinization may be accomplished using IVF containing sodium bicarbonate, often 75 to 150 mEq/L in D5W, to maintain a urinary pH level of >7.5. Caution should be used when providing fluid resuscitation in a chronic intoxication because these patients are more likely to have abnormal renal function and are at higher risk of developing cerebral and pulmonary edema. Hemodialysis is indicated for those with severe toxicity (e.g., SA >100 mg/dl in acute and >60 mg/dl in chronic poisoning, altered mental status, seizures, pulmonary edema, refractory acid-base disturbances, renal failure, and deterioration despite maximal supportive care).

 ## TOXIC ALCOHOLS (ETHYLENE GLYCOL, METHANOL, AND ISOPROPANOL)

Poisoning by ethylene glycol and methanol require early diagnosis and treatment to prevent accumulation of the toxic acid metabolites and subsequent development of profound metabolic acidosis with end-organ complications.

Ethylene glycol has a sweet taste and odor and may be tempting for children to drink. Ethylene glycol is found in antifreeze, coolants, and glass cleaners. Common sources of methanol include antifreeze and windshield washer fluid. The lethal dose of methanol and ethylene glycol is approximately 1 ml/kg; as little as 30 ml may be fatal. Smaller doses may result in end-organ toxicity such as blindness or renal toxicity. Isopropyl alcohol is found in rubbing alcohol and glass cleaners, with the toxic dose approximately 1 ml/kg and the lethal dose between 2 and 4 ml/kg. Toxicity in children can result from direct ingestion or topical exposure (transdermal absorption).

Symptoms
- Early (1 to 12 hours): anorexia, nausea, vomiting, abdominal pain, headache, vertigo, weakness, lethargy, coma (delayed presentation of up to 24 hours has been reported)

- Late (6 to 36 hours): progressive visual disturbances with methanol (e.g., blurred vision, diplopia, scotomata, "snow fields," tunnel vision, blindness), shortness of breath, confusion, lethargy, seizures, coma, hematemesis, flank pain

Signs

- Early: CNS inebriation (e.g., slurred speech, nystagmus, lethargy, coma, ataxia), hypoglycemia (caused by smaller baseline glycogen stores)
- Late: progressive visual field and acuity deficits, optic disc hyperemia, papilledema, mydriasis nonreactive to light, confusion, agitation, delirium, coma, myoclonus, tetany, seizures, tachypnea, hyperpnea, pulmonary edema, ketotic breath, sinus tachycardia, hypertension, hypotension, hematuria, or anuria

Workup

- Obtain measurements of serum electrolytes, BUN/SCr, glucose, amylase, calcium, ketones, osmolality, lactate, ABG, UA, and solvents (e.g., ethanol, ethylene glycol, isopropanol, and methanol).
- Early: Commonly see elevated osmolal gap without anion gap. A normal osmolal gap does not rule out significant toxic alcohol poisoning.
- Late: Commonly see elevated anion gap ± elevated osmolal gap.
  - Anion gap calculation see the previous section on general workup or the poisoned patient.
  - Osmolar gap is defined as the difference between measured serum osmolality and calculated serum osmolality.

$$\text{Osm (mOsm/L)} = 2\,(\text{Na}^+) +$$
$$\left(\frac{\text{glucose}}{18}\right) + \left(\frac{\text{BUN}}{2.8}\right) + \left(\frac{\text{EtOH}}{4.6}\right) + \left(\frac{\text{MeOH}}{3.2}\right) + \left(\frac{\text{EtGly}}{6.2}\right) + \left(\frac{\text{Iso}}{6}\right) + \left(\frac{\text{Acet}}{5.6}\right)$$

For the above equation, sodium is measured as mEq/L and the remaining variables are measured in mg/dl.

- Normal osmolal gap (early or late) does not exclude toxic alcohol poisoning.

- Ketosis (serum and urinary acetone) without acidosis commonly seen in isopropanol poisoning.
- Serum hypocalcemia, urinary calcium oxalate crystals, ATN (microscopic hematuria, proteinuria, oliguria), elevated BUN/SCr, bronchopneumonia on CXR, cerebral edema on head CT may be seen in ethylene glycol poisoning.

Comments and Treatment Considerations

Conventional treatment of ethylene glycol and methanol poisoning includes sodium bicarbonate administration for metabolic acidosis and ethanol or fomepizole (4-MP) infusion to inhibit metabolism to toxic acid metabolites (see Table 35-1 for dosing). Sodium bicarbonate dosed at 1 to 2 mEq/kg/dose IV titrated to serum pH will prevent formic acid entry into the CNS. Vitamin administration for methanol and ethylene glycol ingestions (folinic acid 1 mg/kg/dose IV [max 50 mg/dose] followed by folate 1 mg/kg/dose IV q4h [max 50 mg/dose]) may assist the conversion of formic acid to CO_2 and water for elimination. For ethylene glycol ingestions, thiamine and pyridoxine administration (100 mg of each IV q6h until level is undetectable) is recommended for the conversion of glyoxalic acid.

Fomepizole or ethanol therapy is indicated for those with suspected ingestion by history if no laboratory data are available, for any symptomatic patients, for ethylene glycol or methanol levels >20 mg/dl, or osmolal gap >10 mOsm/L. Ethanol therapy requires serial blood ethanol levels to ensure a concentration between 125 and 150 mg/dl (27 to 32 mmol/L). Fomepizole has the benefit of less CNS depression, smaller volume of fluid administration, less intensive monitoring, and longer duration of action, although the direct cost of therapy is significantly higher. Hemodialysis is typically indicated for those with ethylene glycol or methanol serum concentrations >50 mg/dl (some experts recommend >25 mg/dl), pH ≤ 7.20, and significant end-organ toxicity (e.g., renal insufficiency, visual impairment, seizures).

Pharmacologic measures are generally not effective for isopropyl alcohol ingestions and hemodialysis should be initiated for hypotension unresponsive to fluid boluses, or a blood concentration >400 mg/dl. Some also consider hemodialysis for the pediatric patient with coma and/or respiratory depression.

TRICYCLIC ANTIDEPRESSANTS

Clinical presentation of a tricyclic antidepressant (TCA) ingestion may vary widely due to complex pharmacology. Anticholinergic symptoms usually predominate initially. Children may maintain near-normal hemodynamic parameters and then decompensate suddenly and profoundly.

Symptoms
- Seizures
- Lethargy to coma (children may have paradoxic CNS stimulation initially)

Signs
- Mydriasis (anticholinergic) or miosis (α-adrenergic blockade)
- Dry skin
- Tachycardia
- Lethargy to coma
- Seizures
- Agitated delirium (occasionally)
- Hypotension
- Hypertension (mild, early)

Workup
- ECG may show cardiac conduction disturbances (e.g., prolonged QRS, R in aV_R [rightward axis of terminal 40 ms of limb lead QRS]). These are much more variable in children than adults and they often have a baseline rightward axis deviation. Wide-complex tachycardias (both supraventricular tachycardia [SVT] with aberrant conduction and ventricular tachycardia [VT]) and ventricular fibrillation (VF) can occur.

Comments and Treatment Considerations
All but the most trivial poisonings (<5 mg/kg) require close cardiac monitoring, because patients may rapidly deteriorate in the first few hours after ingestion. If patients remain or become

asymptomatic after 4 to 6 hours of observation, they are unlikely to have a complication related to TCA ingestion. All patients with a cardiac conduction disturbance on ECG should be admitted for cardiac monitoring.

Activated charcoal should be given at a dose of 1 gm/kg PO/NG (max 60 g/dose) and may be repeated every q4-6h as long as gastric motility is evident. Death most commonly results from refractory hypotension or ventricular arrhythmia. QRS > 100 ms or R in aV_R > 3 mm predicts serious toxicity and warrants close monitoring and immediate sodium bicarbonate administration. Sodium bicarbonate (overcomes fast–sodium channel blockade) in 1 to 2 mEq/kg intravenous boluses is recommended until arterial pH is maintained at 7.50 to 7.55. The goal is to decrease the toxic cardiac effects (attenuates conduction disturbance and provides positive inotropic effects). Typical Class Ia and Ic antiarrhythmics are contraindicated in TCA overdose because of the potentiation of the arrhythmias. Lidocaine and β-blockers may also be required to control arrhythmias (see Chapter 35, Tachycardia). Hyperventilation is recommended in those requiring intubation as adjunctive therapy to sodium bicarbonate (target P_{CO_2} ≈30 mm Hg).

 ## CARBON MONOXIDE POISONING

Carbon monoxide (CO) is an odorless, tasteless, and colorless gas produced by the incomplete combustion of any carbon-containing material. CO poisoning typically occurs after exposure to fires from smoke inhalation, automobile exhaust fumes (especially with inadequate ventilation or within an enclosed space), poorly ventilated charcoal, kerosene or gas heaters, and to a lesser extent, cigarette smoke.

The toxicity from CO poisoning is from cellular hypoxia and ischemia. Hemoglobin has a much greater affinity (250 times) to bind CO instead of oxygen, which results in decreased formation of oxyhemoglobin and decreased oxygen-carrying capacity. Furthermore, fetal hemoglobin has even a greater affinity for CO as compared to adult hemoglobin, which puts infants at greater risk after exposure.

Symptoms

Symptoms correlate variably with the carboxyhemoglobin (CoHb) concentration; concentrations up to 9% can be seen in smokers and 2% to 4% in patients living in congested urban areas. In general, the CoHb concentrations listed below roughly correlate to the following symptoms:

- 10% to 20%: headache, dizziness, chest pain, dyspnea
- 20% to 30%: visual disturbances, confusion
- 30% to 40%: syncope
- 40% to 50%: seizures, coma
- >55% or 60%: death

Signs

- PE findings are usually normal
- Cutaneous and mucosal erythema, retinal hemorrhages, and bullae on the skin are all rare

Workup

- CoHb concentration (may be arterial or venous).
- ABG analysis: May show metabolic acidosis. Readings of oxygen saturation will be falsely normal (if calculated from PO_2) unless directly measured by cooximetry.
- ECG: May show nonspecific repolarization or ischemic changes and tachyarrhythmias. May be useful in ruling out other pathologic conditions.
- CXR: CO does not change the CXR itself but may reflect changes resulting from smoke inhalation, such as nonspecific findings of interstitial or alveolar edema, atelectasis, perivascular/bronchial cuffing, and peripheral opacities. May be useful in ruling out other pathologic conditions.

Comments and Treatment Conditions

Treat immediately with 100% O_2. The half-life of CoHb is 4 to 6 hours when breathing room air, 60 to 90 minutes when breathing 100% O_2, and 20 to 45 minutes with hyperbaric O_2 (HBO) at 2.8 standard atmospheres. Do not rely on pulse oximetry. This technique measures CoHb as $O_2 - Hb$ and will be falsely normal. Indications for HBO (not universally agreed on) include CoHb level >25%, pregnancy, end-organ damage (neurologic [mental status changes, seizures, coma] or cardiopulmonary [life-threatening arrhythmias, ischemia]), metabolic acidosis, presence of syncope, and worsening or failure to improve (decreasing CoHb) on 100% O_2 for 4 hours. Newer studies suggest the possible benefit of HBO in preventing neurologic sequelae in patients with lower levels of exposure.

CYANIDE POISONING

Cyanide poisoning is very rare but frequently fatal and is a potentially treatable cause of altered mental status. Routes of exposure include oral ingestion (often suicidal), cutaneous exposure (usually industrial), and inhalation (e.g., smoke from a fire).

Cyanide binds cytochrome oxidase and inhibits oxygen metabolism at the cellular level. The clinical appearance of these patients is therefore similar to those who are hypoxic, except that the blood of patients with cyanide poisoning is well oxygenated; therefore cyanosis does not appear until the onset of respiratory failure. Patients have a severe metabolic acidosis as a result of anaerobic cellular metabolism. An odor of almonds also may be detected.

Symptoms
- Rate of symptom development depends on form, concentration, and route of ingestion: inhalation (seconds to minutes), oral ingestion of cyanide salts (several minutes to 1 hour), organic cyanides (up to 12 hours)
- Initial CNS stimulation followed by a rapid loss of consciousness
- Nausea and vomiting
- Palpitations

Signs

- Agitation, confusion, coma
- Seizures
- Arrhythmias, asystole
- Profound hypotension

Workup

- Clinical diagnosis on the basis on a history of exposure and concordant physical findings.
- ABG, serum lactate concentration, and electrolytes; profound anion gap metabolic acidosis and elevated serum lactate concentration support the diagnosis.
- O_2 saturation and PO_2 are normal.
- Other laboratory results are often too delayed to be helpful in the most serious cases of cyanide poisonings.
- CoHb concentration.

Comments and Treatment Considerations

The patient should receive 100% oxygen. The Lilly Cyanide Antidote Kit (contains amyl nitrite ampule, sodium nitrite, sodium thiosulfate) is the only antidote combination available in the United States and should be administered to all patients with serious symptoms of cyanide poisoning. Nitrites are thought to produce methemoglobin, which subsequently binds to cyanide to produce cyanomethemoglobin. Sodium thiosulfate is given after the more rapidly acting nitrite preparations and enhances endogenous detoxification mechanisms by producing thiocyanate, which is readily excreted by the kidney. Sodium thiosulfate alone (without nitrites) may be the treatment of choice for cases involving smoke inhalation in which CO poisoning may also have occurred; nitrites will worsen oxygenation in CO poisoning and are not recommended.

REFERENCES

Abbruzzi G, Stork CM: Pediatric toxicologic concerns, *Emerg Med Clin North Am* 20:223, 2002.

American Academy of Clinical Toxicology, European Association of Poison Centres and Clinical Toxicologists: Position statements, *J Toxicol Clin Toxicol* 35:695, 1997.

Baud FH, Barriot P, Torris V, et al: Elevated blood cyanide concentration in victims of smoke inhalation, *N Engl J Med* 325:1761, 1991.

Baum CR, Langman CB, Oker EE, et al: Fomepizole treatment of ethylene glycol poisoning in an infant, *Pediatrics* 106:1489, 2000.

Belson MG, Gorman Se, Sullivan K, et al: Calcium channel blocker ingestions in children, *Am J Emerg Med* 18:581, 2000.

Berkovitch M, Matsui D, et al: Assessment of the terminal 40-millisecond QRS vector in children with a history of tricyclic antidepressant ingestion, *Pediatr Emerg Med* 11:75, 1995.

Boyle PJ, Justice K, Krentz AJ, et al: Octreotide reverses hyperinsulinemia and prevents hypoglycemia induced by sulfonylurea overdoses, *J Clin Endocr Met* 76:752, 1993.

Caravati ME: Unintentional acetaminophen ingestion in children and the potential for hepatotoxicity, *J Toxicol Clin Toxicol* 38:291, 2000.

Clark CJ, Campbell D, Reid WH: Blood carboxyhaemoglobin and cyanide levels in fire survivors, *Lancet* 1:1332, 1981.

Edlow J, Macnow L: Headache. In Fleisher GR, Ludwig S, editors: *Textbook of pediatric emergency medicine*, 4th ed, Philadelphia, 2000, Lippincott Williams & Wilkins.

Ely WE, Moorehead B, Haponik EF: Warehouse worker's headache: emergency evaluation and management of 30 patients with carbon monoxide poisoning, *Am J Med* 98:145, 1995.

Erickson SJ, Duncan A: Clonidine poisoning—an emerging problem: epidemiology, clinical features, management and preventative strategies, *J Paediatr Child Health* 34:280, 1998.

Farrar HC, James LP: Characteristics of pediatric admissions for cyclic antidepressant poisoning, *Amer J Emerg Med* 17(5):495, 1999.

Fine JS: Pediatric principles. In *Goldfrank's toxicologic emergencies*, 7th ed, New York, 2002, Appleton & Lange.

Hall AH, Rumack GH: Clinical toxicology of cyanide, *Ann Emerg Med* 15:1067, 1986.

Hecherling PS, Leikin JB, Maturen A: Occult carbon monoxide poisoning: validation of a prediction model, *Am J Med* 84:251, 1988.

Hoffman RS, Goldfrank LR: The poisoned patient with altered consciousness: controversies in the use of a "coma cocktail," *JAMA* 274:562, 1995.

Koren G: Medications which can kill a toddler with one tablet or teaspoonful, *J Toxicol Clin Toxicol* 31(3):407, 1993.

Kulig K, Bar-Or D, Cantrill SV, et al: Management of acutely poisoned patients without gastric emptying, *Ann Emerg Med* 14:562, 1985.

Lee DC, Greene T, Dougherty T, et al: Fatal nifedipine ingestions in children, *J Emerg Med* 19:359, 2000.

Liebelt EL, DeAngelis CD: Evolving trends and treatment advances in pediatric poisoning, *JAMA* 282(12):1113-5, 1999.

Liebelt EL, Shannon MW: Small doses, big problems: a selected review of highly toxic common medications, *Pediatr Emerg Care* 9:292, 1993.

Lifshitz M: Acute poisoning in children, *Isr Med Assoc* 2(7):504, 2000(abstr).

Lis JG: Mental status change and coma. In Fleisher GR, Ludwig S, editors: *Textbook of pediatric emergency medicine*, 4th ed, Philadelphia, 2000, Lippincott Williams & Wilkins.

Litovitz TL, Klein-Schwartz W, Rogers GC, et al: 2001 annual report of American Association of Poison Control Centers: toxic exposure surveillance system, *Am J Emerg Med* 20(5):391, 2002.

Litovitz TL, Manoguerra A: Comparison of pediatric hazards: an analysis of 3.8 million exposure incidents. A report from the American Association of Poison Control Centers, *Pediatrics* 89(6):999, 1992.

Mordel A, Sivilotti ML, Old AC, et al: Octreotide for pediatric sulfonylurea poisoning (abstract), *J Toxicol Clin Toxicol* 36:437, 1998.

Ozanne-Smith J: Childhood poisoning: access and prevention, *J Paediatr Child Health* 37(3):262, 2001.

Perry H, Shannon MW: Acetaminophen. In Haddad L, Winchester J, Shannon M, editors: Clinical Management of poisoning and drug overdose, 3rd ed, Philadelphia, 1998, WB Saunders.

Peterson RG: Management of poisoning. In Yaffe SJ, Aranda JV, editors: *Pediatric pharmacology: therapeutic principles in practice*, 2nd ed, Philadelphia, 1992, WB Saunders.

Pond SM, Lewis-Driver DJ, Williams GM, et al: Gastric emptying in acute overdose: a prospective randomized controlled trial, *Med J Aust* 163:345, 1995.

Proudfoot A: Acute poisoning: principles of management, *Med Int* 61:2499, 1989.

Rumack BH, Matthews H: Acetaminophen poisoning and toxicity. *Pediatrics* 55:871, 1975.

Sadovnikoff N, Varon J, Sternbach GL: Carbon monoxide poisoning—an occult epidemic, *Postgrad Med* 92:86, 1992.

Schonwald S: *Medical toxicology: a synopsis and study guide*, New York, 2001, Lippincott Williams & Wilkins.

Viccellio P, editor: *Emergency toxicology*, 2nd ed, New York, 1998, Lippincott–Raven Press.

Vogel C, Caraccio T, Mofenson H, et al: Alcohol intoxication in young children, *J Toxicol Clin Toxicol* 33:25, 1995.

Woolf AD: Poisoning by unknown agents, *Pediatr Rev* 20(5):166, 1999.

Yuan TH, Kerns WP, Tomaszewski CA, et al: Insulin and glucose as adjunctive therapy for severe calcium channel antagonist poisoning. *J Toxicol Clin Toxicol* 37:463, 1999.

CHAPTER 36

Trauma

MICHELLE M. CARLO

Traumatic injuries account for the majority of deaths in children older than 1 year, exceeding all other causes of death combined. In 1979 Dr. Cowley described the concept of the "golden hour" in the treatment of trauma victims, demonstrating that outcome was significantly linked to the time between initial injury and definitive therapy. In children, this time frame becomes even more relevant when one considers the physiologic differences between adults and children that render them more vulnerable to serious injury after trauma. Although only 10% to 15% of traumatized children have truly life-threatening injuries, the physician must be able to recognize them and subsequently provide appropriate care in an expeditious manner. It has been reported that the overall functional outcome for severely injured children treated at pediatric trauma centers is better when compared to children treated at general hospitals. Therefore, one of the most important roles of the physician caring for an injured child is to anticipate whether the patient will require the immediate care of a surgeon or a subspecialist and to determine the need for transfer to another facility better equipped to handle such an emergency. The pediatric trauma victim may present with severe anxiety even without significant injury or pain, making the initial examination difficult; therefore, the value of serial repeated examinations cannot be overemphasized. Hospital admission for observation of the injured child is recommended if there is concern about potential deterioration and/or adequate supervision.

✳ PREHOSPITAL CARE

The initial phase of resuscitation begins at the scene of the injury. Prehospital preparation is essential and should include ensuring that the first responders are capable of handling pediatric injuries, limiting the time spent on scene before initiation of transfer (ideally within 10 minutes), and C-spine immobilization (stabilization and prevention of additional injuries). A modified immobilization board is needed for the pediatric patient as a result of the enlarged occiput of the pediatric patient that causes the head to flex forward on a flat board (Fig. 36-1). The history surrounding the trauma incident is of particular importance in determining the extent and the nature of the injuries. The physician should obtain as much information as possible regarding the mechanism of injury; the possibility of nonaccidental trauma; if a motor vehicle crash, the extent of damage to the cars and other passengers; the presence of any underlying illnesses affecting care; and estimated blood loss. Once these are known the physician can begin assembling the trauma team and the ancillary services needed to care for the child. Services that may be needed on arrival include

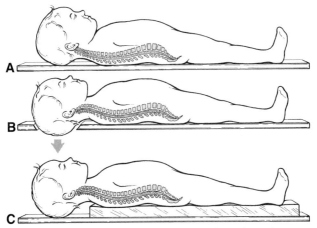

Fig. 36-1   Standard adult backboard. **A,** The enlarged occiput causes the child to flex the head forward. **B** and **C,** Appropriate positioning on a modified board with either the occipital area cut out or a pad under the thorax to prevent flexion of the cervical spine. (From Green N, Swiontkowski M: *Skeletal trauma in children,* 2nd ed, Philadelphia 1998, WB Saunders.)

surgery and surgical subspecialties, blood bank products, radiology, anesthesia, operating room, and transport team if a higher level of care is anticipated.

 INITIAL MANAGEMENT

As in any emergency situation the ABCs of resuscitation should be followed, paying attention to the presence of any life-threatening injury. Whenever possible in parallel with the primary survey of the ABCs, the patient should have two large-bore IV catheters placed, a cardiac monitor applied, and 100% oxygen given as preoxygenation in case intubation is required.

A team leader should be identified and the role for each trauma team member defined. All equipment should be ready and checked for function prior to the patient's arrival including oxygen supply, mask/bag, suction, endotracheal tube (ETT) sizes appropriate for children, stylet, laryngoscope, end-tidal CO_2, oral airways, and medications. The use of the Broselow tape is recommended, particularly for non–pediatric-specific facilities.

PRIMARY SURVEY

As an abnormality is identified it should be addressed in parallel with or before moving onto the next step of evaluation.

Airway

Assume cervical injury and use preventive maneuvers that limit neck movement (jaw thrust vs. sniffing position). Achieving and maintaining airway patency is *vital*, especially because childhood cardiac arrest is usually secondary to respiratory arrest. If trauma involves the airway, consider calling anesthesia or otolaryngology to assist. Evaluate the need for a definitive airway while considering the adequacy of ventilation/oxygenation, need for airway protection, and requirements for the ongoing evaluation of the patient.

Rapid sequence intubation (RSI) is generally the safest and most effective manner to secure an airway. Table 36-1 outlines suggested choices for RSI medications in various circumstances. Succinylcholine should be avoided in patients with trauma older

Table 36-1 Rapid Sequence Intubation Medications

Condition	Drug and Dose	Comments
Normotensive, no head trauma	Etomidate 0.3 mg/kg IV (max 20 mg dose) or Thiopental 4-6 mg/kg IV plus Rocuronium 0.6-1.2 mg/kg IV or Succinylcholine* 1-1.5 mg/kg IV (2 mg/kg for infants), max 150 mg/dose	Atropine 0.02 mg/kg (min 0.1 mg/dose; max 1 mg/dose) premedication is recommended for children younger than 7 years Etomidate lacks analgesic properties, consider adding fentanyl as adjuvant therapy
Hypotensive, no head trauma	Etomidate 0.3 mg/kg IV (max 20 mg dose) or Ketamine† 1-2 mg/kg IV plus Rocuronium 0.6-1.2 mg/kg IV (max 20 mg/dose) or Succinylcholine* 1-1.5 mg/kg IV (2 mg/kg for infants), max 150 mg/dose	Etomidate lacks analgesic properties, consider adding fentanyl as adjuvant therapy Atropine 0.02 mg/kg (min 0.1 mg/dose; max 1 mg/dose) premedication is recommended for children younger than 7 years

Continued

Table 36-1 Rapid Sequence Intubation Medications—cont'd

Condition	Drug and Dose	Comments
Normotensive, head trauma/elevated ICP	Thiopental 4-6 mg/kg IV plus Rocuronium 0.6-1.2 mg/kg IV or Succinylcholine* 1-1.5 mg/kg IV (2 mg/kg for infants), max 150 mg/dose	Lidocaine premedication is recommended for patients with elevated ICP and/or head trauma Atropine 0.02 mg/kg (min 0.1 mg/dose; max 1 mg/dose) premedication is recommended for children younger than 7 years
Hypotensive, head trauma/elevated ICP	Etomidate 0.3 mg/kg IV (max 20 mg/dose) plus Rocuronium 0.6-1.2 mg/kg IV or Succinylcholine* 1-1.5 mg/kg IV (2 mg/kg for infants), max 150 mg/dose	Etomidate lacks analgesic properties, consider adding fentanyl as adjuvant therapy Lidocaine premedication is recommended for patients with elevated ICP and/or head trauma Atropine 0.02 mg/kg (min 0.1 mg/dose; max 1 mg dose) premedication is recommended for children younger than 7 years

ICP, Intracranial pressure.

*Succinylcholine should avoided in patients with trauma older than 24 to 48 hours, in patients with a history of or a family history of myopathies or malignant hypothermia, hyperkalemia, and/or with burns. If no contraindication exists, succinylcholine may be used in place of rocuronium.

†Ketamine is contraindicated in patients with elevated intracranial pressure and should not be used if head trauma is suspected. If using Ketamine IM, dose is 3-7 mg/kg.

than 24 to 48 hours, hyperkalemia, and/or with burns and in patients with a history of or a family history of myopathies or malignant hypothermia. Difficult airways may require use of accessory devices or techniques such as fiberoptic scopes, retrograde intubation, laryngeal mask airway (LMA) use, or a surgical airway. Needle cricothyroidotomy is the "surgical rescue" procedure for children younger than 10 years and may be set up using the adapter of a 3.0 ETT tube attached to a standard IV catheter that is inserted into the airway. High pressures may be needed when squeezing the bag and the "pop-off" valve must be closed so pressure is not released through the valve and adequate time is required for expiration. A needle cricothyroidotomy is a temporizing measure only and is used primarily to provide oxygenation to the patient as ventilation will not be adequate. Emergency cricothyroidotomy, in experienced hands, can be considered for children older than 10 years.

Always consider the patient to have a full stomach and provide cricoid pressure until the airway is secured and orogastric decompression is provided to prevent aspiration of stomach contents.

Breathing

Check for spontaneous breathing and the need for positive pressure ventilation (PPV) as support until endotracheal intubation is accomplished. Observe chest wall movement and auscultate both lung fields to assess air entry. Listen for decreased breath sounds, look for tracheal deviation, and feel for crepitance, which might indicate pneumothorax. If tension pneumothorax is a consideration, rapid needle decompression should be accomplished followed by chest tube placement (see the section Thoracic Trauma, later in this chapter). If the patient is intubated, listen over both axillae and stomach to check tube placement and use a definitive method of confirmation such as end-tidal CO_2 monitoring.

Circulation

Check capillary refill, pulses (both distal and central), and heart rate. Obtain prompt IV access (two large-bore catheters) and hemorrhage control. Remember that in the pediatric population hypotension is a late and ominous sign (see Chapter 20, Hypotension/Shock, for more information on shock states).

Disability

Use the modified Glasgow Coma Scale to determine the degree of neurologic disability (Table 36-2). Check for pupil size and symmetry. Note any abnormal posturing.

Exposure

It is important to completely undress the patient and while maintaining inline stabilization to examine the patient's back. Although new studies suggest that relative hypothermia may be protective in resuscitation, attempt to avoid extreme body heat loss. Remember to remove wet or contaminated clothing.

Comments and Treatment Considerations

In the initial management of the injured child it is important to consider the anatomic and physiologic needs that are different from adults (Fig. 36-2).

Anatomic differences

- The vocal cords when visualized during laryngoscopy are less distant from the mouth and more anterior in children than in adults.
- Children have shorter necks, a short trachea, a large and floppy epiglottis, a small/anterior larynx, and a large tongue.
- Children have larger heads and relatively weak cervical muscles.
- IV access is more difficult. New Pediatric Advanced Life Support (PALS) guidelines suggest that intraosseous (IO) lines can be used in children of all ages. An IO line should be placed in any acutely ill child in whom IV access cannot rapidly be obtained.
  - Placement of an IO line should follow universal precautions. Insertion should be approximately 1 to 3 cm below the tibial tuberosity in the anteromedial aspect of the tibia. The thigh and the knee should be grasped with the nondominant hand to stabilize the site. Needle advancement should proceed at 90 degrees perpendicular to the long axis of the bone in a slightly caudad direction. Needle

Table 36-2 Modified Glasgow Coma Scale

Response	Adults	Children	Infants	Coded Value
Eye opening	Spontaneous	Spontaneous	Spontaneous	4
	To speech	To speech	To speech	3
	To pain	To pain	To pain	2
	None	None	None	1
Best verbal response	Oriented	Oriented, appropriate	Coos and babbles	5
	Confused	Confused	Irritable, cries	4
	Inappropriate words	Inappropriate words	Cries in response to pain	3
	Incomprehensible sounds	Incomprehensible words or nonspecific sounds	Moans in response to pain	2
	None	None	None	1
Best motor response	Obeys	Obeys commands	Moves spontaneously and purposefully	6
	Localizes	Localizes painful stimulus	Withdraws in response to touch	5
	Withdraws	Withdraws in response to pain	Withdraws in response to pain	4

Continued

Table 36-2 Modified Glasgow Coma Scale—cont'd

Response	Adults	Children	Infants	Coded Value
	Abnormal flexion	Flexion in response to pain	Decorticate posturing (abnormal flexion) in response to pain	3
	Extensor responce	Extension in response to pain	Decerebrate posturing (abnormal extension) in response to pain	2
	None	None	None	1
Total Score				3-15

From Nichols GM et al, editors: *Golden hour: the handbook of Advanced Pediatric Life Support*, St. Louis, 1996, Mosby–Year Book.

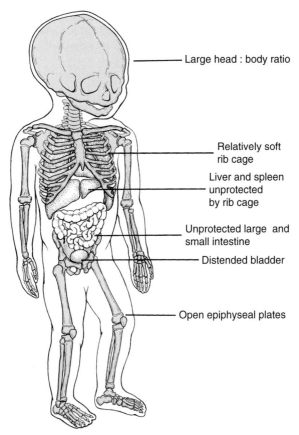

Large head : body ratio

Relatively soft
rib cage

Liver and spleen
unprotected
by rib cage

Unprotected large and
small intestine

Distended bladder

Open epiphyseal plates

Fig. 36-2 Anatomic differences predispose the child to injuries different from those of the adult. These differences include disproportionately large head, pliable rib cage with exposed liver and spleen below its margin, unprotected large and small bowel, distended bladder above the pelvic brim, and open physes. (From Green N, Swiontkowski M: *Skeletal trauma in children,* 2nd ed, Philadelphia, 1998, WB Saunders.)

advancement should stop when there is a sudden decrease in resistance. Stabilize the needle well and test infusion site for ability to infuse fluids without evidence of infiltration.

Physiologic differences

- Oropharyngeal obstructions are common in children.
- A child's initial response to hemodynamic instability is increased heart rate and vascular resistance because of the inability to alter stroke volume.
- Children have greater surface area/mass ratios, predisposing them to greater insensible water losses and placing them at risk of hypothermia.

SCREENING RADIOGRAPHS

The routine use of radiographs without clinical correlation should be discouraged. Traditionally, chest, abdomen, pelvis, and c-spine radiographs were universally obtained in all trauma patients. Many studies suggest that in an alert and cooperative child one can limit the use of x-rays based on physical examination findings. Some authors have proposed that an alert child with no distracting injuries who has no midline cervical tenderness and no pain on neck movement in the absence of any neurologic deficit can have clearance of the cervical spine based on their clinical picture. Other studies have suggested that routine pelvic radiographs have limited value in patients without concerning mechanisms of injury, clinical symptoms referable to the pelvic area, or altered mental status. It is important to note that radiologic studies should not delay the ongoing process of the secondary survey. Ideally, team members can wear lead suits that allow them to continue their work while these radiographs are completed.

Comments and Treatment Considerations

When indicated, three views of the cervical spine are required to evaluate for acute injury: anteroposterior (AP), lateral, and odontoid (Figs. 36-3, 36-4, and 36-5). It is important that all seven cervical vertebrae are visualized, including the C7-T1 junction, and if this is not possible, a CT scan of any question-able areas may be necessary. Anterior pseudosubluxation of C2 on C3 is a common pediatric finding and can be differentiated from true subluxation by Swischuk's posterior cervical line (Figs. 36-6 and 36-7). Swischuk's line should be drawn from the cortex of the spinous process of C1 to C3. Cervical injury is present if the line passes > 1 to 2.0 mm anterior to the spinous process of C2. Always consider the possibility of spinal cord injury without radiographic abnormality (SCIWORA). If cervical

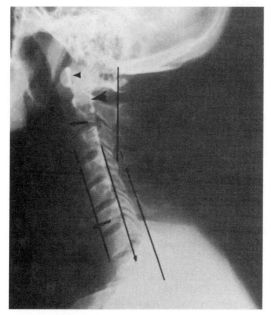

Fig. 36-3   Lateral view of normal cervical spine. Predental space *(arrowhead)*. Harris' ring *(barbed arrow)*. Prevertebral soft tissues *(arrows)*. Posterior cervical line, anterior and pos-terior body lines, and spinolaminar lines *(long arrows)*. (From Davis M, Votey, S, Greenough PG: *Signs and symptoms in emergency medicine,* St. Louis, 1999, Mosby. Courtesy Michael Zucker, MD, Los Angeles, CA.)

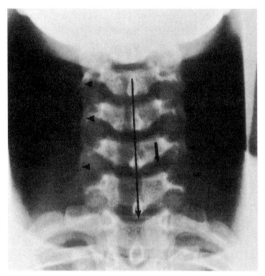

Fig. 36-4 Anteroposterior view of normal cervical spine. Lateral masses *(arrowheads)*. Spinous processes are aligned *(long arrow)*. (From Davis M, Votey, S, Greenough PG: *Signs and symptoms in emergency medicine,* St. Louis, 1999, Mosby. Courtesy Michael Zucker, MD, Los Angeles, CA.)

spine injury cannot be ruled out clinically based on age or altered mental status, the patient should remain in cervical immobilization despite having normal radiographic findings or a cervical MRI scan should be obtained.

CXR will identify the most life-threatening thoracic injuries in children: hemothorax, pneumothorax, aortic injuries, diaphragmatic rupture, and pulmonary contusions (see the section Thoracic Trauma). Rib fractures are rare in children because of increased pliability. If present, they should alert the clinician to the possibility of internal injury and severe trauma. Some studies suggest that the presence of two or more broken ribs in a child younger than 2 years should raise suspicion of abuse.

Pelvic fractures are uncommon in children. If present, they can contribute to major blood loss. Ordering of other

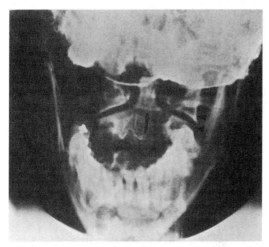

Fig. 36-5 Open-mouth odontoid view of normal cervical spine. Lateral masses C1-C2 are aligned *(arrowheads)*. Dens is unremarkable *(arrow)*. (From Davis M, Votey, S, Greenough PG: *Signs and symptoms in emergency medicine,* St. Louis, 1999, Mosby. Courtesy Michael Zucker, MD, Los Angeles, CA.)

radiographs should be based on history and clinical examination findings.

✻ *EMERGENT LABORATORY STUDIES*

As with screening radiographs, the indiscriminate use of laboratory tests should be avoided. However, the following emergent laboratory tests should be considered:

- CBC: the hematocrit may be normal initially, even in the presence of significant blood loss. It is important to recheck the hematocrit after hydration.
- Type and cross: notify the blood bank of expected need for transfusion.
- PT, PTT: if there is reason to suspect a coagulopathy.
- UA: the presence of gross hematuria should alert the physician to renal damage with the potential for additional

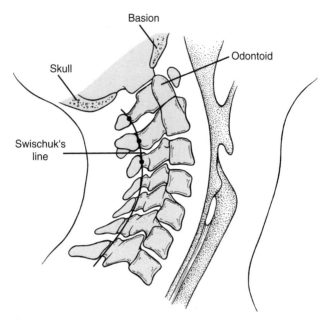

Fig. 36-6 Line drawing of the cervical spine illustrating the basion, odontoid, and Swischuk's line. (From Green N, Swiontkowski M: *Skeletal trauma in children,* 2nd ed, Philadelphia, 1998, WB Saunders.)

abdominal injury. Remember, blood at the urethral meatus is a contraindication to catheterization until the integrity of the urethra is examined (see the later section on abdominal and pelvic injury).
- Pregnancy test for females of Tanner stage IV-V.
- Toxicology testing as indicated.

✷ *SECONDARY SURVEY*

Perform a thorough head-to-toe examination, beginning with reassessment of the ABCs. Specific injuries and treatment con-

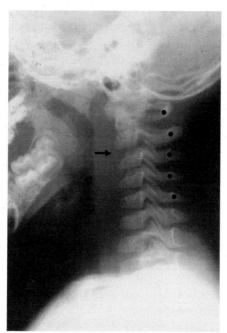

Fig. 36-7   Pseudosubluxation. The arrow points to an apparent subluxation of C2 on C3, which in reality is within normal limits. The arrow is in the retropharyngeal space, which also appears widened but is normal. The dots on the posterior spines are to draw Swischuk's line, which revealed that this spine was normal (see text). (From Green N, Swiontkowski M: *Skeletal trauma in children,* 2nd ed, Philadelphia, 1998, WB Saunders.)

siderations are discussed for each anatomic region. As with all traumatic injuries the presence of bruising, hematomas, external bleeding, lacerations, and deformities should alert the clinician to the presence of underlying serious injury. Children are at particular risk of significant blunt trauma that initially may have few external clues to their presence.

HEAD AND NECK: TRAUMATIC BRAIN INJURIES, FACIAL INJURIES, NECK INJURIES

The incidence of traumatic brain injury in the United States is approximately 100 per 100,000 children. It remains the leading cause of long-term disability among children. Because the signs and symptoms commonly associated with head injury are often absent in children, the clinician should maintain a high index of suspicion when attending to an injured child. CT scan remains the most efficient modality to assess acute head injury and should be obtained as soon as the patient is stabilized. The presence of significant facial trauma and/or neck injuries should prompt the emergency department physician to consult an otolaryngologist or a plastic surgeon early in the course of resuscitation.

Traumatic Brain Injury

Symptoms

- Altered mental status/loss of consciousness
- Vomiting
- Irritability/inconsolability
- Seizures
- Behavior changes

Signs

- Vital signs changes (hypertension, bradycardia, temperature instability)
- Scalp hematomas/step-offs
- Pupillary asymmetry
- Battle's sign/raccoon eyes (suggestive of basal skull fracture)
- Hemotympanum
- Bulging fontanelle
- Otorrhea/rhinorrhea (blood or CSF)
- Abnormal posturing

Workup

- CT scan to identify parenchymal hemorrhage, epidural hematoma (Fig. 36-8), or subdural hematoma (Fig. 36-9)

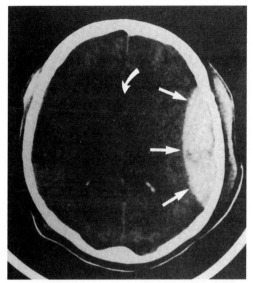

Fig. 36-8   Noncontrast CT scan of epidural hematoma. Convex high-density lesion. (From Rosen P, Doris PE, Barkin RM, et al: *Diagnostic radiology in emergency medicine,* St. Louis, 1992, Mosby.)

should be strongly considered if any of the above signs or symptoms are present, if LOC >1 minute, if patient younger than 2 years, or emesis beginning 4 to 6 hours after injury. CT may not adequately identify fractures and plain radiographs may be needed, particularly if a depressed fracture is suspected. Some authors have proposed using skull radiographs as a screen for injury in asymptomatic children younger than 2 years with minimal or no external evidence of trauma.

- If severe head injury is suspected, it is important to monitor serum sodium and urine osmolarity for the development of diabetes insipidus. These laboratory studies should be checked every 6 hours during the first 48 hours.

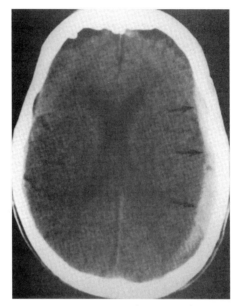

Fig. 36-9 Noncontrast computed tomographic scan of subdural hematoma. High-density region conforming to the convexity of the skull. (From Rosen P, Doris PE, Barkin RM, et al: *Diagnostic radiology in emergency medicine,* St. Louis, 1992, Mosby.)

Comments and treatment considerations

Consider intubation and moderate hyperventilation ($Pco_2 = 30$ to 35) for head injury with mental status changes. Use sedation and pain control once blood pressure is stabilized. Elevate the head of the bed 30 degrees. Lidocaine 1 mg/kg IV and paralysis should be considered before intubation (see Table 36-1 for RSI recommendations). Avoid hypotension; the mean arterial pressure (MAP) goal is >80 mm Hg.

If intracranial injury is suspected, consult neurosurgery for ICP monitoring. Maintain cerebral perfusion pressure (CPP) >50 mm Hg. Consider mannitol dosed at 0.5 to 1 g/kg intravenously given over 20 minutes if there is evidence of increased

ICP or herniation (blown pupil, posturing) as a bridge to surgical intervention. Results should be evident within 15 minutes and doses may be repeated at 0.25 to 0.5 g/kg/dose intravenously q4h as needed provided the patient does not become hypotensive. Furosemide may be considered as an adjunct to or a replacement for mannitol when contraindicated. Furosemide is commonly dosed at 1 mg/kg/dose intravenously q6h. Monitor serum osmolality with a goal of 310 to 320 osm. If ICP is persistently elevated >15 mm Hg, consider barbiturate therapy after intubation. Thiopental and pentobarbital infusions can result in severe hypotension and respiratory depression, requiring intubation of the patient. Seizures are common in children after head injury. Seizure prophylaxis with fosphenytoin or lidocaine (neuroprotective) is controversial. Avoid hyperthermia. Antibiotic prophylaxis, such as cefazolin 75 to 100 mg/kg/day intravenously divided q8h (max 6 g/day), for any open fractures is suggested. Tetanus prophylaxis should be provided if necessary (see Chapter 5, Bites, for dosing).

Facial Injuries
Facial injuries can affect the patency of the airway, and in circumstances in which loss of airway may occur, intubation should be accomplished (see the earlier section Primary Survey, Airway).

Symptoms
- Facial pain
- Pain or discomfort with bite (malocclusion)
- Visual disturbances

Signs
- Bleeding
- Facial asymmetry/deformities
- Step-offs or focal pain
- Extraocular muscle palsy/dysconjugate gaze
- Septal hematoma
- Broken teeth
- Conjunctival hemorrhage or retinal hemorrhage (consider nonaccidental trauma if mechanism of injury is inconsistent)

- Facial petechiae (consider nonaccidental trauma if mechanism of injury is inconsistent)

Workup
- Facial CT scan is the study of choice (better than plain radiographs).
- Panorex for dental trauma.

Comments and treatment considerations
Repair of facial trauma can be delayed until life-threatening injuries have been addressed. Consider consultation with otolaryngology, plastic surgery, or oral surgery as indicated. May consider starting prophylactic antibiotics, ensuring adequate gram-negative coverage if the sinuses are involved. Ampicillin-sulbactam dosed at 200 mg ampicillin/kg/day intravenously divided q6h (max 8 g ampicillin/day) is a good empiric choice. Tetanus prophylaxis should be provided if necessary (see Chapter 5, Bites).

Neck Injuries
Signs and symptoms of neck injuries in children may be subtle. If a neck wound is evident, consider damage to airway or cervical spine. Penetrating neck injuries can potentially injure major structures such as arteries, spinal cord, trachea, and esophagus. Penetrating injuries require emergency surgical consultation and should never be blindly explored.

The neck is divided into three anatomic zones when discussing penetrating trauma. Zone I is the area between the thoracic inlet and cricoid or sternal notch, zone II is the area between the cricoid/sternal notch and the ankle of the mandible, and zone III is the area above the angle of mandible.

Symptoms
- Hoarseness
- Dysphagia
- Dyspnea

Signs
- Bleeding
- Hematoma

- Stridor
- Bruits
- Hemoptysis
- Subcutaneous emphysema
- Absent pulses
- Horner's syndrome

Workup
- C-spine radiograph.
- CT scan of neck.
- CXR.

Comments and treatment considerations
A surgeon should be consulted immediately because many penetrating injuries will require exploration. The patient may also require subspecialty consultation for bronchoscopy and/or esophagoscopy if tracheal or esophageal injury is suspected. Four- vessel angiography is emerging as an important adjunct to the evaluation of penetrating neck injuries (particularly zone I and II).

THORACIC TRAUMA

Intrathoracic injuries are less common but more deadly than abdominal injuries. According to the National Pediatric Trauma Registry, this is the second most common cause of death after CNS injury. Eighty-five percent of these injuries are a result of motor vehicle crashes and/or blunt trauma. Children may have significant intrathoracic damage without external signs. Potential injuries include flail chest, open/penetrating wounds, pneumothorax, hemothorax, tracheobronchial disruption, esophageal injuries, pulmonary and cardiac contusions, great vessel injuries, and diaphragmatic rupture (see Chapter 30, Respiratory Distress).

Symptoms
- Respiratory difficulty
- Chest pain or tightness
- Anxiety

Signs

- Chest wall deformities
- Bruising
- Flail chest or asymmetric chest expansion (rib fracture)
- Hypoxemia
- Decreased breath sounds and/or asymmetric chest rise (pneumothorax)
- Distended neck veins (rare in children)
- Tracheal deviation (tracheobronchial disruption, tension pneumothorax)
- Bowel sounds in chest (diaphragmatic rupture)
- Subcutaneous emphysema (tracheobronchial disruption, pneumothorax)
- Hemoptysis (great vessel injury, pulmonary injury)
- Tachycardia, arrhythmias, hypotension, shock

Workup

- CXR: The following findings in a chest radiograph should prompt investigation and further imaging: widened mediastinum, loss of aortic knob contour, depression of left main bronchus (>40 degrees below horizontal), deviation of trachea or esophagus to the right of T4 spinous process, left pleural cap, left hemothorax.
- Chest CT scan if any abnormalities on x-ray (see below).
- ECG and echocardiogram if cardiac injury suspected.

Comments and Treatment Considerations

Address the ABCs. If a tension pneumothorax is suspected, immediate decompression is required with a needle or catheter in the second intercostal space at the midclavicular line. A chest tube should be placed after decompression. Do not wait for radiograph results to confirm diagnosis (see Chapter 30, Respiratory Distress).

If a hemothorax is present, tube thoracostomy is indicated. Use a size appropriate for age. Location of insertion is the fifth intercostal space at the anterior axillary line. Direct the tube posteriorly and use an autotransfuser if available. Transfer to the operating room for thoracotomy is indicated if initial tube drainage is >20 ml/kg or continued drainage >2 ml/kg/hr for >2 hours.

Rib fractures are uncommon because a child's rib cage is pliable. If present, they should serve as a marker for the severity of trauma. Beck's triad (muffled heart sounds, jugular venous distention, and hypotension) is not commonly present in children with pericardial tamponade. Suspect pericardial tamponade if there is unexplained hypotension and a penetrating chest wound. Definitive treatment is pericardiocentesis (see Chapter 36, Respiratory Disease). Treat with aggressive fluid resuscitation. Cardiac echocardiogram (if available) is both sensitive and specific for diagnosis.

 ## ABDOMINAL AND PELVIC TRAUMA

Abdominal injuries are common in children and usually occur secondary to blunt trauma. Mechanism is an important indicator, as in the case of seat-belt or handlebar trauma. Although overall mortality is low (5%), approximately one third of children with major trauma will have significant intraabdominal injuries that require treatment. Injuries usually involve solid organs. The spleen is most commonly injured, followed by the liver and then the kidney. It is important to consider that children have a large abdominal cavity and a proportionally small pelvis. Abdominal contents begin as high as the nipple line and their location can vary with diaphragmatic excursion. Recent studies support the nonoperative and conservative management of most blunt abdominal injuries. Some injuries such as pancreatic pseudocyst and duodenal hematoma will present days to weeks after initial injury (see Chapter 1, Abdominal Pain).

Serial abdominal examinations are invaluable in the evaluation of children, because their level of anxiety and crying can hamper the initial examination. Injuries to consider include solid organs such as renal, splenic, or liver contusions, lacerations, and/or fractures; hollow viscus injury such as duodenal hematoma, bladder rupture, vascular injury, pelvic fracture; and/or diaphragmatic rupture.

A recent study showed six findings that had a high association with intraabdominal injuries: low systolic blood pressure, femur fracture, AST > 200 or ALT > 125, urinalysis with >5 RBCs/hpf, and initial hematocrit <30%.

Symptoms
- Abdominal pain
- Nausea
- Vomiting
- Hematemesis
- Hematochezia
- Hematuria

Signs
- Tenderness to palpation (note location for clues to internal damage)
- Bruising (in particular, seat-belt marks)
- Abdominal distention
- Absent bowel sounds
- Guarding
- Rebound tenderness
- Pelvic girdle instability
- Scrotal hematoma (associated with pelvic injuries)
- Hemodynamic instability

Workup
- Abdominal CT scan is the imaging of choice for intraabdominal injuries.
- Pelvic x-rays to identify fractures.
- Ultrasound: Numerous studies have shown that in children focused abdominal sonography for trauma (FAST) is not as reliable to detect peritoneal free fluid as CT and has a high rate of false-negative results.
- The use of peritoneal lavage in children remains controversial and should be reserved for children requiring immediate surgical intervention (no time for imaging).
- Foley catheter unless suspicion of pelvic injury and urethral disruption. Retrograde urethrogram should precede Foley catheter placement when these diagnoses are being considered.

- Laboratory testing:
  - Urinalysis for hematuria. Studies show gross hematuria associated with abdominal symptoms is a reliable marker for intraabdominal injury (spleen 37%, liver 33%, kidney 26%). In children the bladder is an intraabdominal organ and is thus exposed to injury.
  - Obtain aspartate transaminase (AST)/alanine aminotransferase (ALT), amylase, and lipase if liver or pancreas injury suspected.

Comments and Treatments Considerations

Support the ABCs and consult surgery emergently. See Chapter 20, Hypotension/Shock, for management of hemorrhagic shock, remembering that vasopressor therapy should be avoided in hemorrhage and, if used, should be chosen to preferentially increase systemic vascular resistance. Early gastric decompression is beneficial. If pulseless and penetrating injury present, the patient may require emergent thoracotomy. If blunt trauma, thoracotomy rarely indicated. Emergent laparotomy, especially if peritoneum is violated or flank wound present, is generally required for gunshot wounds, impaled objects, evisceration, diaphragmatic injury, pneumoperitoneum, or persistent gastrointestinal tract bleeding. Suspect hollow viscus injury if a pancreatic injury is present; the only CT finding may be free fluid. Penetrating abdominal injuries will likely require preventive broad-spectrum antibiotic therapy. Options may include triple coverage with ampicillin 100 to 200 mg/kg/day intravenously divided q6h (max 12 g/day), gentamicin 4-7.5 mg/kg/day intravenously divided q8-24h (dose and frequency dependent on age) and metronidazole 30 mg/kg/day intravenously divided q6-8h (max 4 g/day). Clindamycin 30 mg/kg/day intravenously divided q6-8h (max 4.8 g/day) may be used in place of metronidazole. Alternatively, a β-lactamase–stable antibiotic such as piperacillin-tazobactam 300 mg piperacillin/kg/day intravenously divided q6-8h (max 18 g piperacillin/day) ± gentamicin may be used.

Conservative management in an intensive care unit of stable patients with solid organ blunt trauma injuries is common. The patient should be observed closely for 24 to 48 hours because most injuries requiring intervention will become evident within the first 18 hours. Consider abuse in all perineal trauma.

 ## SPINAL CORD INJURY

Spinal cord injury in children is uncommon, yet the associated morbidity and mortality make it a diagnostic priority in the face of an injured child. Most of these injuries are associated with motor vehicle crash or car versus pedestrian. A unique entity associated with pediatric trauma is spinal cord injury without radiographic abnormality (SCIWORA). It presents as a brief sensory or motor deficit followed by delayed and progressive onset of severe neurologic deficits up to 4 hours after injury. Some studies suggest that up to one third of children with cervical bony injury will have neurologic deficits and only half of them will have radiologic abnormalities. It is therefore important to perform a thorough neurologic examination in any injured child, even in the face of normal imaging study findings.

Symptoms
- Weakness
- Pain
- Paresthesias
- Paralysis
- Electrical shock–like sensations
- Numbness

Signs
- Abnormal deep tendon reflexes
- Priapism
- Abnormal rectal tone

Workup
- C-spine (as discussed previously).
- CT scan if bony cervical spine not adequately visualized or abnormal neurology examination findings.
- MRI is the study of choice for the diagnosis of spinal cord injury because it provides greater detail of the soft tissue of

the cord itself. Consider MRI in any patient with significant injury or neurologic abnormality, particularly if radiographs and CT scans are normal.

- If a child's cervical spine cannot be clinically cleared 72 hours after injury, an MRI scan of the spine is indicated to evaluate for ligamentous injuries.

Comments and Treatment Considerations

Immobilize spine with cervical collar/backboard if injury is suspected. Support the ABCs as indicated; neurogenic shock is classically seen as hypotension, bradycardia, and peripheral vasodilation. (see Chapter 20, Hypotension/Shock.)

Though controversial, high-dose steroid treatment for spinal cord injury should be considered in consultation with neuro-surgery given as a 30-mg/kg IV bolus of methylprednisolone over 15 minutes, followed 45 minutes later by a continuous infusion of 5.4 mg/kg/hr. Pediatric patients with spinal cord injuries should be admitted to an intensive care unit setting with pediatric neurosurgical consultation. Consider lumbar fracture or chance fracture (L2-L4) in young children wearing lap belt.

 ### *EXTREMITY TRAUMA*

Initial consideration should be given to life- or limb-threatening injuries. Secondary survey extremity injuries include fractures, dislocations, lacerations, punctures, crush injuries, compartment syndrome, neurovascular injury, and soft-tissue injuries. Identify patterns suggestive of inflicted injury (see Chapter 2, Abuse/Rape). Provide protection with a splint until evaluated by orthopedics.

Symptoms
- Pain
- Deformities
- Decreased use or range of motion
- Numbness
- Paralysis
- Pallor

Signs

- Pulselessness distal to injury (emergency)
- Paresthesias
- Paralysis

Workup

- Plain radiographs.
- Doppler if vascular injury suspected.
- Angiography (if available).
- Compartment pressure measurement if concern for compartment syndrome.

Comments and Treatment Considerations

Suspect an open fracture if there is a laceration of the extremity. Make note that the laceration may be quite far from the fracture site. Open fractures are an orthopedic emergency and may require the patient to be taken to the operating room for irrigation and reduction. Prophylactic IV antibiotics with good staphylococcal and streptococcal coverage such as cefazolin 75 to 100 mg/kg/day intravenously divided q8h (max 6 g/day) should be started. Tetanus prophylaxis should be provided if necessary (see Chapter 5, Bites).

Compartment syndrome is a surgical emergency. Signs may include pain, pallor, pulselessness, paresthesias, and paralysis. Not all these symptoms will be present or readily apparent in children. Persistent pain may be the only symptom. Critical compartment pressure depends on MAP, but generally treatment is indicated when compartment pressure is >30 to 45 mm Hg. If symptoms do not improve within 30 to 60 minutes, a fasciotomy is indicated. Emergent consultation with orthopedics and/or plastic surgery is recommended.

REFERENCES

Bracken MB, et al: A randomized, controlled trial of methylprednisolone or naloxone in the treatment of acute spinal cord injury, *N Engl J Med* 322:1405, 1990.

Coley BD, Mutabagani KH, Moore LC, et al: Focused abdominal sonography for trauma (FAST) in children with blunt abdominal trauma, *J Trauma* 48:902, 2000.

Fabian TC: Infection in penetrating abdominal trauma: risk factors and preventative antibiotics, *Am Surg* 68:29, 2002.

Garcia VF, Gotscall CS, Eichelberger MR, et al: Rib fractures in children: a marker for severe trauma, *J Trauma* 30:695, 1990.

Greenes DS, Schutzman SA: Clinical indicators of intracranial injury in the head-injured child, *Pediatrics* 104:861, 1999.

Holmes JF, Sokolove PE, Brant WE, et al: Identification of children with intra-abdominal injuries after blunt trauma, *Ann Emerg Med* 39(5):110, 2002.

Mehall JR, Ennis JS, Salrzman DA, et al: Prospective results of the standardized algorithm based on hemodynamic status for managing pediatric solid organ injury, *J Am Coll Surg* 193:347, 2002.

Nance ML, Keller MS, Stafford PW: Predicting hollow organ injury in the pediatric blunt trauma patient with solid visceral injury, *J Pediatr Surg* 35:1300, 2000.

Patel JC, Tepas JJ, Mollih DL, Pieper P: Pediatric cervical spine injuries: defining the disease, *J Pediatr Surg* 36:373, 2001.

Potoka DA, Schall LC, Ford HR: Improved functional outcome for severely injured children treated at pediatric trauma centers, *J Trauma* 51:824, 2001.

Pozner C, Cranmer H, Lewiss R: Approach to trauma and burns. In Davis et al, editors: *Signs and symptoms in emergency medicine*, St. Louis, 1999, Mosby.

Quayle KS: Minor head injury in the pediatric patient, *Pediatr Clin North Am* 46(6):1189, 1999.

Ralston ME: Role of flexion-extension radiographs in blunt pediatric cervical spine injury, *Acad Emerg Med* 8(3):237, 2002.

Sanchez JI, Paidas CN: Trauma care in the new millennium, *Surg Clin North Am* 79(6):1503, 1999.

Stafford PW, Blinman TA, Nance ML: Practical points in evaluation and resuscitation of the injured child, *Surg Clin North Am* 82(2):93, 2002.

Taketomo CK, Hodding JK, Kraus DM, editors: *Pediatric dosage handbook*, 8th ed, Hudson, Ohio, 2001, Lexicomp.

Taylor GA, Eichelberger MR, Potter BM: Hematuria: a marker of abdominal injury in children after blunt trauma, *Ann Surg* 208:688-693, 1998 (abstr).

Tepas JJ III, Ramenofsky ML, Barlow B, et al: National pediatric trauma registry, *J Pediatr Surg* 24:156, 1989.

CHAPTER 37

Vaginal Bleeding

KAREN EILEEN DULL

Vaginal bleeding during childhood is abnormal after the first week of life and before menarche. After menarche, pregnancy status must be obtained in all females (and empirically considered in children older than 8 years) with vaginal bleeding. Regardless of possible pregnancy and gestational age, physicians should initiate standard ABCs and supportive care in the bleeding patient. After stabilization, attention can then be turned toward the cause of the bleeding.

PREGNANCY

Regardless of the gestational age, pregnant patients should be initially treated as any patient who presents to the ED with vaginal bleeding. This includes evaluation for hypovolemia including baseline hematocrit, remembering that the hematocrit even in the face of active bleeding may be normal until the dilutional effects of time or rehydration occur. Performance of a pelvic examination to assess the severity of the bleeding is required.

Pregnant patients have an increase in blood volume, which may mask the classic signs of shock. If the patient is hypotensive, orthostatic, or tachycardic, the physician should assume the blood loss is severe and treat these patients for shock. Two large-bore intravenous catheters should be placed and a 1-L bolus of crystalloid fluid should be rapidly infused. If no response is seen, additional boluses should be given and blood transfusion may be required. Rapid treatment of the underlying cause of bleeding, with appropriate consultation to gynecology, is required.

After initial evaluation and stabilization of the patient, fetal heart activity should be assessed using a Doppler stethoscope or sonography. Normal fetal heart rate ranges from 120 to 160 beats per minute. Persistent tachycardia should be considered an early sign of fetal distress. Fetal bradycardia or late decelerations with contractions suggest fetal distress and should be managed as a dire emergency. Continuous fetal monitoring is the most sensitive way to evaluate the hemodynamic status of the mother and fetus in advanced pregnancy.

ECTOPIC PREGNANCY

Vaginal bleeding or pelvic pain in the early stages of pregnancy should be considered an ectopic pregnancy until proven otherwise. External vaginal bleeding, though commonly present in ectopic pregnancy, is generally not profuse. Patients with ruptured ectopic pregnancy may occasionally present with syncope without other significant complaints.

Symptoms
- Vaginal bleeding ++++
- Localized or diffuse abdominal pain ++++
- Amenorrhea +++
- Nausea and vomiting ++

Signs
- Pelvic tenderness ++++
- Adnexal tenderness ++++
- Adnexal mass +++
- Normal uterine size +++

Workup
- Qualitative urine pregnancy test +++++.
- Quantitative serum pregnancy test (if qualitative test result is positive).
- Transvaginal or transabdominal ultrasound +++++.
- Hematocrit with type and crossmatch (required).
- Rh assay (required).

Comments and Treatment Considerations

Pregnant patients with vaginal bleeding or pelvic pain in early pregnancy require evaluation for the potential for ectopic pregnancy. Ruling out the diagnosis of ectopic pregnancy generally uses a combination of two tests: a quantitative β-human chorionic gonadotropin (β-hCG) and a transvaginal ultrasound. At a quantitative β-hCG level of >1500 mIU/ml (this number is institution specific), a transvaginal ultrasound will demonstrate definitive signs of intrauterine pregnancy (IUP) if present (e.g., yolk sac, fetal pole, "double-ring sign," or more advanced findings such as a fetal heart beat). In the absence of history or findings demonstrating a spontaneous abortion or other diagnosis such as missed abortion, failure to demonstrate definitive signs of IUP with levels of β-hCG >1500 mIU/ml indicates a diagnosis of ectopic pregnancy.

If a patient has signs of shock, operative management is emergently indicated. In the stable patient treatment may be medical (methotrexate) or surgical. Consultation with an obstetrician/gynecologist should occur from the emergency department.

Stable low-risk patients with β-hCG levels <1500 mIU/ml and without definitive signs of IUP on ultrasound generally can be managed as outpatients. These patients require definitive follow-up with an obstetrician/gynecologist for reevaluation and a recheck of a β-hCG in 48 hours. For comparison, in a normal IUP, the β-hCG should double every 2 days between days 2 and 40 after conception.

Mothers who are Rh negative should receive one prefilled syringe of $Rh_o(D)$ immune globulin IM (RhoGAM) *minidose* through the twelfth week of gestation. If spontaneous or induced abortion or tubal rupture occurs after the thirteenth week of gestation, the dose is one prefilled standard-dose syringe of $Rh_o(D)$ immune globulin. Ideally the dose is given within 3 hours of the abortion or tubal rupture, although it can be given within 72 hours of termination of the pregnancy.

SPONTANEOUS ABORTION

Spontaneous abortion is the involuntary expulsion of products of conception during the first 20 weeks of gestation.

Classification of abortions include complete abortion (passage of fetus with a closed cervical os), incomplete abortion (passage of some tissue but without closure of the cervical os), missed abortion (nonviable fetus without passage), and septic (uncommon in the United States).

Symptoms
- Pelvic pain ++++
- Appropriately sized uterus

Signs
- Vaginal bleeding ++++

Workup
- As above for evaluation of possible ectopic pregnancy.

Comments and Treatment Considerations
Treatment options include surgical evacuation, medical treatment, and expectant management. If there is evidence of cardiovascular compromise, persistent vaginal bleeding, or signs of infection, obstetric consultation is essential for possible dilation and curettage. Completion of abortion is defined by the status of the cervical os. Increasingly, obstetricians manage patients with incomplete abortions expectantly. Obstetric consultation should be obtained, particularly if outpatient management with very close follow-up is being considered. $Rh_o(D)$ immune globulin should be given if indicated, see previous section for dosing.

PLACENTAL ABRUPTION
Placental abruption is disruption of the uteroplacental bond that can cause fetal and maternal death. Severe pain, particularly in the setting of cocaine use, should suggest diagnosis.

Signs
- Abdominal and pelvic pain ++++
- Vaginal bleeding ++++ (blood may be trapped between the placenta and uterus)

Signs

- Hypertonic and tender uterine ++++
- Vaginal bleeding ++++
- Back pain +++
- Fetal distress (tachycardia, bradycardia)
- Preterm labor ++
- Maternal shock
- Fetal demise
- Disseminated intravascular coagulation (DIC)

Workup

- Diagnosis is clinical.
- PT/PTT and DIC panel.
- US is often nondiagnostic even in critical cases +++.
- Hematocrit is frequently normal +++.
- Type and crossmatch blood.
- Rh status.

Comments and Treatment Considerations

Oxygen, two large-bore intravenous lines and hemodynamic support. Continuous maternal and fetal monitoring is crucial. Cessation of contraction, a rapidly enlarging uterus, or board-like rigidity may be suggestive of increasing severity of abruption. $Rh_o(D)$ immune globulin should be given for mothers who are Rh negative (see earlier discussion). Emergent obstetric consultation and hospital admission are required.

PLACENTA PREVIA

Placenta previa should be considered in all patients with vaginal bleeding in the third trimester (particularly "painless vaginal bleeding"). An ultrasound should be obtained before an invasive pelvic examination is performed.

Symptoms

- Vaginal bleeding, often sudden, painless, and profuse

Signs

- Vaginal bleeding

Workup
- Ultrasound is diagnostic +++++.
- Hematocrit.
- Type and crossmatch blood.

Comments and Treatment Considerations

Oxygen, two large-bore intravenous lines, hemodynamic support, and fetal monitoring should be initiated. Emergent obstetric consultation is required. $Rh_o(D)$ immune globulin should be given for mothers who are Rh negative (see earlier discussion).

MOLAR PREGNANCY

Hydatidiform mole occurs in 1:200 to 1:2000 pregnancies in the United States. Invasive model (chorioadenoma destruens) occurs in 1:12,000 pregnancies. This is a progressive form of hydatidiform mole that has invaded the myometrium or other structures. Choriocarcinoma is an epithelial tumor that occurs in 1:40,0000 pregnancies. Timely diagnosis of molar pregnancy is important because early treatment is highly effective.

Symptoms
- Molar pregnancy often has no specific clinical characteristics to distinguish it from a normal pregnancy in the early stages of gestation
- Vaginal bleeding +++++
- Abdominal pain ++

Signs
- Absent fetal heart tone +++++
- Uterine enlargement may be disproportionate to the expected gestational age +++
- Preeclampsia in pregnancy <24 weeks of gestation ++
- Enlarged ovaries caused by theca lutein cysts ++
- Hyperemesis gravidarum, which is frequently severe and protracted compared to normal pregnancy ++
- Anemia secondary to vaginal bleeding +++, with occasional manifestation of what appears to be hydatid vesicles from the vagina

- Signs of hyperthyroidism + and pulmonary trophoblastic emboli +

Workup
- Continuous disproportionate rise in serum β-CG levels.
- Ultrasonography is the technique of choice to confirm the diagnosis of a mole.
- Rule out metastases (chest x-ray; consider head CT).

Comments and Treatment Considerations
Treatment of hydatidiform mole consists of dilation and curettage. Patients who have vigorous bleeding and a uterine size >20 weeks of gestation should be treated in an area where abdominal hysterectomy can be performed in an emergency. Chemotherapy, primarily methotrexate, is used for invasive and metastatic disease. Consultation with a gynecologist and oncologist is required.

TRAUMA

Trauma is one of the most common causes of vaginal bleeding during childhood. Vaginal bleeding after trauma may be an indication of rectal, bladder, or abdominal viscera injury. Sexual assault or abuse should always be considered.

Symptoms
- Vaginal bleeding +++
- Lower abdominal pain ++

Signs
- Lower abdominal pain ++
- Vaginal or rectal lacerations +++

Workup
- Vaginal examination. May require conscious sedation (see Chapter 2, Abuse/Rape).
- Baseline hemoglobin.

- Urinalysis.
- Pregnancy test (in all Tanner III and above classified females).
- Sexual assault protocols if indicated (see Chapter 2, Abuse/Rape).
- Ultrasound should be obtained in any pregnant patient.

Comments and Treatment Considerations

Hematomas of the vaginal tract can potentially cause necrosis of overlying vulvar skin and require a thorough evaluation. Most minor lacerations will heal without immediate intervention. Larger lacerations or persistent bleeding from smaller lacerations should be referred to a gynecologist for possible exploration and repair in the operating room. If history is not consistent with the injury, then a social service evaluation is required and the child must be kept safe until an investigation can be completed (see Chapter 2, Abuse/Rape).

 ## BLEEDING DIATHESIS

Patients with blood dyscrasias usually have other signs of bleeding such as epistaxis, bruising, or bleeding gums; however, bleeding diathesis such as von Willebrand's disease, aplastic anemia, idiopathic thrombocytopenic purpura, or liver dysfunction may rarely present initially during menarche with excessive bleeding (see Chapter 6, Bleeding and Bruising).

 ## PELVIC INFLAMMATORY DISEASE

Patients with pelvic inflammatory disease (PID) usually present with nonbloody vaginal discharge and pelvic/abdominal pain. Some patients may have a slightly bloody discharge, although frank bleeding is uncommon. Most first episodes of PID in adolescents are the result of an infection with *Neisseria gonorrhoeae* or *Chlamydia trachomatis* (see Chapter 1, Abdominal Pain).

VAGINAL FOREIGN BODY

Symptoms
- Vaginal bleeding ++
- Abdominal pain +
- Foul-smelling discharge +++

Signs
- Vaginal discharge +++
- Abdominal tenderness +

Workup
If a vaginal foreign body is suspected but the vagina cannot be visualized, the patient should undergo gentle vaginal lavage. Radiographs are unhelpful because most foreign bodies are radiolucent. The most common intravaginal foreign body is toilet paper, but retained tampons, beads, crayons, pins, and batteries have also been found.

Comments and Treatment Considerations
A foreign body may be removed in the emergency department using a cotton-tipped applicator or warm saline irrigation if the patient is cooperative. Sedation may be necessary. After removal, the child should perform sitz baths at home. Patients should be reminded to change tampons frequently; maximum time is 8 hours per tampon.

 URETHRAL PROLAPSE

Urethral prolapse refers to the protrusion of the urethral mucosa through its meatus. The prolapsed segment becomes constricted by the smooth muscle layers at the meatus, impairing venous blood flow. It is most common in African American girls between the ages of 4 and 10 years.

Symptoms
- Painless "vaginal bleeding" that represents bleeding from the urethra ++++

Signs
- Red or purplish soft, doughnut-shaped mass in child's vulva

Workup
- If diagnosis is uncertain, a urinary catheter may be inserted into the bladder.

Comments and Treatment Considerations
If only a small segment has prolapsed and does not appear to be necrotic, sitz baths and topical estrogen cream is recommended. Commonly Premarin 0.0625% cream is used and a small amount is applied two times per day. Resolution takes 1 to 4 weeks. If the mucosa appears necrotic, urology should be consulted for surgical correction.

 ## *DYSFUNCTIONAL UTERINE BLEEDING*

Dysfunctional uterine bleeding is defined as excessive, prolonged bleeding from the endometrium without an identifiable pathologic condition. In adolescents anovulation is the most common cause of dysfunctional uterine bleeding.

Symptoms
- Painless vaginal bleeding +++++

Signs
- Vaginal bleeding
- Normal pelvic examination findings

Workup
- Pregnancy test.
- Hematocrit, type and crossmatch.
- Gonococcal and *Chlamydia* tests.

Comments and Treatment Considerations
The treatment for most dysfunctional uterine bleeding resulting from anovulation in a patient with a normal hematocrit is supplemental iron and gynecologic follow-up. Supplemental elemental

iron is dosed at 2 to 3 mg/kg/day PO divided qd–tid (max 65 mg elemental iron/dose). Patients with mild anemia and who are hemodynamically stable should be treated with hormonal therapy such as oral contraception. A common regimen includes Lo/Ovral, one tablet qid for 4 days, then one tablet tid for 3 days, then one tablet bid for 2 weeks. Patients should be advised that they will likely experience "withdrawal bleeding" after completion of the hormonal therapy. The patient should also be given an antiemetic, such as ondansetron or prochlorperazine, which may be needed for the first few days. If the patient is unstable or has severe bleeding, gynecologic consultation should be sought for possible intravenous hormonal treatment, blood transfusion, or dilation and curettage.

 ## NEONATAL BLEEDING

During the first few weeks of life the normal female newborn may have sloughing of the endometrial lining in response to declining maternal estrogen levels. The bleeding should stop within the first 7 to 10 days of life. No treatment is required.

REFERENCES

Anveden-Hertzberg L, Gauderer MWL, Wlder JS: Urethral prolapse: an often misdiagnosed cause of urogenital bleeding in girls, *Pediatr Emerg Care* 11:212-214, 1995.

Berkowicz RS, Goldstein DP, DuBeshter B, Bernstein MR: Management of completed molar pregnancy, *J Reprod Med* 32:634, 1987.

Bravender T, Emans SJ: Menstrual disorders. Dysfunctional uterine bleeding, *Pediatr Clin North Am* 46:545, 1999.

Brennan DF: Ectopic pregnancy—part II: diagnostic procedures and imaging, *Acad Emerg Med* 2:1090, 1995.

Brennan DF: Diagnosis of ectopic pregnancy, *J Florida MA* 84:549, 1997.

Clark SL, Koonings PP, Phelan JP: Placenta previa/accreta and prior cesarean section, *Obstet Gynecol* 66:89, 1985.

Combs CA, Nyberg DA, Mack LA, et al: Expectant management after sonographic diagnosis of placental abruption, *Am J Perinatol* 9:170, 1992.

Dowd MD, Fitzmaurice L, Knapp JF, Mooney D: The interpretation of urogenital findings in children with straddle injuries, *J Pediatr Surg* 29:7, 1994.

Ellis MH, Beyth Y: Abnormal vaginal bleeding in adolescence as the presenting symptom of a bleeding diathesis, *J Pediatr Adolesc Gynecol* 12:127, 1999.

Emans SJ: *Pediatric and adolescent gynecology*, Philadelphia, 1998, Lippincott–Raven Press.

Falcone T, Desjardins C, Bourque J, et al: Dysfunctional uterine bleeding in adolescents, *J Reprod Med* 39:761, 1994.

Flanagan J, Cram J: Index of suspicion, *Pediatr Rev* 20(4):137-140, 1999.

Grisoni ER, Hahn E, Marsh E, et al: Pediatric perineal impalement injuries, *J Pediatr Surg* 35:702, 2000.

Kahn JG, Walker CK, Washington E, et al: Diagnosing pelvic inflammatory disease, *JAMA* 266:2594, 1991.

Lavin C: Dysfunctional uterine bleeding in adolescents, *Curr Opinion Pediatr* 8:328-332, 1996.

Lowe TW, Cunningham FG: Placental abruption, *Clin Obstet Gynecol* 33:406, 1990.

McEvoy GK, editor: *Rh$_o$ (D) immune globulin. AHFS drug information 2002*, Bethesda, Md, 2002, American Society of Health-Systems Pharmacists.

McKennett M, Fullerton JT: Vaginal bleeding in pregnancy, *Am Fam Physician* 51:639, 1995.

Nadukhovskaya L, Robert D: Emergency management of the nonviable intrauterine pregnancy, *Am J Emerg Med* 19:495, 2001.

Paradise JE, Willis ED: Probability of vaginal foreign body in girls with genital complaints, *Am J Dis Child* 139:472-476, 1985.

Peipert JF, Boardman L, Hogan JW, et al: Laboratory evaluation of acute upper genital tract infection, *Obstet Gynecol* 87:730, 1996.

Poirier MP, Friedlander LR: Pediatric vaginal bleeding. Urethral prolapse, *Acad Emerg Med* 6:527, 1995.

Ricketts V: Vaginal bleeding. In Davis MA, Votey SR, Greenough PG, editors: *Signs and symptoms in emergency medicine,* St. Louis, 1999, Mosby.

Szulman AE, Sutri U: The syndrome of hydatidiform mole. I. Morphologic evolution of the complete and partial mole, *Am J Obstet Gynecol* 32:20, 1978.

Valerie E, Gilchrist BF, Frischer J, et al: Diagnosis and treatment of urethral prolapse in children, *Urology* 54:1082, 1999.

Walker CK, Kahn JG, Washington AE, et al: Pelvic inflammatory disease: meta-analysis of antimicrobial regimen efficacy, *J Infect Dis* 168:969, 1993.

Watson EJ, Hernandez E, Miyazawa K: Partial hydatidiform moles: a review, *Obstet Gynecol* 42:540, 1987.

CHAPTER 38

Vomiting

MARK L. WALTZMAN

Vomiting is a highly coordinated reflexive process that begins with involuntary retching. This is in contrast to regurgitation, which is the effortless movement of stomach contents into the esophagus and mouth.

The various etiologies of vomiting range from the ominous, such as increased intracranial pressure (ICP) or sepsis, to the benign, such as mild infection. Bloody emesis or hematemesis is addressed in Chapter 16, Gastrointestinal Bleeding.

NEUROLOGIC

Increased ICP from any etiology can cause vomiting. Vomiting is often the presenting complaint in a child with increased ICP from a malfunctioning ventriculoperitoneal shunt (see Chapter 3, Altered Mental Status).

APPENDICITIS

Vomiting is a relatively common presenting symptom in a child with appendicitis +++. Careful history will usually indicate that vomiting developed after the onset of abdominal pain (see Chapter 1, Abdominal Pain).

TESTICULAR TORSION

Vomiting may be present in up to two thirds of boys with testicular torsion (see Chapter 31, Scrotal Pain or Swelling).

GASTROINTESTINAL OBSTRUCTION

Vomiting is a common symptom in many types of intestinal obstruction including malrotation, volvulus, intussusception, incarcerated inguinal hernia, and small bowel obstruction. In the case of obstruction emesis may be bilious (see Chapter 1, Abdominal Pain).

 METABOLIC/ENDOCRINE

There are a number of metabolic and endocrine causes of vomiting. Routine laboratory tests are usually not required for most patients with vomiting. However, in patients for whom the etiology of the vomiting is not clearly attributed to mild GI tract infection, further testing may occasionally demonstrate a significant abnormality suggestive of an inborn error of metabolism. In addition, an abnormal glucose concentration may be indicative of new-onset diabetes.

INBORN ERRORS OF METABOLISM

In the newborn period inborn errors of metabolism will often present as an exaggerated episode of "gastroenteritis." Frequently the evaluation will demonstrate a child who is "sicker" than expected. The patient will appear significantly dehydrated and ill. Laboratory analysis may demonstrate a severe acidosis with or without hypoglycemia. Newborn screening may show a defect; however, newborn screens vary from state to state and a more complete metabolic evaluation may be indicated. This workup should be considered in any child who presents with significant hypoglycemia (serum glucose <50 mg/dl) and include serum amino acids, urine organic acids, and ammonia level, as well as a serum insulin level. Consultation with a pediatric metabolic specialist is recommended.

NEW-ONSET DIABETES MELLITUS

Diabetes mellitus should be considered in the vomiting child with a history of polyuria, polydipsia, and polyphagia. Often these symptoms are not volunteered by the family; however, documented weight loss in a child without known illness should raise the suspicion and lead to further questioning. Screening with urine "dipstick" should be performed (see Chapter 1, Abdominal Pain).

 ## TOXINS

There are multiple toxic ingestions that lead to vomiting. These toxins include environmental exposures (organophosphates and carbamates, epoxy resins, copper, fumes, and solvents) and ingestions of organic material (acorns, buttercups, cactus, catnip, chamomile, chili pepper, chrysanthemum, holly berry, jimson-weed, poinsettia, poison ivy, etc.) (see Chapter 35, Toxic Ingestion, Approach To).

 ## MEDICATIONS

Various prescription medications can also cause vomiting as a side effect, such as chemotherapeutic agents, opioids, SSRIs, and digitalis. An antiemetic can be prescribed as a short-term intervention when toxicity is ruled out, the medication cannot be discontinued, and a suitable alternative is not available.

 ## PYLORIC STENOSIS

Classic hypertrophic pyloric stenosis occurs in the first-born male between 4 to 6 weeks of life. However, it may occur in any infant younger than 3 months and is due to a hypertrophic pylorus. Pyloric stenosis is manifested by the gradual onset of progressively worsening nonbloody nonbilious emesis that may be projectile. The term *projectile* is very subjective. Emesis associated with pyloric stenosis is expelled with significant force, not an increased frequency of "spitting up." The infant with pyloric stenosis will be hungry after the emesis and feed vigorously. Signs and symptoms are usually due to the severity of dehydration associated with the progressive emesis.

Symptoms
- Nonbloody, nonbilious emesis, which may be projectile ++++
- Decreased urine output
- Weight loss

Signs
- Evidence of clinical dehydration +++
- "Olive" type of mass felt on abdominal examination (may be difficult to palpate in the unrelaxed infant with a distended abdomen)
- Wasted appearance in severe cases
- Visible peristalsis

Workup
- Electrolytes to assess for a metabolic alkalosis +++.
- KUB (if obtained to rule out intestinal obstruction, will often show a distended stomach).
- US is usually the study of choice (demonstrates an elongated, thickened pylorus) ++++.
- Upper GI study may be diagnostic if needed to rule out other anatomic abnormalities.

Comments and Treatment Considerations
Treatment is primarily surgical with a pyloromyotomy. The surgery is relatively simple and curative. Most children are feeding normally within 2 to 3 days after surgery. Medical therapy with chronic administration of atropine is reported but not routine. Surgery is not emergent and should be delayed until fluid and electrolyte abnormalities are corrected.

 ## STAPHYLOCOCCAL FOOD POISONING

Staphylococcal food poisoning is the most common type of food poisoning seen in the United States. Symptoms are caused by the ingestion of preformed staphylococcal enterotoxin from contaminated foods. Contaminated food sources are usually those that come in contact with food handlers and are then left at room temperature for a number of hours before being eaten:

Custards, pastries, mayonnaise-containing salads, and cold meats are common sources. Symptoms usually develop within 2 to 4 hours of ingestion.

Symptoms
- Nausea/vomiting
- Known ingestion of a "risky" food
- Known contacts with similar symptoms

Signs
- Nausea
- Vomiting
- Abdominal pain
- Prostration
- Diarrhea
- History of other infected individuals eating same food

Workup
Laboratory testing is usually not indicated. In large outbreaks either the suspected food source, more than two infected individuals' stool samples, or emesis may be cultured for large amounts of the same colony of *Staphylococcus aureus* for epidemiologic purposes.

Comments and Treatment Considerations
Antibiotics are not indicated. Care is supportive but may require intravenous fluids and possible need for hospitalization.

 PANCREATITIS

Vomiting is a very common symptom in a patient with pancreatitis (see Chapter 1, Abdominal Pain).

 GASTROENTERITIS

Gastroenteritis is a broad term that describes infections of the intestinal tract by viral, bacterial, or parasitic organisms. These infections are usually self-limited and can be caused either by fecal-oral spread or from contaminated food and water. The severity of disease depends on the quantity of infectious agents in the food or water, virulence factors of the specific agent, immune factors of the host, and age and general health of the patient. Younger children will often have more severe disease, primarily because of their inability to maintain adequate hydration, whereas older children and adults often have a brief self-limited course of illness. Whether the infection is due to person-to-person spread or contamination can be determined by epidemiologic and symptomatic presentation.

Because vomiting and diarrhea may also be indicative of more concerning etiologies, it is important to have a high index of suspicion for other causes when abdominal pain is focal, systemic symptoms are present, or signs specific to other etiologies are present. If there is focal tenderness in the right upper quadrant, acute cholecystitis or cholangitis should be considered. If there is tenderness in the epigastrium or either upper quadrant, acute pancreatitis should enter the differential. Right lower quadrant tenderness may indicate acute appendicitis (see Chapter 1, Abdominal Trauma). Costovertebral angle tenderness, with or without dysuria, urgency, or frequency should lead the clinician to include pyelonephritis in the differential (see Chapter 18, Hematuria). If there is evidence of arthritis, arthralgia, or rash, inflammatory bowel disease must also be considered.

Symptoms
- Vomiting: initially nonbilious but may turn bilious or bloody if prolonged
- Diarrhea: usually follows the vomiting but may precede it; is normally nonbloody, nonmucoid, and watery
- Crampy abdominal pain

Signs
- Fever: usually low grade <39° C (102° F)
- Tachycardia: depending on hydration status
- Soft abdomen ± hyperactive bowel sounds

Workup
- Stool culture is usually not indicated in children with minimal fever and nonbloody diarrhea. In patients with

protracted symptoms, high fever, and bloody diarrhea or who are immunocompromised, consider stool cultures for *Escherichia coli* O157, *Salmonella, Shigella, Yersinia,* and *Campylobacter* infection.

- Urinalysis to exclude possible infection and to assess hydration status.
- Consider testing for ova/parasites for children with a pertinent travel history.
- Electrolytes are generally not required but may be obtained to evaluate for metabolic acidosis and hypoglycemia. Electrolytes, blood urea nitrogen, and creatinine may be considered in patients who appear clinically dehydrated.

Comments and Treatment Considerations

Most cases of gastroenteritis can be treated with oral rehydration therapy. If moderate to severe dehydration is present, intravenous hydration may be necessary and possible hospitalization until symptoms resolve. Usual fluid management in an otherwise healthy patient includes 10 to 20 ml/kg of normal saline or lactated Ringer's solution as a bolus, which may be repeated. If required, maintenance fluids with D5½NS or D5¼NS may be given as follows: 4 ml/kg/hr for the first 10 kg of weight, then 2 ml/kg/hr for the next 10 kg of weight, and then 1 ml/kg/hr for each additional kilogram >20 of weight.

Because most cases of gastroenteritis are of viral etiology, initial antibiotic therapy is not warranted and may prove harmful. Patients with *E. coli* O157 infections should *not* be routinely treated with antibiotics because therapy appears to increase the risk of hemolytic uremic syndrome (see Chapter 10, Diarrhea).

Oral or parenteral ondansetron (Zofran) may be effective in alleviating nausea and vomiting associated with viral gastroenteritis, particularly when the patient is unable to tolerate a PO challenge. Dosing for parenteral ondansetron in gastroenteritis is usually initiated at 0.15 mg/kg IV × 1 dose (max studied dose is 4 mg, but lower doses may be as efficacious; please note these doses are significantly less than those commonly needed if the drug is used as an antiemetic for chemotherapy) and is associated with improved outcome in patients receiving intravenous hydration. Successful oral dosing has also been reported at 1.6 mg PO q8h for children 6 months to 1 year of age, 3.2 mg PO q8h for children aged 1 to 3 years, and 4 mg PO q8h for children aged 4 to 12 years (Ramsook et al, 2002). In this study the oral ondansetron regimen was continued for 48 hours on an outpatient basis. A significant increase in the episodes of diarrhea was noted in the oral ondansetron group compared with the placebo group.

Patients with nontyphoidal salmonella infection do not benefit from antimicrobial treatment unless they are at increased risk of invasive disease (younger than 3 months, persons with malignant neoplasms, hemoglobinopathies, or immunocompromise either caused by disease process or medications, persons with chronic GI disease, or in cases of severe colitis). Salmonella infection contracted in the United States is usually susceptible to amoxicillin dosed at 25 to 50 mg/kg/day PO divided q8h (max 500 mg/dose) × 7 days or trimethoprim (TMP)-sulfamethoxazole dosed at 6 to 12 mg TMP/kg/day PO divided bid (max 160 mg TMP/dose) × 7 days. For more severe cases ampicillin dosed at 200 mg/kg/day IV divided q6h or a third-generation cephalosporin such as ceftriaxone dosed at 50 mg/kg/day IV q24h (max 2 g/day) or cefotaxime dosed at 150 mg/kg/day IV divided q8h (max 6 g/day) × 7 days may be used. Fluoroquinolones may be considered in resistant cases, particularly those contracted in developing countries.

Patients with *Shigella* infection should be treated with antibiotics for a duration of 5 days, because antibiotics have been shown to shorten the duration of disease, eradicate organisms from feces, and decrease the progression to dysentery. Optimally, antibiotic choice should be directed by sensitivities. TMP-sulfamethoxazole is a common first-line choice; see earlier discussion for dosing. Amoxicillin is less effective and is generally not used. Resistant strains may require parenteral third-generation cephalosporin (as discussed earlier) or a fluoroquinolone, such as ciprofloxacin dosed at 20 mg/kg/day PO divided bid (max 500 mg/dose).

Antibiotic treatment benefit for otherwise healthy patients with *Yersinia* enterocolitis has not been established.

Campylobacter infections may be treated with erythromycin base dosed at 30 to 50 mg/kg/day PO divided q6-8h (max 2 g/day) × 5 days or azithromycin dosed at 10 mg/kg/dose (max 500 mg/dose) PO × 1 day, then 5 mg/kg/day (max 250 mg/dose) PO every day × 4 days if still symptomatic at time of culture results. Antibiotic therapy appears to shorten the duration of illness and prevent relapse.

 ## GASTROESOPHAGEAL REFLUX DISEASE

Gastroesophageal reflux disease (GERD) is in fact regurgitation. When the lower esophageal sphincter (LES) is not competent, excessive and passive movement of stomach contents occurs and causes symptoms. Several factors contribute to the competency of the LES such as position, angle of insertion of the esophagus into the stomach, and sphincter pressure. The causes of reflux vary. Reflux may occur across a lax LES or when pressure across the LES is increased, such as with coughing, crying, or defecating. Infants have smaller reservoir capacity of the esophagus; therefore vomiting caused by reflux is more common than in adolescents or adults. Overfeeding must also be considered in the differential diagnosis along with GERD.

Symptoms
- Nonbloody, nonbilious emesis
- Emesis that is not forceful nor projectile
- Emesis that worsens when intraabdominal pressure is increased (siting up position, crying, coughing, or stooling)
- Chronic cough may be associated with GERD and microaspiration

Signs
- Well appearing
- Gaining weight
- Epigastric discomfort or tenderness
- Chronic wheezing: may be associated with esophagitis and/or microaspirations

Comments and Treatment Considerations
The evaluation of GERD in an infant should be based on the severity of the symptoms. For mild symptoms with evidence of

appropriate weight gain, no specific evaluation is needed. For infants with irritability/pain, a trial of feed thickening with 1 tablespoon of rice cereal/4 ounces of formula, placement at a 30-degree angle after feeding and an H_2-blocker such as ranitidine dosed at 4 mg/kg/day PO divided bid may alleviate symptoms. For persistence of symptoms, despite symptomatic interventions, radiographic evaluation should be considered to confirm diagnosis and to rule out other possible etiologies. Upper GI with small bowel followthrough will help to provide anatomic pathology. Specific studies for reflux include pH probe, radiolabeled "mild scan," or for evaluation of esophagitis and endoscopy. Infants with severe GERD are often difficult to manage and should be referred to a pediatric gastroenterologist.

 ## RUMINATION

Rumination, as a disorder, is potentially dangerous condition. It usually appears between 3 and 14 months of age and is more common in males. Repeated regurgitation of food without nausea or associated GI illness may lead to poor weight gain or weight loss. GERD has been thought to be one explanation of rumination, although other theories exist. Psychogenic rumination occurs in otherwise developmentally normal infants who may have a disturbed parent-child relationship.

Self-stimulating rumination is usually seen in the mentally retarded and can be identified at any age. Rumination can be considered a spectrum. On one end is GERD with little psychiatric illness, and on the other end is severe psychiatric illness in poor parent-child relationship or mental retardation.

Symptoms
- "Frequent vomiting"
- Posturing with an arched back "Sandifer's maneuver"
- Rhythmic tongue sucking

Signs
- Weight loss
- Poor weight gain

- Foul odor from the mouth (because of frequent regurgitation, which may not be followed by emesis)
- Poor dentition (seen in older patients, because of acidity of stomach contents in contact with the teeth)

Comments and Treatment Considerations

The evaluation of rumination disorder should include exploring the stressors in the infant relationship. It is important to evaluate for signs of GERD as well. In some infants the disorder is believed to remit spontaneously. However, electrolyte imbalance, weight loss, and dehydration have been associated with persistent rumination.

 STREPTOCOCCAL PHARYNGITIS

Streptococcal pharyngitis can cause vomiting and mild abdominal pain and should be considered when the patient complains of sore throat or dysphagia (see Chapter 26, Mouth and Throat Pain).

 URINARY TRACT INFECTIONS/PYELONEPHRITIS

Urinary tract infections commonly cause vomiting in pediatric patients. A urinalysis to rule out a possible infection should be considered in any young girl or a male infant younger than 6 months with fever and persistent vomiting (see Chapter 14, Fever, and Chapter 18, Hematuria).

 PREGNANCY

Pregnancy as a cause of vomiting should be considered in any female of childbearing age.

REFERENCES

Behrman R, Kliegman R, Arvin A: *Nelson: textbook of pediatrics*, 15th ed, Philadelphia 1996, WB Saunders.

Flanagan CH: Rumination in infancy—past and present, *J Am Acad Child Psychiatry* 16:140-149, 1977.

Herbst J, Friedland GW, Zboraliski FF: Hiatal hernia and rumination in infants and children, *J Pediatr* 78:261-265, 1971.

Hernanz-Schulman M, Sells LL, Ambrosino MM, et al: Hypertrophic pyloric stenosis in the infant without a palpable olive: accuracy of sonographic diagnosis, *Radiology* 193:771, 1994.

Kent R, Olson: *Poisoning and drug overdose*, 2nd ed, New York 1994, Appleton & Lange.

Lourie RS: Experience with therapy of psychosomatic problems in infants, In Hoch PH, Zubin J, editors: New York, 1954, Grune & Stratton.

Pickering LK, editor: *2000 red book: report of the Committee on Infectious Diseases*, 25th ed, Elk Grove Village, Ill, 2000, American Academy of Pediatrics.

Ramsook C, Sahagun-Carreon I, Kozinetz CA, Moro-Sutherland D: A randomized clinical trial comparing oral ondansetron with placebo in children with vomiting from acute gastroenteritis, *Ann Emerg Med* 39(4):397-403, 2002.

Reeves JJ, Shannon MW, Fleisher GR: Ondansetron decreases vomiting associated with acute gastroenteritis: a randomized controlled trial, *Pediatrics* 109(4):e62, 2002.

Sheinbein M: Treatment for the hospitalized infantile ruminator: programmed brief social reinforcers, *Clin Pediatr* 14:719-724, 1975.

Wong CS, Jelacic S, Habeeb RL: The risk of the hemolytic-uremic syndrome after antibiotic treatment of *Escherichia coli* O157:H7 infections, *N Engl J Med* 342(26), 2000.

CHAPTER 39

Weakness/Fatigue

ANDREA E. C. SHAH

Weakness and fatigue are generalized symptoms that may be caused by disorders anywhere along the pathway from brain to neuron to peripheral nerve to neuromuscular junction to muscle. Causative illnesses may range from minor viral infections that will resolve spontaneously to severe life-threatening conditions that require immediate attention. This chapter discusses potentially serious and more common diagnoses that may cause weakness or fatigue.

 ## TRAUMA

Weakness may be caused by various types of trauma, including spinal cord injury and head trauma. The diagnosis of trauma is usually obvious based on history and physical examination findings with the exception of child abuse in which case the presentation may not correlate with the history (see Chapter 2, Abuse/Rape; Chapter 3, Altered Mental Status; Chapter 27, Neck Pain/Masses; and Chapter 36, Trauma).

 ## TOXINS

Numerous toxins can cause neuropathies presenting with fatigue or paralysis, including organophosphates and heavy metals (see Chapter 35, Toxic Ingestion, Approach To). In addition, various envenomations can present with weakness, particularly pit viper bites and scorpion stings (see Chapter 5, Bites).

✤ *GUILLAIN-BARRÉ SYNDROME*

Guillain-Barré syndrome (GBS) is an acquired neuropathy secondary to inflammation resulting in demyelination and in severe cases axonal injury. Acute illness can progress to involve respiratory muscles, causing respiratory failure. An antecedent infection is present in 50% to 70% of cases, often upper respiratory tract infection or diarrhea. Specific associated agents include *Campylobacter jejuni*, Epstein-Barr virus (EBV), cytomegalovirus (CMV), and *Mycoplasma*. GBS is the most common cause of acute generalized paralysis and typically presents with a symmetric ascending paralysis that is rapidly progressive.

Symptoms

- Symmetric weakness usually beginning in the distal legs (may present as gait disturbance in young children) and spreading to the arms
- Pain in the extremities, which in young children may present as irritability
- Possible cranial nerve involvement causing facial weakness (Bell's palsy) and difficulty swallowing in up to 40% of patients
- Miller Fisher variant (5% of cases) involves the specific triad of ophthalmoplegia, ataxia, and hyporeflexia
- Older children may complain of paresthesias and numbness

Signs

- Symmetric weakness in distal muscle groups
- Bilateral hyporeflexia or areflexia
- Autonomic dysfunction, including labile heart rate (supraventricular tachycardia, bradycardia) and blood pressure (including orthostatic hypotension) in about 6% of patients
- Respiratory muscle weakness (15% to 20% may require mechanical ventilation)

Workup

- Diagnosis is primarily clinical.

- Evaluation of cerebrospinal fluid (CSF), although not necessary for diagnosis, reveals elevated protein with normal cell count (20% may maintain normal protein levels through the first week of illness).
- Careful assessment of respiratory function, including oximetry and forced vital capacity.

Comments and Treatment Considerations

Because of the high risk of respiratory compromise and autonomic dysfunction, all patients with suspected GBS should be admitted with frequent monitoring of vital signs and respiratory function. All patients with continuing progressive symptoms should be admitted to an ICU setting. The typical course of GBS involves progression over days to weeks followed by gradual recovery over several months, with 80% obtaining full recovery by 12 months. There is inconclusive evidence that plasma exchange or intravenous immune globulin (IVIG) may hasten recovery. IVIG dosed at 2 g/kg IV × 1 dose is used more often in children due to ease of administration.

 ## TRANSVERSE MYELITIS

Transverse myelitis is an autoimmune-mediated inflammation of the spinal cord, affecting both sensory and motor tracts. It is a unifocal process of varying lengths, affecting both sides of the cord. Involvement of C3, C4, and C5 can lead to diaphragmatic paralysis and respiratory failure. Often there is an antecedent infection, and in some cases there may be an underlying autoimmune disease (e.g., systemic lupus erythematosus [SLE]). Symptoms may present over hours to days, with 80% reaching a peak within 10 days. Transverse myelitis may involve any level of the spinal cord, with the thoracic region affected nearly 80% of the time.

Symptoms

- Local back pain is often an initial complaint
- Leg paresthesias

- Lower extremity weakness, may be asymmetric
- Urinary retention
- Fever, nausea, and muscle pain may precede neurologic symptoms

Signs

- Decreased muscle tone initially, followed by spasticity later in the disease course
- Hyporeflexia initially, followed by hyperreflexia with positive Babinski's sign later in the disease course
- A specific sensory level may be discerned in older children

Workup

- MRI may show widening in the area of involvement. More importantly MRI rules out other lesions, specifically abscess or tumor.
- CSF may reveal lymphocytic pleocytosis and elevated protein.

Comments and Treatment Considerations

All patients with transverse myelitis should be admitted to the hospital. Treatment is primarily supportive. Systemic cortico-steroids, such as pulse dose intravenous methylprednisolone, have often been used in treatment, but there is no definitive evidence of efficacy. The natural course of transverse myelitis demonstrates improvement beginning after several weeks. Function may be regained as late as 2 years after onset, but as many as 50% have persistent deficits.

 MALIGNANCY

Weakness and fatigue can be among the complaints that accompany various malignancies, either as a primary function of the cancer or as part of a paraneoplastic syndrome. Detailed history and physical examination can direct the need for further testing to make the specific diagnosis (see Chapter 28, Pallor).

BOTULISM

Botulism is characterized by a descending paralysis caused by a toxin produced by *Clostridium botulinum*. Botulinum toxin blocks the release of acetylcholine at the neuromuscular junction, resulting in flaccid paralysis. Illness can progress to involve the respiratory muscles, leading to respiratory failure and the need for mechanical ventilation in as many as 60% to 70% of patients. The toxin may be ingested in contaminated food or be produced by *C. botulinum* infection in a contaminated wound. Infant botulism, most common in infants 2 to 4 months of age, is caused by toxin produced in the GI tract by ingested *C. botulinum* spores. The spores can be found in contaminated soil or honey, although a source is often not identified.

Symptoms
- Descending paralysis beginning with the cranial nerves: ptosis, diplopia, blurred vision, dysphagia, and dysarthria followed by upper extremity, respiratory muscle, and lower extremity paralysis progressing proximally to distally
- Infant botulism presents with ptosis, poor feeding, weak suck, drooling, loss of head control, and lethargy
- Constipation often precedes neurologic symptoms in infantile botulism
- Nausea, vomiting, abdominal pain, and diarrhea develop 12 to 36 hours after ingestion of contaminated food and may precede neurologic symptoms in food-borne botulism; constipation then typically follows

Signs
- Ptosis and extraocular muscle weakness
- Hypoactive gag reflex
- Hypotonia and muscle weakness
- Dilated pupils that may be poorly reactive or nonreactive
- Hyporeflexia (a later sign)

Workup
- Diagnosis is clinical.
- Stool culture positive for *C. botulinum* is confirmatory.

- Botulinum toxin may be detected in serum or stool approximately 50% of the time.
- A full septic workup should be performed in infants, because the presentation is similar to sepsis, meningitis, and dehydration.

Comments and Treatment Considerations

All patients should be admitted to the hospital. Treatment is primarily supportive, including careful respiratory support. With the exception of wound botulism, antibiotics are not helpful and are not indicated. If antibiotics are given in a case in which botulism is considered but not certain, aminoglycosides should definitely be avoided because this class of antibiotics potentiate neuromuscular blockade. Botulinum antitoxin is available from the Centers for Disease Control and Prevention (CDC) (1-404-329-2888) and should be given as soon as possible to slow disease progression and shorten the course of disease in patients with food-borne or wound botulism. Botulinum antitoxin should *not* be given for infant botulism because it has not been proven effective and may be harmful. Botulinum immune globulin (Baby BIG) is recommended for the treatment of infant botulism and may reduce the time to recovery. As with the antitoxin, Baby BIG should be requested and given as soon as the diagnosis is suspected, without waiting for laboratory confirmation. Baby BIG is available from the California Department of Health Services (CDHS) Infant Botulism Treatment and Prevention Program (1-510-540-2646). All cases must be reported to the state health department.

 ## *TICK PARALYSIS*

Tick paralysis is a rapidly progressive (over 12 to 36 hours) ascending paralysis caused by toxin produced by certain species of ticks. In the United States the illness occurs most frequently in the Southeast, Pacific Northwest, and Rocky Mountain regions. There are six species of ticks that can cause paralysis in the United States, with the Rocky Mountain wood tick (*Dermacentor andersoni*) and American dog tick (*Dermacentor variabilis*) most common. The illness is more severe in Australia where the scrub tick (*Ixodes holocyclus*) is the primary cause.

Symptoms
- Ascending weakness/paralysis
- Paresthesias

Signs
- Lower extremity and possible upper extremity paralysis
- Cranial nerve palsies
- Normal sensory examination

Workup
All patients with acute ascending paralysis should be examined closely for attached ticks.

Comments and Treatment Considerations
Removal of the complete tick is curative. If the tick is not removed, mortality is 10% to 12%.

 ## MYOSITIS/RHABDOMYOLYSIS

Myositis, inflammation in the muscle tissue, may be caused by viral or bacterial infections. Common infectious agents include influenza, human immunodeficiency virus, coxsackievirus, EBV, adenovirus, and *Mycoplasma*. Additional causes in children include autoimmune diseases, particularly juvenile dermatomyositis and polymyositis, which tend to have a more insidious onset. Muscle breakdown (rhabdomyolysis) may also be caused by compression injury, seizures, or alcohol ingestion and may lead to renal dysfunction.

Symptoms
- Muscle pain
- Weakness

Signs

- Fever (with both infectious and autoimmune myositis)
- Muscle weakness more often seen in the gastrocnemius and soleus muscle groups with infectious causes and in the proximal muscle groups with autoimmune causes
- Characteristic rash involving face (heliotropic) and extensor surfaces of extremities is associated with dermatomyositis
- Characteristic Gottron's papules (flat-topped red papules over the knuckles) are common with dermatomyositis

Workup

- Diagnosis is supported by elevation of creatine phosphokinase levels in serum.
- Urinalysis may reveal myoglobinuria.
- Electrolytes, blood urea nitrogen, and creatinine levels should be obtained to evaluate renal function.
- Electromyograms can aid in diagnosis.
- Muscle biopsy may be needed to diagnose particular disorder.

Comments and Treatment Considerations

Aggressive intravenous fluid management including alkalinization may be necessary to minimize potential renal damage. Pulse systemic corticosteroid treatment is effective in virtually all cases of dermatomyositis and many cases of polymyositis. When the diagnosis of dermatomyositis or polymyositis is suspected, involvement of a rheumatologic specialist is helpful for treatment plan and follow-up.

 ## *ELECTROLYTE DISTURBANCES*

Electrolyte disturbances of various etiologies may cause weakness and fatigue in children.

HYPERMAGNESEMIA

Hypermagnesemia causes diminished or absent reflexes and weakness. It may occur in patients with altered renal function who are taking magnesium-containing antacids or laxatives.

Severe magnesium toxicity has also been reported in children who have received excessive doses of magnesium-containing antacids or laxatives. Elevated serum magnesium levels also occur in mothers and their newborns after the treatment of preeclampsia with magnesium sulfate. Treatment includes discontinuation of magnesium. Severe magnesium toxicity and subsequent respiratory and cardiac arrest may respond to administration of intravenous calcium gluconate dosed at 60 to 100 mg/kg/dose (max 3 g/dose) via a large peripheral or preferably central line. Occasionally intubation may be needed for respiratory support for severe acute hypermagnesemia.

HYPOKALEMIA

Hypokalemia may also cause diminished or absent reflexes and weakness. Low serum potassium levels, regardless of the etiology, cause flattening or inversion of T waves and appearance of U waves on ECG.

- Familial periodic paralysis is an inherited disorder causing episodes of flaccid paralysis associated with hypokalemia that occur after a period of rest following strenuous exercise. Episodes may self-resolve or can be treated with oral potassium supplementation dosed at 2 to 5 mEq/kg/day (max 100 mEq/day).
- Thyrotoxic periodic paralysis is most common in Asian males and presents with evidence of thyrotoxicosis and hypokalemia. Treatment includes potassium supplementation and may require β-blockade, propylthiouricil (PTU), and/or methimazole. A pediatric endocrine consult is strongly recommended.
- Renal disorders, particularly renal tubular acidosis, may present with hypokalemic paralysis.

 ## INFECTIONS

Any infection may cause weakness or fatigue in children. It is important to distinguish simple viral illnesses that require no treatment from potentially severe infections such as sepsis or meningitis. This distinction can often be made clinically but may, especially in the very young infant, require laboratory evaluations (see Chapter 14, Fever). In addition, some viruses, particularly influenza and mononucleosis (EBV), are more commonly associated with weakness and fatigue.

INFLUENZA
Symptoms
- Abrupt onset of illness
- Chills or rigors
- Headache
- Malaise
- Myalgia (young children may refuse to walk)
- Respiratory tract involvement including cough, sore throat, and nasal congestion
- May have abdominal pain, nausea, and vomiting

Signs
- High fever (typically lasts 2 to 4 days)
- Pharyngitis
- Conjunctivitis
- Rhinitis
- Cervical lymphadenopathy
- Myositis with calf tenderness (particularly with influenza B)

Workup
- Viral cultures, if needed.
- Rapid antibody tests are now available.

Comments and Treatment Considerations
Influenza is a self-limited illness with only supportive care required. Disease course tends to be more severe in the very young, the immunocompromised, or patients with underlying pulmonary disease. Antivirals may be considered to treat influenza if diagnosis is made within the first 2 days of illness.

MONONUCLEOSIS
Symptoms
- Prodrome of malaise, anorexia, and chills
- Sore throat

- Fatigue
- Headache

Signs

- Fever, which may be high and may last 1 to 2 weeks
  ++++/+++++
- Tonsillopharyngitis with exudates
- Anterior and posterior cervical adenopathy
- Splenomegaly +++
- Hepatomegaly ++/+++
- Jaundice +/++

Workup

- Rapid Monospot test result may be negative early in illness
  and is unreliable in children younger than 4 years.
- EBV titers can be used for younger children and can
  distinguish acute from previous infections.
- CBC may reveal atypical lymphocytosis.
- Liver function test results and bilirubin level may be
  elevated.

Comments and Treatment Considerations

Mononucleosis is a self-limited illness with complete recovery
expected. Fatigue can be pronounced and slow to resolve, lasting
months in some patients. The pharyngitis may be indistinguishable from streptoccocal pharyngitis without testing and some
patients may have bacterial superinfection or coinfection.
Corticosteroids such as dexamethasone may be useful for severe
tonsillar enlargement with potential airway compromise but
should not be routinely used because they may interfere with the
body's immune response. Patients with evidence of bacterial
superinfection should be treated with antibiotics as appropriate.
However, amoxicillin administration should be avoided because
up to 80% of patients with EBV infection will develop a rash
upon receiving amoxicillin.

Patients with mononucleosis and splenomegaly should be
advised to avoid contact sports for at least 4 weeks and until
cleared clinically. Though rare, cases of splenic rupture in
patients with EBV infection have been documented.

CHRONIC FATIGUE SYNDROME

Patients with chronic fatigue syndrome (CFS) may present with any of a variety of symptoms with persistent or relapsing fatigue as a hallmark. Symptoms must have an acute onset and be present for at least 6 months to make the diagnosis. Patients with CFS are predominantly white females. The etiology of CFS is unknown, although there is some evidence that infectious, immunologic, and psychologic factors may play a role. The symptoms are frequently debilitating and in children often cause a significant amount of school absenteeism.

Symptoms

Fatigue for 6 months or more, new onset, not caused by ongoing exertion, with reduction in activity level and at least four of the following:

- Impaired cognition (children may show drop in school performance)
- Sore throat
- Tender cervical or axillary nodes
- Muscle pain
- Multi-joint pain
- Headaches
- Unrefreshing sleep
- Postexertional malaise
- Children also frequently have low-grade fever and abdominal complaints

Signs

- Tender cervical or axillary lymph nodes, as above
- May have orthostatic intolerance with abnormal tilt-table testing findings
- Generally, examination findings are otherwise normal

Workup

- Diagnosis is clinical and is a diagnosis of exclusion.
- Exclude psychiatric disorders, collagen vascular disease, malignancy, hypothyroidism, sleep apnea, chronic infections, etc.

- Laboratory work to eliminate other organic diseases may include complete blood cell count, erythrocyte sedimentation rate, thyroid function tests, liver function tests, electrolytes, blood urea nitrogen, creatinine, glucose, albumin, globulin, calcium, and phosphorus.

Comments and Treatment Considerations

There is no specific treatment for CFS. Psychologic follow-up may be helpful. Pediatric patients may present earlier in the course of illness than adults (sometimes earlier than 6 months). The outcome of CFS in children is better than in adults, with most patients having significant improvement or complete resolution in 1 to 6 years.

REFERENCES

American Academy of Pediatrics: Influenza. In Pickering LK, editor: *2000 red book: report of the Committee on Infectious Diseases*, 25th ed, Elk Grove Village, Ill, 2000, American Academy of Pediatrics.

American Academy of Pediatrics: Epstein-Barr virus infections. In Pickering LK, editor: *2000 red book: report of the Committee on Infectious Diseases*, 25th ed, Elk Grove Village, Ill, 2000, American Academy of Pediatrics.

American Academy of Pediatrics: Botulism and infant botulism. In Pickering LK, editor: *2000 red book: report of the Committee on Infectious Diseases*, 25th ed, Elk Grove Village, Ill, 2000, American Academy of Pediatrics.

Ahlawat SK, Sachdev A: Hypokalaemic paralysis, *Postgrad Med J*, 75:193, 1999.

Anderson PB, Rando TA: Neuromuscular disorders of childhood, *Curr Opin Pediatr* 11:497, 1999.

Anderson TD, Shah UK, Schreiner MS, Jacobs IN: Airway complications of infant botulism: ten year experience with 60 cases, *Otolaryngol Head Neck Surg* 126(4):234, 2002.

Arnon SS, Schechter R: Botulism. In Behrman, Kliegman, Jenson, editors: *Nelson's textbook of pediatrics*, 16th ed, Philadelphia, 2000, WB Saunders.

Bond GR: Snake, spider, and scorpion envenomation in north America, *Pediatr Rev* 20(5):147, 1999.

Caserta MT, Hall CB: Antiviral agents for influenza, *Pediatr Ann* 29(11):704, 2000.

Cawkwell GMD: Inflammatory myositis in children, including differential diagnosis, *Curr Opin Rheumatol* 12:430, 2000.

Centers for Disease Control and Prevention: Infant botulism—New York City, 2001–2002, *MMWR Morb Mortal Wkly Rep* 52:21-24, 2003.

Centers for Disease Control and Prevention: Measles—United States, 1995, *JAMA* 275(19):1470, 1996.

Centers for Disease Control and Prevention: Tick paralysis—Washington, 1995, *JAMA* 275(19):1470, 1996.

Cheng TL: Infant botulism, *Pediatr Rev* 21(12):427, 2000.

Cox NC, Hinkle R: Infant botulism, *Am Fam Phys* 65(7):1388, 2002.

Evans OB, Vedanaryayanan V: Guillain-Barré syndrome, *Pediatr Rev* 18(1):10, 1997.

Fukuda K, Straus SE, Hickie I, et al, and the International Chronic Fatigue Syndrome Study Group: The chronic fatigue syndrome: a comprehensive approach to its definition and study, *Ann Intern Med* 121(12):953, 1994.

Graf WD, Katz JS, Eder DN, et al: Outcome in severe pediatric Guillain-Barré syndrome after immunotherapy or supportive care, *Neurology* 52:1494, 1999.

Grattan-Smith PJ, Morris JG, Johnston HM, et al: Clinical and neurophysiological features of tick paralysis, *Brain* 120:1975, 1997.

Gutman L: Periodic paralyses, *Neurol Clin* 18(1):195, 2000.

Haslan RHA: Transverse myelitis. In: *Nelson's textbook of pediatrics*, 16th ed, Philadelphia, 2000, WB Saunders.

Hughes RA, van Der Meche FG: Corticosteroids for treating Guillain-Barré syndrome (abstract), *Cochrane Database Syst Rev* CD001446(3), 2000.

Hughes RA, Raphael JC, van Doorn PA: Intravenous immunoglobulin for Guillain-Barré syndrome (abstract), *Cochrane Database Syts Rev* CD002063(2), 2001.

Index of suspicion, *Pediatr Rev* 16(6):223, 1995.

Jenson HB: Epstein-Barr virus. In: *Nelson's textbook of pediatrics*, 16th ed, Philadelphia, 2000, WB Saunders.

Jenson HB: Chronic fatigue syndrome. In: *Nelson's textbook of pediatrics*, 16th ed, Philadelphia, 2000, WB Saunders.

Jones HR: Childhood Guillain-Barré syndrome: clinical presentation, diagnosis, and therapy, *J Child Neurol* 11(1):4, 1996.

Knubusch M, Strassburg HM, Reiners K: Acute transverse myelitis in childhood: nine cases and review of the literature, *Dev Med Child Neurol* 40:631, 1998.

Krilov LR, Fisher M, Friedman SB, et al: Course and outcome of chronic fatigue in children and adolescents, *Pediatrics* 102(2):360, 1998.

Natelson BH: Chronic fatigue syndrome, *JAMA* 285(20):2557, 2001.

Pascuzzi RM: Drugs and toxins associated with myopathies, *Curr Opin Rheumatol* 10:511, 1998.

Pascuzi RM, Fleck JD: Acute peripheral neuropathy in adults: Guillain-Barré syndrome and related diseases, *Neurol Clin* 15(3):529, 1997.

Pachman LM: Juvenile dermatomyositis. In Behrman, Kliegman, Jenson, editors: *Nelson's textbook of pediatrics*, 16th ed, Philadelphia, 2000, WB Saunders.

Peter J, Ray CG: Infectious mononucleosis, *Pediatr Rev* 19(8):276, 1998.

Poehling KA, Edwards KM: Prevention, diagnosis, and treatment of influenza: current and future options, *Curr Opin Pediatr* 13:60, 2001.

Poirer MP, Causey AL: Tick paralysis syndrome in a 5-year-old girl, *Southern Med J* 93(4):434, 2000.

Sarnat HB: Guillain-Barré syndrome. In: *Nelson's textbook of pediatrics*, 16th ed, Philadelphia, 2000, WB Saunders.

Schexnayder SM, Schexnayder RE: Bites, stings, and other painful things, *Pediatr Ann* 29(6):354, 2000.

Shapiro RG, Hatheway C, Swerdlow DL: Botulism in the United States: a clinical and epidemiologic review, *Ann Intern Med* 129(3):221, 1998.

Singh U, Scheld M: Infectious etiologies of rhabdomyolysis: three case reports and review, *Clin Infect Dis* 22:642, 1996.

Wright P: Influenza viruses. In Behrman, Kliegman, Jenson, editors: *Nelson's textbook of pediatrics*, 16th ed, Philadelphia, 2000, WB Saunders.

Index